Praise for

ASHTANGA, EMBODIMENT AND COMPLEX SYSTEMS

Upon diving into Iain's book, I found myself fully absorbed and unable to put it down. Having shared similar experiences with influential figures like Sharathji Jois and Rolf Najokat, I felt a strong connection to Iain's narrative, resonating deeply with his insights and reflections. The book chronicles his journey from his initial trip to Mysore to his later practice at Sharath's shala in Hebbal, offering a fascinating glimpse into the evolution of his thoughts and perceptions over time. Yoga instructors will appreciate Iain's candid exploration of the realities and mysteries of yoga, while practitioners will find inspiration in his honest and relatable account, which serves as a roadmap for their own potential journey.

—Clayton Horton, Senior Ashtanga Yoga Instructor, Greenpath Yoga

Iain Grysak's 'Ashtanga, Embodiment, and Complex Systems' offers a profound and timely contribution to yoga literature. The author's lived experience shines through in his writing, providing dogma-free insights into the practice that resonate deeply with my own twenty-year journey with Ashtanga yoga and meditation. What struck me most about this collection was its ability to put into words sensations and experiences I've had but struggled to articulate. Iain's clear, vivid descriptions helped me connect the dots between my practice, my sense of self, and the world around me. This book is more than just a personal reflection—it offers a quiet hope that through authentic embodied encounters with reality, we can find a viable path forward for both individuals and our species. The release of 'Ashtanga, Embodiment, and Complex Systems' is a gift to the Ashtanga community, which is currently navigating a period of healing. But its significance extends far beyond this community, speaking to anyone interested in yoga, meditation, or personal growth. I believe this book will continue to give back to readers for years to come, offering a rich source of inspiration and guidance on their own paths towards greater awareness and understanding.

—Gregory Steward, Senior Ashtanga Yoga Instructor, Ashtanga Vidya

Iain Grysak shares his unique worldview and intimate experience with Ashtanga yoga in this collection of essays. With vulnerability, authenticity, love, and hope, he opens up about his journey as a student, teacher, and disciple of Guruji Sharath Jois. Through his writing, Iain shows that consistent dedication to an Ashtanga practice can restructure both body and mind. Moreover, by embracing difficulties with an open heart, we can navigate the challenges that arise on our spiritual paths. Iain's essays offer a powerful reminder that humanity has the potential for growth and positive change. His work is a testament to the transformative power of yoga and meditation, and his message is one of hope and encouragement. By sharing his insights and experiences so openly, Iain invites readers to embark on their own journey of self-discovery and spiritual exploration.

—Sérgio Ramos, Ashtanga Yoga Nazare

Iain Grysak's 'Ashtanga, Embodiment and Complex Systems' is a remarkable and sensitive book that weaves together a rich narrative about the embodied experience. Drawing on diverse resources from yoga to vipassana, systems theory, biology, psychology, environmental science, and phenomenology, it offers a nuanced exploration of what it means to be human. Despite the theoretical depth, Grysak's focus remains firmly grounded in practice, examining how we live, move, breathe, heal, listen, and respond to ourselves and others. A core insight that emerges is that relationships between entities are more significant and real than individual components alone. Starting from various postures or concepts within Ashtanga yoga, these essays expand into a comprehensive vision of bodily and earthly experience. I highly recommend this book to anyone interested in yoga, meditation, nature, or embodiment, as it offers a unique and thought-provoking perspective on the interconnectedness of human experience.

—Andrew Alexander Davis, Professor of Philosophy, Belmont University

This collection of essays bears witness to Iain's ongoing evolution, exploring the intricate complexities of a practitioner's personal and collective realities, embedded within the dynamically interconnected systems shaping our world. Rather than adhering to any cultural narrative or echo chamber, Iain advocates for developing one's unique organic and adaptive identity, at the intersection of decentralized processes that challenge the pursuit of an unattainable perfect state. Instead, he leans towards self-realizing embodied paths which naturally reconcile apparent contradictions. Interconnectedness has it that in 2003 I introduced Iain to Ashtanga yoga after meeting at a meditation retreat. After just a few sessions with an early Western teacher in the Mysore-style practice, he fully committed himself to this path and has since become one of today's most profound and knowledgeable yogis.

—Sébastien Arcand-Tourigny D.O., Osteopath, Yogi and Musician

ASHTANGA, EMBODIMENT & COMPLEX SYSTEMS

Reflections during my years
of practice with **Sharath Jois**
(2014–2024)

IAIN **GRYSAK**

DISCLAIMER

The author and the publisher are not responsible for any injury resulting from the practice of instructions included in this book. The described activities, physical or other, could be tiresome or dangerous for certain individuals and so the reader should consult a medical professional beforehand.

Discovery Publisher

Copyright © 2025 by Iain Grysak
All rights reserved.
First paperback edition, 2025

Chapters "A Conversation Between Andy Davis & Iain Grysak" and "Wellbeing on the Edge: Learning From Mysore-Style Ashtanga Yoga," Copyright © Andy Davis and Iain Grysak

In chapter "Reflections on Todd Hargrove's *A Guide to Better Movement* in the Context of Ashtanga Yoga practice," quotes from *A Guide to Better Movement*, Copyright © Todd Hargrove, under Fair Use Copyright

Drawings, *Urdhva Danurasana*, *Samasthiti*, *Utpluthi*, Copyright © Allen Enrique

Cover Artwork © Discovery Publisher

Title: *Ashtanga, Embodiment & Complex Systems: Reflections during my years of practice with Sharath Jois (2014–2024)* / Iain Grysak

Subjects: Yoga | Mind-Body Relations | Metaphysical

No part of this book may be reproduced in any form or by any electronic or mechanical means including information storage and retrieval systems, without permission in writing from the publisher.

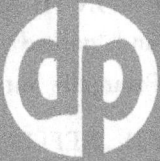

616 Corporate Way
Valley Cottage, New York
www.discoverypublisher.com
editors@discoverypublisher.com

New York • Paris • Dublin • Tokyo • Hong Kong

CONTENTS

INTRODUCTION	3
A NEW CHAPTER: REFLECTIONS FROM MYSORE, SIX WEEKS IN	11
On "orthodox Ashtanga" and whether traditional practice instructions should be strictly followed without modification	20
"YOU STOP THERE.": LESSONS FROM SHARATH JOIS AND REFLECTIONS ON THE MYSORE METHOD	23
On my statement about Sharath having gone further in his own practice that anyone else in this lineage and system	33
On Iyengar and Ashatanga	34
On my experience with Rolf vs. with Sharath	35
THOUGHTS ON DEEPENING AN AUTHENTIC YOGA PRACTICE	37
PERCEIVING & BEING PERCEIVED: THE RECIPROCAL RELATIONSHIP WITH THE NON-HUMAN WORLD	47
On the divide between "us" and "nature"	62
On some interpretations of Patanjali's Sutras	64
"YOU STOP THERE." [PART II]: REFLECTIONS ON MY SECOND TRIP IN MYSORE WITH SHARATH JOIS	65
On the nature of the injury in this trip in Mysore	86
STARTING THIRD SERIES [AGAIN]: REFLECTIONS ON AN ELEVEN-YEAR RELATIONSHIP	89
On "all [Ashtanga] methods are good" and "all paths lead to the same goal"	111

BECOMING ANIMAL: USING ASHTANGA VINYASA YOGA AND MEDITATION AS EMBODIMENT PRACTICES FOR THE CULTIVATION OF ORGANIC INTELLIGENCE — 115

On the "future of humanity" — 131
On Vipassana meditation — 132
On long sittings in Vipassana meditation — 133

FURTHER REFLECTIONS ON ORGANIC INTELLIGENCE, ANIMISM, GAIA & RELATIONSHIP WITH THE NON-HUMAN — 137

SUKHA — 149

THE GEOMETRY OF BANDHA — 151

SOME THOUGHTS ON ALIGNMENT — 155

A SYSTEMS-THINKING PERSPECTIVE ON THE RESOLUTION OF PAIN IN ASHTANGA YOGA PRACTICE — 157

On structure, systems and reductionism — 177
On diet — 178
On commenting on an injury experienced by a practitioner that I have not specifically known or worked with — 180
On practicing with more serious types of injury — 181

BRAHMACHARYA: EXPLORING RELATIONSHIP FROM AN ANIMIST AND SYSTEMS PERSPECTIVE — 183

On the term "brahama" — 198
On duality and separateness being a cross to bare — 198
On yoga being about transcending the physical — 200
On being judgmental — 202

NATURE SPIRITS — 205

TEACHING VS. PREACHING: EMBODIMENT AS THE GATEWAY TO AUTHENTIC UNDERSTANDING AND INTEGRATION — 209

WELLBEING ON THE EDGE: LEARNING FROM MYSORE-STYLE ASHTANGA YOGA — 221

Introducing the edge — 221
Sensation and imagination — 224
Mysore-style Ashtanga — 227
Bringing out the edge — 229
Discomfort and wellbeing — 233
Learning at the edge — 235

THE TREE OF BANDHA: MOVING IN EMBODIED RELATIONSHIP WITH THE EARTH	239
REFLECTIONS ON TODD HARGROVE'S "A GUIDE TO BETTER MOVEMENT" IN THE CONTEXT OF ASHTANGA YOGA	261
"MOVEMENT HOMEOPATHY" IN ASHTANGA YOGA	273
REFLECTIONS ON THE NEW SHALA AND MY FIFTH TRIP OF PRACTICE IN MYSORE WITH SHARATH JOIS	285
On diet; more specifically on fungus, mold, or cultured/fermented foods, yeasts, etc., and soy products	312
On developing your own lifestyle	313
On practicing the same sequence every day over a long period of time	315
THE ROLE OF THINKING IN ASHTANGA YOGA PRACTICE: A CONVERSATION WITH ANDY DAVIS	317
THE ENERGETIC DYNAMICS OF ASHTANGA ADVANCED A (THIRD SERIES)	329
Surya Namaskar A & B and standing sequence	330
Lateral extensions and leg behind the head variations (Visvamitrasana to Durvasana)	335
Arm balances (Urdhva Kukkutasana to Astavakrasana)	343
Transitions and peak backbending (Purna Matsyendrasana to Supta Trivikramasana)	350
Standing balances and final backbending (Digasana to Eka Pada Rajakapotasana)	357
Final backbending sequence	366
SUSTAINING A DAILY PRACTICE OF THE ASHANGA SYSTEM	371
INDEX	375

ASHTANGA,
EMBODIMENT
& COMPLEX
SYSTEMS

ASHTANGA, EMBODIMENT & COMPLEX SYSTEMS

Reflections during my years
of practice with **Sharath Jois**
(2014–2024)

IAIN GRYSAK

ASHTANGA,
EMBODIMENT
& COMPLEX
SYSTEMS

INTRODUCTION

I WAS APPROACHED IN EARLY NOVEMBER 2024 with the idea of collecting various essays I had written and publishing them in a book format. At the time, I was busy preparing for what would be my seventh trip to practice with my teacher, Sharath Jois, in Mysore, India. Less than one week after I agreed to the book project, we received the shocking news of the sudden and untimely passing of Sharathji.

My departure for Mysore was less than two weeks away and I grappled to come to terms with the massive void that had suddenly opened up in my own life and in the heart of the Ashtanga community. The implications of the sudden departure of Sharathji weighed heavily on both the future of the lineage of practice and on short-term considerations for my upcoming trip.

As did many of my peers who were due to practice in December and January, I decided to take the scheduled flight to India as planned, arriving in Mysore just in time to attend a memorial ceremony for Sharathji.

Still groggy and disoriented from a night of air and bus travel, the memorial ceremony allowed for the reality of the situation to permeate deeper into my being. The subsequent days felt empty and pointless, as I went through the motions of getting my belongings out of storage, setting up my apartment, meeting old friends and doing the needful things to prepare for a two-month stay in Gokulam. Under normal circumstances, this would include going to SYC to register for practice, which always felt like a homecoming and an affirmation of the central purpose for making the trip to Mysore. Daily afternoon walks around Kukkarahalli Lake have also been a ritual and form of practice in itself during my Mysore trips.

Fortunately, there was no need for this to change, and my first walk there and meeting of the resident Indian pariah dogs, both new and familiar from previous trips, provided a sense of normalcy and comfort for me to open up to the new reality that this trip would constitute.

I first came to practice with Sharathji in October of 2014. At that stage, I had maintained a daily Ashtanga practice for 11 years, and had completed Fourth series with my previous teacher, Rolf Naujokat in the early months of that same year. The years 2013–2014 represented a major transition phase in my life. I had left my previous home of Whitehorse, in the cold, dry and sparsely populated Yukon Territory of Northern Canada, where I had lived and taught Mysore-style Ashtanga from 2004 to 2013. I had settled in Ubud, in humid, tropical and densely populated Bali in 2014, and founded a new Mysore program, which I have maintained and still teach today.

Prior to 2014, I identified as a Theravada Buddhist and was a prominent member of the Goenka Vipassana organization, sitting annual long courses of 30–60 days and having been appointed as an assistant teacher responsible for conducting 10-day retreats. For 10 years, the Theravada Buddhist cosmology and practice provided the foundational framework for my life, in spite of certain aspects of the Goenka organization which had always generated internal friction and dissonance for me.

In 2013, I read the seminal book *The Guru Papers* by Joel Kramer and Diana Alstad. The clarity with which their apodictic arguments were presented stimulated a fundamental shift in my worldview, which resulted in a natural shedding of the Buddhist cosmology and a departure from the Goenka organization. It was a joyful experience, and I found the absence of a rigid worldview and framework to be refreshing and stimulating.

While I maintained the practice of Vipassana meditation itself (and still consider it to be an essential technique), I found myself instinctively gravitating back to my original spiritual inspiration, which was that of untamed nature. I was drawn back into Animism, as expounded by one of my favorite philosophers, David Abram, deep ecology, embodiment and the science of complex systems, all of which I had previously explored in my university education prior to first traveling to India in 1998.

I also felt that Indian philosophy, spirituality and religion had reached their expiration date in terms of my interest and their ability to exert influence on my life and I was invigorated by developing a fresh perspective on the roots of my spirituality and understanding of life.

The essays in this book represent the evolution of my practice, teaching and worldview for the 10-year period that began with a new teacher, a new home, and a new philosophical and spiritual framework in 2014. Four of the essays were specifically written about my first, second and fifth trips to practice in Mysore with Sharathji. The other essays explore physical, energetic and philosophical dimensions of Ashtanga practice, reinterpreted through my own animistic and complex systems oriented worldview.

The essays are presented in chronological order, the first two having been inspired by my first trip to Mysore with Sharathji in 2014, and the final essay compiled at home in Ubud, Bali during the dark time period of 2020–2021.

Re-reading some of them for the first time since they were written has been an interesting experience. Some of my perspectives have evolved considerably between then and now and I found myself wanting to change aspects of some of the essays. I decided to leave them untouched, as representative snapshots in time of the evolution of my thought processes and worldview.

The political events of 2020–2023 affected me deeply and had profound implications for practical aspects of my day-to-day life. I began to suffer from burnout and chronic stress, due to the situation that had been imposed on me, and I found it necessary to devote my spare time and energy to researching and understanding the political forces that shape the structure of human civilization. Prior to 2020, I considered politics to be an utterly boring and mundane subject and hence I had avoided it for the entirety of my life up to that point. When politics began to affect my own life in such an adverse way, it became unavoidable for me to dedicate myself to understanding the forces that are at play. The results of my research were distressing, and the net result of both the physiological and psychological burnout and adversity was that I stopped writing about yoga and the other themes contained in these essays from 2021 to present. I have no shortage of ideas, and it is very likely that I will eventually return to writing about these themes. Perhaps there will be a second volume to this book one day.

It is now mid-December 2024, and I have been in Mysore for three weeks. The central purpose of coming to Mysore to practice with Sharathji has always been to cultivate depth in my practice. I felt that the best way I could honor Sharathji would be to continue to cultivate the sort of depth in my practice that he had stimulated in me over the years. On my final trip in 2023, Sharathji had given me the first couple of postures of Fourth series. I had previously completed Fourth series with Rolf Naujokat in 2013, but I had stopped practicing it for most of the 10-year period that I was with Sharathji, as I felt he was giving me more than enough to work on as he moved me through Intermediate and Third series, one posture at a time. Once he started me on Fourth series at the end of my last trip in 2023, I decided that it was time to reintroduce it to my daily home practice, as I anticipated working through it fully with him over the next several Mysore trips. Over the past eight months or so, I have been practicing about three quarters of Fourth series, twice per week, as part of my daily routine, and slowly adding the remaining postures one by one.

Although my body was still familiar with the fourth series asanas, reintroducing them into a regular practice after such a long period of abstaining from them resulted in a necessary stage of structural shifting and integration, which I feel I am just starting to come into a place of stability with at present. I therefore felt that continuing with the practice routine I had developed over the past year would be ideal.

I considered staying in Mysore and simply practicing at home, perhaps with a small group of friends who could help each other with *catching*, etc. During my first days here, a friend told me about a new shala that had opened up in Gokulam. The teacher is Rakesh Jain, who is also authorized by Sharathji. I went to practice there for a couple of days and immediately felt at home and comfortable. Rakesh is in the same lineage under Sharathji, holds a beautiful and humble practice space, and gives excellent adjustments in *catching*, etc. So, I have continued with my own daily practice there and feel quite happy with that decision. It has been nice to continue working on reintegrating Fourth series in a focused shala environment, in the presence of a capable and humble teacher, and I already feel deep benefits in my personal practice. I have settled into a rhythm that is consistent with my previous Mysore trips. I go to the shala for practice in the morning, walk around the lake in the afternoons, cook nourishing food and spend a lot of time on my own. I feel happy to be here and confident that this is the best way for me, personally, to honor Sharathji.

I've always held a massive amount of respect for Sharathji, which I expound on in my essays that specifically address my trips to Mysore to practice with him. He exemplified the qualities of discipline and devotion and did an admirable job of taking over the Ashtanga lineage from his grandfather, Sri K. Pattabhi Jois, as it continued to grow in size and scope.

Sharathji and I didn't share many words with each other, but we had a deep mutual respect and understanding. His role in my life was that of the one teacher who could clearly see exactly where I was at, in my practice and my life, and to relentlessly push my edge to bring me to my full potential. I have always been a capable and disciplined self-practitioner and I will have no problem with continuing the process of deep and evolutionary practice on my own, but the unexpected departure of the only teacher who could push me just that little bit further will be something I mourn for a long time to come.

I will conclude by sharing one of the last interactions that I had with Sharathji in class on my final trip to practice with him in 2023. One of the main features of my trips with Sharathji was his relentless pushing of my limits in *catching*. Each season I spent with him, he would take me deeper and deeper into it, obliterating my erroneous preconceptions of my own limits. On my final two trips with him, and especially the last one, he was consistently putting my hands above my kneecaps, something I previously had never dreamed possible.

The interaction I am thinking of occurred in the final led intermediate class of the season. At the end of each led intermediate class, after we completed three drop backs, Sharathji would walk around and do *catching* with each student who practices full intermediate series, one by one. I would always position myself on the right side of the front row for led intermediate class, because he usually started the *catching* process there, and I always preferred to be one of the first people; it is easier for me when I am still warm from my drop backs and I prefer not to wait around getting cold and stiff.

In this final led class of the season, I did my first drop back and saw him walking to my side of the room. "Oh, good," I thought, "I'll be one of the first ones." As I did my second drop back, he came towards me and was already getting into my personal space. I started to arch for my third drop back and he suddenly stepped in to grab my arms and commanded, "Go!" I was one third of the way to the ground in a drop back, and in a split second, I had to switch mentally from "my hands are going to drop to the ground" to "my hands are now going to catch my knees." There was no time to resist, so I simply surrendered and relaxed as best as I could, which was the essence of what he had taught me over the years. It ended up being very easy as he put my hands above my kneecaps and it was actually one of the nicest *catching* adjustments I had ever experienced.

Whether Sharathji did it on purpose, or just because he was in a hurry to start *catching* doesn't matter; it turned out to be the final experience of something he had done to me many times—catching me off guard and unprepared in order to shatter my self-imposed limitations.

Iain Grysak
Mysore, India
December 2024

A note about the structure of the book

The essays are arranged chronologically, according to the date they were written. Most of them generated feedback and questions from readers at the time they were written. I often find that feedback stimulates further thought on the subject at hand. I decided to include some of my replies to the initial feedback on each essay when I felt they provided additional relevant information and perspective to the essay itself. These replies are included at the end of each essay, with the subheading **"ANSWERS TO QUESTIONS."** The original questions posed by readers are not included.

ASHTANGA,
EMBODIMENT
& COMPLEX
SYSTEMS

A NEW CHAPTER

Reflections from Mysore, six weeks in

— November 2014 —

I DON'T OFTEN PUBLICLY EXPRESS opinions or viewpoints until I have fully digested and integrated the experiences that lead to their formation. I realize that this has become increasingly rare in today's world of social media where we can impulsively broadcast all of our experiences and opinions instantly. It is not uncommon for photos, quotations and reactions from a certain experience to be uploaded to thousands of people on social media, before the experience itself is even finished.

Often, this sharing creates a fabricated picture of a fairy tale life rather than a representation of the reality as it is. I find this fascinating, disturbing and bizarre, all at once. Even before the era of social media and widespread use of the internet, I never owned or carried a camera, much to the disappointment of friends and family who wished to see visual documentation of my travels and experiences. I felt that the act of taking a picture was already turning the experience into a false representation of itself and removed me from actually participating in and experiencing it fully. I feel the same way about social media these days and so I do not tend to publicly share many representations of my day-to-day life.

Yet, I have been touched by the number of emails and messages I have received over the past seven weeks from friends and acquaintances who are genuinely interested to know how my time here, in Mysore, is going. After writing a similar description numerous times in email replies, I decided to write a longer reflection of my time here to share with others.

In order to do that, a bit of background to the current situation is required.

Though I have been drawn to practice in Mysore a few times over the 16 years that I have been practicing yoga and the 11 years that I have had a daily Ashtanga practice, for the most part I have not felt it to be a strong priority. Not coming to Mysore had become a conscious choice, as I worked my way through the Ashtanga series and became a Mysore-style Ashtanga teacher. The next logical step for most people pursuing this track is to come to Mysore, practice at the KPJAYI and receive authorization.

In fact, I did come to Mysore in 2000, while I was still an Iyengar Yoga practitioner who had a strong draw to the flow and breathing in the Ashtanga method. After finding the old AYRI shala in Lakshmipuram, I knocked on the door and met Sri K. Pattabhi Jois briefly. He asked me two or three questions and then advised me to watch a Mysore-style session the following morning. My Iyengar biases did not lead to a favorable opinion about what I saw that morning and I happily left Mysore to return to my Iyengar teacher in North Goa.

In 2003, I met Mark Darby, and was inspired to switch my personal practice to the Ashtanga method, learning Primary and Intermediate series from him. As I was already teaching yoga in the Iyengar style at the time, it was natural for my teaching to follow this shift in my personal practice. By 2006, my teaching had completed the transition that my personal practice had taken three years earlier to the "correct" Mysore-style method. As I was living in a remote part of Northern Canada at that time, without access to a senior teacher, I had to use my instinct and intuition to guide both my practice and teaching of the method as I founded an Ashtanga community there.

In 2007, I decided that things were serious enough that I should emerge from my Northern isolation and connect to the global Ashtanga community.

Coming to practice in Mysore seemed to be the most appropriate way to do that and I began to seriously plan for this.

During a course I took with Richard Freeman, a fellow student happened to recommend to me that I should visit Rolf Naujokat if I was intending to go and practice in India. She felt that Rolf and I would be a good match for each other. I instantly felt a strong draw to go and see Rolf and registered for classes with him that same winter. So, I had revised my plan to include a winter of practice with Rolf before I started going to Mysore. That was 2007.

That first winter with Rolf became seven winters. When you know you have met your teacher, it is clear.

Rolf initially took away my self-taught Third series practice and insisted on teaching it to me in the correct way, which meant a certified teacher giving me the postures one by one. He retaught me Third series over 3 winters, and then taught me Fourth series over 4 winters, which we completed in April 2014.

As I progressed through the advanced series and began to place more emphasis on my career as a Mysore-style teacher, I would question from time to time whether I was doing the right thing by choosing not to go to Mysore. It would help me a lot as a teacher to get authorized and to "prove" myself to the greater global Ashtanga community in this way.

Yet, inside, I had no desire for the Mysore experience. I was spending 3–5 months each year with Rolf and also sitting an annual 30–60 day Vipassana retreat. I felt completely devoted to Rolf as my teacher. I had no desire or need for another teacher, and felt I was getting a truly authentic transmission of the Ashtanga lineage from Rolf. It seemed counterproductive to fragment my time and my *Bhakti* by trying to develop a relationship with Sharath at the same time as I was practicing with Rolf. If I had been to Mysore during those years, it would only have been for the authorization certificate, which to me was not an authentic or appropriate reason to go.

In making life choices, I have always tried to allow my heart and my connection to my deeper yearnings to lead the way. Often, this went counter to what logic or reason dictated. I have always chosen the experiences that lead to deeper fulfillment inside me over experiences that might give me a strategic advantage in some superficial realm of life.

Many things in my life and inside me changed during the years of 2012–2014. One of those things was my feelings about Mysore.

In many ways, my relationship with Rolf came to a form of completion when we finished Fourth series in April 2014. While nothing about my feelings for him changed, the superficial aspects of our relationship did. There were no new postures to learn after that, as he had taught me as far as he had learned himself. While that did not mean I could no longer benefit from and enjoy practice with him, there were other aspects of his yoga shala that were less than ideal for me. These had become increasingly difficult to ignore.

In fall 2013, I was teaching for what would be the last time in my previous home of the Yukon in Northern Canada. I was starting to get ready for what would be my final trip to Goa to finish Fourth series with Rolf. I was researching something online and came across a blog post from a well-known certified Ashtanga teacher. I casually read the post, which ended up being a description of some aspects of her experience in the shala on her previous trip to Mysore. She was learning the end of Fourth series with Sharath and it happened to be about the same place in the series as I was at in my learning with Rolf. Though her description was brief, I had a powerful visceral reaction to how she described learning that part of Fourth series with Sharath. I could literally feel the intensity and focus of the shala in her description and I could sense how it would be to practice what I was practicing if I were in the shala in Mysore with Sharath.

And so, it was awakened—a deep authentic yearning to practice in Mysore. Not for authorization, not to prove myself to anyone, but simply to come and feel what it was like to practice there. And for me, that was the right reason to go.

Fourteen months later, it is November 2014, and here I am—seven weeks into my first practice session with Sharath Jois in Mysore, which brings me back to how things are going here.

I came with a very open mind, with as little expectations as possible as to what I might experience and how it might be here.

I've heard all the negative stories about Mysore—the superficial competitiveness and aggressive attitudes of some folks, the anonymity, the inexperienced assistants giving poor or dangerous adjustments, etc.

I also knew that I would have to let go of my Fourth series practice for my time here, and start over as a beginner, surrendering to the pace that Sharath would deem appropriate for me to progress through the system again under his guidance.

Thus far, I haven't felt negatively affected by any of these factors. I do see that some practitioners are competitive and superficial. They are desperate for some form of recognition from Sharath—chasing after the next posture, or authorization, and this forms the basis of their actions and experience here. It doesn't seem like a pleasant experience for them.

Yet, I don't find it to be anywhere near the degree that other people have reported. I also don't experience the social discussions about practice to be geared in that direction either. Which posture or series one is on has only been given a passing mention in most of the conversations I've had with other practitioners, and that also in a non-judgmental way.

It's also a fact that I am my usual hermit self here, and socialize very little. Most of the socializing I have done is with people I already know from other places and already feel some sense of like-mindedness with. So, it's possible that I'm just blind to certain attitudes in the general student population. Nonetheless, I think the important point is that it is not a part of my own experience here, which shows that it is avoidable.

Another factor in this is that I have arrived in Mysore at an ideal time in my own journey. Having completed Fourth series with Rolf, I have my practice. It is something that no one can take away from me, and after 11 years of daily practice, I am beyond needing to prove anything to anyone. Whatever postures Sharath gives me has no bearing on the practice that my teacher taught me over the past 7 years.

I am also an established and respected Ashtanga teacher. Whether I get authorized and certified or not has no bearing on the opinion of the many students who have practiced with me as their teacher over the past decade.

So really, I have nothing to chase after here — only to enjoy what is given as a bonus to what I already have. If I had come even 3 or 4 years ago, I might have felt more caught up in the chasing after recognition part of some other people's experience here.

In terms of safety, I could not feel more at ease, and I think that is the experience of many people. All the stories of bad alignment and frightening adjustments are not true, from what I have observed. In fact, I think more of this goes on in other studios around the world, and amongst teachers who have misinterpreted the Ashtanga method or feel as they, as teachers, have something to prove to their students.

Sharath runs a very tight and clean ship. He has an excellent sense of how and what each student should be practicing, and he keeps a close eye on his assistants and what they are doing. He is very good at making sure each student develops the protective factors of strength and alignment in the practice.

The only posture I have been adjusted in here is catching the legs in the final backbend. Sharath is truly masterful at this adjustment, and he continues to take me much deeper into it than I have ever experienced before. When he adjusts me in this posture, it feels almost effortless and very safe and well aligned. This morning he moved my hands to hold my knees for the first time ever. It was intense, but didn't feel like a struggle. It was relatively easy for something that seven weeks ago I would have said was impossible for my body. When I came up from the backbend, he was smiling broadly at me.

When the assistants adjust me, it is obviously without the level of skill and experience that Sharath has, but it is usually very good and I have yet to have a "bad adjustment."

I could see the potential for less experienced practitioners who are also very enthusiastic and less aware of their own bodies and limitations to use the heat and intensity of the room here to push themselves too far in certain postures—but overall I would not say it is an unsafe place to practice, in fact, it is the very opposite.

Coming from a daily practice of Fourth series, followed by several hours of teaching on most days, I was looking forward to my time here as a bit of an easy ride. I knew I would be practicing Primary series only for at least a few weeks, and then adding on Intermediate postures one by one. As I completed both of these series 9 or 10 years ago, I assumed it would mean three months of relaxed, easy practice. I looked to it as a restorative yoga holiday of sorts.

The heat and intensity were the first things that struck me here. I arrived at the very beginning of the season and Sharath started off with a series of 5 led Primary series classes for everyone. I've never practiced with so many people at once—80 people in the room. Sharath's pace and vinyasa count was also quite strong for me and I felt humbled to be struggling in Primary series during those first five classes. I enjoy hot, sweaty practices very much, but it has been a long time since I practiced in the kind of heat that I arrived to here. I've also done fast Primary series practices, but holding *chatwari* was not something I was used to.

Ever attentive, Sharath called me out on several things during the first led classes, including holding the entire class up in *chatwari* for some time while he yelled at me from the stage to "do it properly." I had no idea what he meant until he finally told me to "go lower." I had been accustomed to keeping my upper arms parallel to the ground, but he insisted that I go down until my chest was nearly touching the ground.

Since I've adapted to his specifics and to the heat, I've enjoyed practicing Primary series here thoroughly. I have taken the opportunity to develop more strength in some of the transition vinyasas and my focus on *mula bandha* more deeply. As the postures themselves are all very accessible for me, I've taken the opportunity to challenge myself more in other areas of the practice.

By the second or third week, my upper body felt noticeably bigger and stronger, but not in a way that was making me tighter. I still felt tired in my breathing muscles (due to being extra precise and clean in the vinyasa) by the end of each practice until the end of the first month.

After practice at the shala, I come home and do my 45-minute pranayama practice in the open air on our balcony and I was surprised at first to find that this was also challenging due to the extra workout I was experiencing on the muscles of breathing and stabilizing. It was also a month before my pranayama practice regained its usual ease.

Sharath started me on Intermediate series at the end of my third week. He gave me a few postures every few days for a couple of weeks and then held me on *Kapotasana* for a week. This week he gave me the go-ahead to start *Supta Vajrasana*.

Now that I feel fully adapted to all aspects of practice here, it is really a sweet practice experience. To be able to flow through postures that have long ago been integrated into my body and nervous system is now giving me that restorative experience that I thought I would feel in the first month. To be able to take the time to deepen the meditative and strengthening aspects of vinyasa, breath and *mula bandha* in Primary and Intermediate series is a nice experience after all these years of putting my focus on the advanced series.

Sharath is an excellent teacher in all ways. He is truly a master of this system, and he understands all of its aspects from the physical, to the psychological, to the spiritual. His ability to be present and keep track of 200–300 students per day every day is stunning. He doesn't memorize exact details about everyone, but he does know each person and where they are at. He also knows how to work with each person as an individual based on that understanding, and what each person is and isn't ready for. The fact that he keeps this up for six months continuously, perhaps seeing 600–800 different people over these six months is truly astounding. He has my full respect.

His talks and the way he answers questions in conferences are also very good. I was happy to discover that he does talk about yoga and what is important in the same way that I have come to understand. His storytelling and references reflect a context of traditional Indian philosophy—something I've moved away from in the past year or two—but the essence of the meaning and his understanding of it are similar enough to my understanding for me to enjoy his talks thoroughly.

Sharath tirelessly expounds the same essential messages to all the students. "The yoga has to happen inside you." He says this several times during each and every conference. He regularly reminds us that he has woken up at 1 a.m. every day for the past 25 years, not to self-aggrandize, but rather to convey the message of *bhakti*. He wants all students to understand that focus and dedication are essential ingredients for true understanding and experience of "the yoga happening inside you."

In his physical adjustments, Sharath knows how to take you deeper into a challenging posture in a way that feels both safe and effortless. I've noticed he does not adjust very much. Only catching the legs in the final backbend (or working up to that for those who cannot yet catch), and a few other key postures from each series. Nothing that is not necessary. He spends a lot of time sitting on the stage, surveying the entire room, quietly watching.

A few mornings ago as I walked out of the shala after practice, Sharath happened to be standing near the door about to help someone in a backbend. He'd been up since 1 a.m., done his own practice, and was probably about halfway through his daily task of supporting and teaching 200–300 students for 6 hours.

"Thank you, Sharath," I said quietly as I walked past him. He turned his head and for a moment met my gaze and smiled a true and authentic smile. He showed no tiredness, no impatience, no patronizing—neither of us wanted anything from the other. "Thank you," he replied, and turned back to his next backbending adjustment.

I have little doubt that I have found my new home for developing my own practice, and my next teacher.

ANSWERS TO QUESTIONS

❧ On "orthodox Ashtanga" and whether traditional practice instructions should be strictly followed without modification

I believe the backlash against "orthodox Ashtanga" has been created by practitioners and authors who have misunderstood the system. Those who took a strongly fundamentalist and narrow-minded interpretation of the system, and later abandoned it because it did not work for them or their students, can tend to be very outspoken against what they see as a very rigid system. I think this shows more about the inner tendencies of these practitioners than it does about the system itself.

Sharath's approach to teaching the system does not fall into this narrow-minded category, from what I have observed. Sharath treats each student as an individual, and sets different standards for physical expectations based on the individual's unique characteristics of age, injury, health, etc. He may set stronger standards for a young, healthy or physically capable student to achieve perfection in a difficult asana before moving them on in the series. With other students who are older, injured, or simply do not have the physical capacity, he will move them on without having achieved the same degree of perfection that other students may be expected to have. He may grant teaching authorization to someone who is less advanced in the physical practice, while someone who is further along may not be authorized.

In conference talks, Sharath constantly emphasizes that physical development in asana is only a doorway to the real yoga, which must happen inside oneself. He reminds us that someone who "only" does half of Primary series can be a real yogi, while someone practicing advanced series may not attain this inner understanding and transformation of yoga. Sharath expounds the message that yoga is the transformation of the entire person, and that physical attainments in asana are not a guarantee of this inner transformation.

I have never met or practiced with an Ashtanga teacher who falls into the narrow-minded, fundamentalist category. Although I am sure such teachers do exist, I think they are by far a minority, and the greater Ashtanga community (especially those who seek training from Sharath) do not fall into this category.

My own personal approach, and the approach taken by other teachers and peers that I respect and have worked with, is to adapt the system to bring healing and transformation to each student—on all levels of the being. A 65-year-old with various chronic pains and injuries can practice the same system as a 25-year-old who is strong and healthy. They can learn the same sequences. What will be very different is how they practice these sequences. The older, less physically capable student will likely move more slowly and possibly with some temporary or permanent modifications of challenging hip rotations, etc. The younger student may move more quickly, but be asked to stay at certain postures until the requisite physical changes to complete the postures come about. I have taught numerous students in the older and less physically able category, and found that they can attain great benefits from the practice, without having to change very much about the postures or sequences. Due to their maturity, their focus and understanding of the inner aspects of the practice are often much deeper than that of the younger and more physically able students.

As a teacher, I try to work intuitively and in direct relationship with each student as they really are, from moment to moment, rather than placing them in a certain category and following a formula. I try to see how the set sequence of the Ashtanga system can be made to work for each practitioner and their unique individual characteristics, so that the real yoga can happen on the inside. This allows for endless possibilities.

Following rigid interpretations of "Patanjali yoga," "meditation" and "pranayama" can become just as dogmatic and unhealthy as rigid interpretations of the physical aspects of asana. All of these aspects of yoga have dual potential as either tools to help us deepen our relationship with ourselves, or as rigid dogmas which only serve to take us deeper in bondage and delusion. The difference lies in the intention and awareness that we bring to whichever practice or scripture it is.

"YOU STOP THERE."

Lessons from Sharath Jois and reflections on the Mysore method

— January 2015 —

I RECENTLY RETURNED FROM MY FIRST three-month trip to practice with Sharath Jois in Mysore. I am not a newcomer to the Ashtanga system—I completed the Fourth series with my previous teacher Rolf Naujokat earlier in 2014, and have maintained a daily Ashtanga practice for nearly 12 years. I knew that when I went to Mysore for the first time, none of this would matter.

When I went to register at the beginning of my three months, Sharath asked me his standard question, "Who is your teacher?" I replied that I had been with Rolf for the past eight years and first learned the system from Mark Darby a few years before that. Sharath didn't ask which posture or series I had learned, nor did I volunteer this information; he had no further questions for me.

Regardless of a person's background, Sharath has everyone start over from the beginning when they come to Mysore for the first time. There are good reasons for this. The way the practice has been taught in Mysore has changed over the years. The practice itself and the method remain the same, but one thing that has changed, and continues to change, is how quickly and under what circumstances people are taught new postures and series. Each Ashtanga teacher also has their own interpretation of how SKPJ or Sharath taught them.

Due to all this variation, the level of integrity in the practice of a first-time student in Mysore can vary. Sharath takes everyone back to the beginning, and observes their practice based on his own standards.

What stood out to me right away is that Sharath has high standards, demanding great integrity from the students who come. These perhaps arise from Sharath's own high standards that he sets for himself.

Sharath has been a part of the Ashtanga lineage in Mysore longer than any other living person. Although he was only a small boy when the first Western students came to practice in Mysore, he began his life in SKPJ's house, and lived and breathed alongside his grandfather until his death. Sharath's connection to the lineage is quite different from a few trips to Mysore—or even many trips—punctuating an otherwise separate life on the other side of the world.

Sharath has completed 25 years of "serious practice" as he calls it—not counting the years he learned asanas for fun before the age of 19. He has been teaching for nearly as long, and in recent years has taught hundreds of students per day, every day of his teaching season. Sharath witnessed firsthand how SKPJ's teaching method changed over the years, and how different types of bodies and minds responded to those methods. He has spent 25 years applying his own evolving interpretation of the method to many different types of bodies and minds.

Sharath has also gone further in his own practice that anyone else in this lineage and system, and still maintains his daily personal practice in spite of having enormous personal responsibilities of family and institution.

Sharath Jois has had more direct experience with the practice on his own body, and in the bodies of thousands of students, than anyone else alive.

His perspective on the practice is unique in its macro and universal, as well as micro and personal aspects.

For my own first trip in Mysore, Sharath had me do Primary series only for the first three weeks. He began giving me Intermediate series postures in the fourth week, one or two or three at a time. He would wait for a few days or a week and then would give me the next set of postures. This started to become a familiar routine during the second month. At the end of the second month, he told me to practice up to *Eka Pada Sirsasana* and the next day he instructed me to join the led intermediate class.

During my first Led Intermediate class, after completing *Eka Pada Sirsasana* I began to roll up my mat and make my way to the change room for finishing postures. As I stood up, Sharath came over and said, "You try *Dwi Pada*." I had to unroll my mat in a hurry, and was still setting it back up as Sharath started counting the five breaths for the posture. I quickly tried to zip myself into *Dwi Pada*. During the exiting vinyasa, Sharath stood in front of me and said, "You stop there." I nodded in understanding and as I moved through upward and downward dog, he looked at me again and repeated for emphasis, "You stop there."

I wasn't surprised. Out of all four series that I have learned and practice, two of my most challenging postures are still in Intermediate series — *Dwi Pada Sirsasana* being one of them.

My previous teachers had deemed those postures to be good enough to move beyond, and for the past 7 years I have only been practicing Intermediate series once per week, devoting the main days of the week to practicing the Third and Fourth series.

Although I have been well aware that two of my Intermediate postures are not up to the standard of all my other postures, the fact that I only encounter them once per week has allowed me to avoid doing the necessary work to go deeper into them. When I would occasionally reflect on this, I would chalk it up to the fact that my 6 ft 3 body and its natural lordosis would not be capable of doing those two postures to the degree of perfection that I have observed other advanced practitioners doing. "Everyone has one or two weak postures," I told myself. I continued to gloss over these postures in my once a week Intermediate practice.

While just about any other senior teacher would judge my *Dwi Pada* to be good enough, Sharath has higher standards. And even if it was good enough, Sharath knew that it could still improve.

"You stop there."

Once he gave me that instruction, I knew the now-familiar pattern of me getting new postures regularly was broken. There would be no new set of postures later that week, or the following week. In fact, he kept me on *Dwi Pada* for the entire third month until the end of my trip. I was not surprised. Each week, before the Monday Led Intermediate class, my girlfriend Susan would say, "I think Sharath will move you on this week." I would smile and say, "We'll see."

It wasn't so difficult for my ego to accept that I had been stopped in Intermediate series. I knew I wouldn't get beyond Intermediate series on my first trip, and expected my two challenging postures to be noticed by Sharath. What was difficult was that I had to actually do the work on *Dwi Pada*!

Nothing changed in my *Dwi Pada* for the next few days, so I decided to give it a little more examination at home. I asked Susan to adjust me more deeply into it, to the degree that I felt Sharath wanted me to be able to do on my own. She did this once or twice so I could get the feeling of the posture.

For the rest of that week, I played around with it at home, trying to find my way into what it felt like when I was adjusted more deeply by Susan. I started to have some degree of success in what I had previously considered to be impossible for my body. In class at the shala, I would also spend more time on it, doing it 2 or 3 times before moving into my finishing postures. Within two weeks of Sharath's "you stop there" instruction, my *Dwi Pada* had improved significantly and visibly. I could feel a whole new level of extension in my upper thoracic spine, ease in lifting my head, and evenness throughout my body.

Still, it was not yet as good as it could be. As I was leaving the shala after practice one morning, Sharath asked: "Iain—you did *Dwi Pada*?" "Yes," I replied. "OK," he smiled and left it at that.

It was during my third or fourth led Intermediate class that Sharath came up behind me during *Dwi Pada*. "Lift your head more!" he exclaimed. I tried. "Iain—lift the head, spread your feet more!" He half-heartedly pulled my left foot to the side. He clearly was not going to adjust me; he wanted me to do the work myself. As I rolled up my mat to leave after *Dwi Pada*, he again said, "The head must be more up—spread the feet!" He looked perplexed, as if I was ignoring his instructions on purpose. "I'm trying," I assured him.

Day by day, *Dwi Pada* became deeper and fuller. I no longer needed to play around with it at home outside of regular practice time, the transformation of the posture had taken on a life of its own and was steadily moving in a particular direction. In the three weeks since I have left Mysore, it has continued to improve, and the new state of the posture now feels very natural. It's been so enjoyable for me to see the changes in a posture in which I previously assumed I had already reached my maximum potential that I have continued to practice Intermediate series only instead of immediately going back to my regular Third and Fourth series practices. It's nice to spend some more time with what Sharath has taught me.

For this change to occur, I needed no technical instruction, and I only needed two adjustments from Susan. I didn't need a two-hour workshop, breaking down the mechanics of the posture, or a special adjustment clinic. I didn't need bodywork. I didn't even need to be adjusted by Sharath in the posture. All I needed was to hear the words "You stop there," in order to begin to focus and develop the posture myself.

This clarifies and validates some of my understanding of how the Ashtanga system works, both as a practitioner and as a Mysore-style Ashtanga teacher.

I am now based in Ubud, Bali and I am exposed to a wide range of students, coming from all over the world and coming from many different teachers. This is quite interesting and a great experience for me. I can now understand much more clearly why Sharath takes everyone back to Primary series when they start with him.

My perspective is that a significant percentage of students who come to practice with me are practicing further into the series than is appropriate for them. I have frequently felt the need to pull people back when they join practice with me, pointing out which postures they have not yet properly integrated or developed, and asking them to stop their practices there. Some students are quite open to this, some are not so happy. It's a bit tricky as a teacher, to be able to do this in a compassionate way so that it doesn't feel as I am taking something away from the student. The reality is, I am giving them something, by showing them where they need to work.

By saying "You stop there" at *Dwi Pada*, Sharath didn't take away the second half of Intermediate, Third and Fourth series away from me. I still have all those postures, and I can still practice them whenever I want (just not in Mysore yet). But what Sharath did is to give me *Dwi Pada*, and that is a real gift. By being asked to stop and do the work, I now feel what *Dwi Pada* should really feel like, for the first time — 11 or 12 years after I first learned it.

Having realized this, I am now finding it easier as a teacher to ask students to "stop there." And if the student is receptive to it, within a matter of days, I can see, and they can also feel, how the posture I have stopped them on starts to transform and change.

There is also the potential to take this concept to an extreme and demand an ideal of perfection that is unattainable. As in anything else, it takes skill and experience to find the middle path, and to find the middle path with compassion. Becoming rigid and overly idealistic will be just as detrimental as being the opposite way.

Each student is an individual, and each individual has their own unique capacity for the different types of movements. As I worked on *Dwi Pada* in the shala in Mysore, I couldn't help but look around and start to compare. Especially during Led Intermediate, I noticed that some of the people who were allowed to move on past *Dwi Pada* and do more postures were not doing *Dwi Pada* any better than I was. In fact, some were significantly worse than me.

I would sometimes grumble to Susan later in the day about this. She would remind me that they had probably also been stopped on *Dwi Pada* for some time, and that Sharath had eventually decided that they had reached their maximum potential and moved them on. "He knows that you can still do it better," she told me. Of course, I knew she was right.

The act of stopping students at a particular posture in the Ashtanga system is not to force everyone to conform to a set standard, but to make sure that each individual develops the posture to their own maximum potential, in a way that is healthy for them.

This is why the standards are different for each individual. The expectations for *Marichyasana D* are going to be very different for an older person who has had five knee surgeries, compared to a younger person who is healthy, but just a bit stiff. The young and stiff person will likely be asked to stop there until they open up and can bind the posture, whereas the older person with damaged knees may be given different expectations.

It takes perceptiveness, skill, and experience on the part of a teacher to do this kind of analysis well. This is the correct application of the Ashtanga system, what I believe is the most important insight we as teachers should be trying to develop in ourselves.

It's my observation that some Ashtanga teachers can get involved in other aspects of teaching at the expense of this insight. It's especially easy to get caught up in teaching that makes the students feel good on a superficial level. Examples of this are giving great adjustments, giving students new postures, and displaying a lot of intellectual knowledge around the anatomy and physiology of the body and how it works in the postures.

When you hear praises being spoken about some Ashtanga teachers, often "he/she gives great adjustments" is a part of this description. And almost everyone feels good when they come away from a few weeks with a senior teacher and have been given a bunch of new postures to work on. And teachers who have a lot of intellectual understanding of anatomy and physiology, and can give long workshops discussing and expounding this understanding are also given a great deal of respect. These are all good recipes for popularity and influence for the teacher. It's an understandable challenge for teachers to resist focusing on these aspects of teaching. The result, however, can be to lose perspective on what the actual point of the practice is.

Receiving a quality adjustment can be very transformative. In fact, it is often an essential ingredient in instigating a transformative process. As I mentioned earlier, when I started to explore *Dwi Pada* more, the first thing I did was ask Susan to adjust me more deeply into it, so I had a bodily experience to work towards. Getting a good adjustment can help to open things up, but more important it gives the mind and nervous system an organic experience of what the end result should FEEL like in the body, so that one can try to recreate it when working on one's own.

Though I asked Susan to adjust me in *Dwi Pada*, I only needed her to adjust me two times. Once I had that experience, I knew my job was to then recreate it myself. It just gave me an understanding of what I was looking for. Sharath never attempted to adjust me in *Dwi Pada*. He merely verbalized in the simplest terms what was lacking in the posture, and then left it up to me to figure it out.

This is how the most skillful teachers will work with students—give them the minimum amount of input necessary for them to understand where they should be going, and then leave it up to them to work it out for themselves. This approach produces the strongest, most stable and most integrated result in the students, and it gives the students greater strength, confidence and power in the long run.

All good teachers know this. When I was practicing Iyengar yoga 15 years ago, I also had this experience. One day I was trying to do an arm balance, struggling and falling over again and again. My teacher (who also happened to be named Sharat) was standing a few feet away quietly watching me. After a lengthy period of time, one of the other students asked, "Sharat, why won't you help Iain?" My teacher replied, "As a teacher, you have to watch, and see how far your student can go." This wisdom is there in all good teachers, from all traditions of yoga, and other forms of practice as well.

Over-adjusting takes power away from the students, and gives it to the teacher. The students become dependent on the teacher for those "great adjustments" to help them feel good. They never develop the ability to make themselves feel good. This dependency serves the teacher by giving them more popularity, student numbers and income, so it can be difficult for the teacher to resist giving out "great adjustments" like candy. I remember my first Iyengar teacher describing this dynamic. He said, "I could give you all an amazing buzz in class every day, and make you addicted to me. I have the power to do this. But my job is to teach you independence, so you can rely on yourselves. This is real yoga."

Understanding of anatomy and physiology is also important. To know how the joints should be rotating, where a particular movement should and shouldn't be coming from, what specific part of the body is actually stuck, and similar categories of knowledge are helpful and important, especially for protection against injury. But—they do not replace the real work that needs to be done to get unstuck.

Years ago I attended a couple of workshops with senior Ashtanga teachers. In these workshops, the teachers broke down the mechanics of *Eka Pada* and *Dwi Pada*. It was interesting and illuminating—intellectually. But these workshops did not change my experience of *Dwi Pada* even slightly. I came away feeling as if I had just spent hours with a teacher who had a lot of knowledge—but my *Dwi Pada* did not change one bit from it. Years later, it was only when Sharath told me, "You stop there" that I finally did the work to change my own *Dwi Pada*.

Teachers who give out a lot of new postures can also be very popular. Some students may attend a two- or four-week workshop or a few weeks of Mysore classes with a "posture-happy" teacher coming away with a handful of new postures to "work on," whether the student is ready for them or not. At the same time, the teacher might be giving "great adjustments" in the difficult postures that are already part of the students' practice repertoire—instead of stopping them there and asking them to work more deeply. This dynamic can breed misunderstanding of how the system works on the body-mind, what the job of the teacher is and what the goals of the practice actually are.

Other, less experienced teachers—with little or no traditional Ashtanga training—develop liberal interpretations of the Ashtanga method and offer Mysore style and Led classes under the Ashtanga name. These teachers are giving out as many postures as a student can handle without collapsing from exhaustion. The goal is to give a strong workout. The result is usually very little integration and a lot of pain and injury. This is also a gross misinterpretation of the method.

The Ashtanga practice is here to help us see where we are stuck. This can manifest on the physical, energetic, mental or emotional plane (or most likely all four at once). Stopping at the postures that force us to encounter where we are stuck is how we actually get to work through some of this, and this is how the practice transforms us as people—physically, energetically, emotionally, and mentally.

The very best Ashtanga teachers will be the ones who show us where we are stuck, and where we need to stop and do the work. The best Ashtanga teachers will be the ones who don't keep giving us great adjustments every day, or spend hours explaining to us the anatomical details, or hand out new postures that we are not ready for. The best Ashtanga teachers will encourage or even force us to stop there, give us minimal guidance, and ask us to do it ourselves. This, in my humble opinion, is the role of the Mysore-style Ashtanga teacher, and the correct application of the method.

ANSWERS TO QUESTIONS

❧ On my statement about Sharath having gone further in his own practice than anyone else in this lineage and system

When I say Sharath has been a part of the Ashtanga lineage longer than anyone, I am referring to multiple levels, beyond the *asana* practice. By taking birth in SKPJ's house, Sharath was exposed, since birth to the entire lifestyle of a master yogi, including all the non-*asana* limbs of practice and lifestyle. Observing Sharath's own lifestyle today—everything from his basic lifestyle choices to his consistency of practice—it is clear that he has absorbed and integrated all these other limbs for the duration of his life. Also, if one counts "time" in terms of, say, number of hours with SKPJ, then there could not be anyone else who has spent more hours, more continuously with SKPJ than Sharath. That is why SKPJ passed the lineage on to Sharath, and not one of the old school Western teachers. As I wrote in this essay, there is a big difference between making annual trips for a few months of the year, and living the life with SKPJ full time since birth.

Sharath has been teaching or assisting in a daily Mysore program for 6 months of the year for almost 25 years. Given that continuity, and given the number of students he has seen each day for that period of time, I think it is quite safe to say that Sharath has much more experience in terms of sheer numbers of students he has taught than any other senior teachers.

In terms of practice, Sharath completed Fifth series, as far as we know. I'm not sure whether it is known or not how far he got into sixth series. I am quite sure that no one else practiced that far.

I don't mean to discredit the practice or teachings of any other senior advanced teachers. Anyone who has practiced for decades has my full respect and is obviously doing something very right. And I have absolutely no doubt that they all have much to offer as teachers.

This essay is not at all about "old school teachers" vs. Sharath. In fact, I learned to the end of the Fourth series from an old school teacher (Rolf Naujokat), and will cherish this experience for the rest of my life. When I went to practice with Sharath for the first time this year, I was filled with natural awe and respect at the level of integrity he carries in every realm of his life, practice and teaching. He impressed me deeply. In my eyes he is truly a master teacher and has integrated and distilled all the elements of a yogic life and the physical Ashtanga Vinyasa practice.

This essay is about what I learned from Sharath, which is mainly a validation of my own understanding of the Mysore method, gained through self-study and self-observation.

❧ On Iyengar and Ashtanga

When I first went to visit Pattabhi Jois's shala in Lakshmipuram in 2000, he allowed me to watch part of a class. It was the last hour or so of the Mysore practice, and it was mostly beginners practicing. At that time I had never tried Ashtanga and had inherited my Iyengar teachers' very strong ideas about what *asana* should and should not look like. Iyengar practitioners and teachers tend to be very rigid in their approach. They tend to write off anything that does not conform to their understanding as being completely useless at best, and detrimental to the practitioner's wellbeing at worst. So, I was watching SKPJ and Sharath teaching Mysore style to beginners with these eyes. My main concern with what I saw was that it seemed very sloppy and the alignment of the postures seemed very unhealthy.

I still place a lot of importance on "good alignment" in practicing the postures and vinyasas now. However, my idea of what alignment is, how it should be taught, and what the essential features of it are, have changed significantly. How it is applied and will manifest in each individual will vary quite a bit. We all have completely different physical and psychological makeups. What constitutes "good alignment" will not be the same for each person.

❦ On my experience with Rolf vs. with Sharath

I am certain that Sharath saw the level of experience I had in my practice with Rolf, and this prompted him to be a little more strict with me, as he knew I would be capable of filling in whatever little holes in my practice had been overlooked by myself and my previous teachers. In many ways, I consider his treatment of me in my two trips to be a compliment and an acknowledgment of the level of development that I do have in my practice.

In this essay, I explain in more detail why I feel it is good that Sharath takes everyone back to the beginning when they start practice with him for the first time. The way the practice has been taught has changed greatly over the past 30–40 years. Sharath has developed his own understanding of how the practice works best for people, and the standards with which he teaches reflect that understanding. This is very different from how the teachers who learned from SKPJ 20 or 30 years ago were taught. To be honest, many of the practitioners I see who have been trained by some of the older senior teachers do not have a very strong practice. They have been allowed to gloss over the difficult parts, and these weak spots in their practices stand out quite a bit to me. In contrast, most practitioners I know who have been trained by Sharath have a very strong practice, with few holes or weak spots, as he requires people to stop and work on those weak spots, sometimes for years at a time.

The whole process is also a very good exercise in humility, which is a quality that can always be deepened by advanced practitioners.

THOUGHTS ON DEEPENING
an authentic yoga practice
— April 2015 —

AUTHENTIC YOGA PRACTICE IS AN exploration in relationship. One who is practicing yoga as *sadhana* (rather than yoga as entertainment) has a relationship with their teacher, a relationship with the practice method or tradition, and most importantly a relationship with the self.

Ultimately, the real work of yoga is to deepen and strengthen these relationships. A solid and stable relationship with the teacher and with the tradition of practice are essential factors in a healthy and transformative yoga practice, but ultimately those relationships are meant to serve as the foundation and support for the deepening of the practitioners' relationship with the self. A deepening of practice always involves a deepening of relationship.

It can be helpful to keep this in mind when we are seeking out ways to deepen our yoga practice.

There are many yoga experiences for sale these days, and many of them are marketed very well. These experiences may include some or all of the following: A famous and charismatic teacher (or several famous teachers);

a certificate of completion, perhaps conferring one with the title of "teacher"; exposure to new postures and/or innovative techniques, knowledge, information, tricks, etc.; a paradise-like setting; and perhaps supplementary forms of quasi-spiritual entertainment.

These types of yoga retreats and events may look exciting and feel stimulating, but when considering this kind of experience, I feel it is important to ask oneself if it will really deepen one's practice—if it will really strengthen one's relationship with a teacher, a tradition, and with oneself—or if it is simply a quasi-spiritual form of entertainment, yet another distraction in the world of commodities competing for a piece of our increasingly weakened attention span.

It is common Western thinking that deepening comes through accumulation. The more we can accumulate, the more we have, and the more we have to offer.

A quick glance at the website of an average Western yoga studio (and Eastern studios which mimic the Western yoga studio model) will exemplify this type of thinking. A popular studio usually offers classes in a number of different styles or forms of yoga. Something is there for everyone, and the potential student is welcome to choose whatever suits their particular mood: Hot or cool, fast or slow, gentle or vigorous, etc. Glancing at the teacher roster will usually show a large number of teachers. The biographies of the teachers usually include a list of several different styles of yoga that they have "studied" and an even longer list of well-known teachers that they have "studied with." There are even multidisciplinary teacher training programs where over a span of one month, potential teachers are "trained" in several different styles of yoga, by several different mentors, and then left to decide which particular form they want to start teaching.

It is increasingly rare to see a yoga school which gives thorough and structured instruction in one tradition or system of yoga, and even rarer to see a teacher's biography which states something along the lines of "I am qualified to teach yoga because I spent 20 years practicing under Master teacher X and went really deep with him."

In any long-term relationship, we need to continue to adjust and recalibrate in order to keep it healthy. The same goes for a long-term relationship with a teacher and a tradition of practice. This commitment and constant adjustment and recalibration can be a strong stimulus for healthy self-evolution, if done with intention and awareness. Ultimately, this provides a stable foundation to take us deeper into relationship with ourselves and to evolve into healthier and more functional people.

A relationship by definition involves an interaction or exchange between two entities. If we are having a "relationship" with ourselves, and deepening that relationship through yoga practice, it implies that there are two different aspects of ourselves that need to communicate with each other.

Canadian author Matthew Remski recently wrote an article in which he attempted to define the concept of "meditation." Part of his definition included:

It can be helpful to view meditation as the gradual process of improving numerous layers of internal conversation between the "feeling-self" and the "conscious-self."

I found this to be quite helpful in clarifying my own concept of how we use yoga practice to deepen communicate with ourselves.

Modern human society has created the possibility for our conscious minds to exist almost entirely in a world of ideas, conceptions and creations. We really don't need to feel very much if we prefer not to. Much of the conceptual world of the conscious mind makes little or no sense to the innate intelligence of the feeling body—yet we have trained ourselves to stop hearing the feeling body as we drag it along through the conceptual universe the mind has created.

Only in times of extreme pleasure or extreme discomfort, when the feeling body shouts out so loudly that it can no longer be ignored do we start to listen. Even in these times, that listening rarely represents healthy discourse or dialogue between the conscious mind and feeling body. Usually it involves doing the quickest and easiest thing possible to satisfy the cravings or remove the cries of pain of feeling body, so that it retreats back into the shadows and we can return to our fabricated mental world of ideas and concepts.

My various practices have evolved and intertwined over the past 15–20 years to the stage where they are united by one process: To improve the communication and deepen the relationship between my conscious mind and my feeling body. In other words, my practice is a vehicle to deepen my relationship with myself.

The different forms of formal practice that I take on a daily basis—including Vipassana meditation, Ashtanga Vinyasa yoga, Pranayama, the Buddha's *pancha sila* or Patanjali's *yamas* and *niyamas* (the practice of investigating the ethics of our relationships with the world), dietary observations, etc.—are all different lenses through which I examine and tinker with this central theme. Each of these practices is necessary for me, as any one of them alone will not suffice to cover the entire field of my own experience, my own feeling body.

Just as "science" is divided into separate categories of exploration, such as physics, biology, chemistry and psychology, so that the entire field of publicly observable, objective reality is covered, so the different spiritual practices of seated meditation, asana, pranayama, ethics, diet, etc., are all there to cover the entire field of the introspective, subjective reality of the feeling body.

According to some interpretations of the Buddha's teaching, the unconscious mind is constantly in contact with the sensations of the feeling body. Not only that, but the unconscious mind is constantly generating a reaction of craving or aversion to the sensations of the feeling body. We remain mostly unaware of this ongoing process of reaction to sensation, but its long-term effects become deeply embedded in our psyches. These reactions are the foundations of all our mental complexes, habit patterns, tendencies and the general issues that most people are aware, to some degree, that they have and that perhaps they should "work on." The Buddha termed them "sankhara" (in the Pali language) and Patanjali termed them "*samskara*" (in Sanskrit). According to both teachers they are the source of all our suffering, both internally and externally as we reflect them into our relationships with the world.

The first step to working on these reactive habit patterns is to become consciously aware of them. The most effective way to do this is to go straight to the source where they are generated—the interaction of the mind with the feeling body. The essence of the Buddha's Vipassana practice is to be aware of the feeling body without generating any reaction to it as continuously as possible.

In the *Satipatthana Sutta*, the Buddha claimed that if we can stay aware of the sensations of the feeling body and we manage to not generate any reaction of craving or aversion to those sensations and feelings and we can do this continuously, without interruption, not missing that awareness for even a moment, then we will become fully liberated from all of our *sankhara* patterns (enlightened) within a period of 7 days to 7 years. Whether it takes 7 days or 7 years would depend on the level and degree of accumulation of *sankhara* patterns, which is unique in each individual.

It may sound fairly simple to become liberated. We just have to do one thing for somewhere in between 7 days and 7 years. Unfortunately, observing the feeling body objectively is not an easy thing to do. In fact, it is epically hard work.

Any authentic practice that takes us deeper into this experience is not likely to be an easy sell. It is an immense challenge to face what is happening inside without flinching or turning away. Yet, my own explorations have led me to believe that this is the most direct way to becoming the most consistent, integrated, functional and meaningful beings that we can possibly be. It is really the only way to strengthen and deepen our relationship with ourselves. It is the most honest communication there is.

Once the conscious mind and feeling body have learned how to communicate with each other more harmoniously, we start making healthier life choices on all levels, from what we choose to eat and how we spend our time, to how we tend to react and interact on a deeper level with everything around us, including other beings.

I have observed these benefits grow in myself over 15 years of steady and consistent practice. It is my understanding of what Sharath Jois often refers to in conferences as "the yoga happening inside you." While I do have doubts and reservations about whether these benefits can be extrapolated to the Buddha's definition of total liberation, I have no doubt that the benefits exist and continue to increase with long-term practice.

Yoga and meditation practices that are for sale are often touted as bringing about "bliss," "peace," "happiness," etc. There is little doubt that a deeper sense of contentment, consistency and functionality should be the long-term results of these practices. We may very well also experience short-term effects that can be both blissful and intoxicating as we practice.

However, for one who is practicing authentically, by which I mean using the practice as a means to deepen their awareness of and communication with the feeling body, there is soon enough going to be some unpleasant experiences and feelings to encounter. In fact, this can sometimes be the dominant experience for extended periods of time along the way.

All of our negative and unpleasant *sankhara* patterns need to come into the light of the conscious mind, via the feeling body. We need to see them and look them in the eye and learn how to be completely comfortable and OK with them. Only then will the patterns weaken and begin to dissipate.

The good news is that we don't need anything aside from our own steady awareness to achieve this. We don't need protection or help from deities. We don't need mantras, blessings, incense or prayers. We don't need *shak-*

tipat. We don't need a body worker or an exorcist. It's all within our own reach—all we have to do is be willing to know and feel our own *sankhara* patterns completely, by using an authentic practice to take us there. Then, the transformation happens naturally, without force or being contrived by the conscious mind.

Once we've created non-reactive union between the conscious mind and the feeling body, the realignment happens automatically. For 99 percent of people, having a stable relationship with one tradition and one guide will also be a necessary support network to this work.

This is simple, but epically challenging. Human beings are hard-wired to seek pleasure and avoid pain. So, if we are engaging in a practice that brings us into conscious contact with some potentially unpleasant experiences in the feeling body, our natural instinct will be to run away. It requires comprehension of the process, determination, focus and faith to stay with it and override our instinctual response to avoid. We must also do this in a balanced way, encountering only as much as we have the capacity to process and integrate into our lives. Not so many people are willing to do this deeper work, which is why spending 20 years with a master teacher in one particular practice remains an uncommon phenomenon.

When people are working authentically and they do start to encounter deeper layers of themselves through practice, I have observed that there are three things that tend to happen:

1. Stop practice—turn away and repress *sankhara* patterns

This is the most common occurrence. Stopping practice can mean quite literally quitting. Stopping Ashtanga (or whatever practice it may be) and moving on to another form of yoga or practice.

But it can also manifest in subtler ways. For example—a teacher holds a student on a particular posture because it is not yet mastered there is still some deep work to do. The posture is challenging as it is bringing up some unpleasantness in the feeling body and the mind is reacting to that. The student decides that he has had enough of this particular teacher and moves on to find another teacher who is less demanding and allows them to avoid, modify or even skip that posture. The student hasn't quit Ashtanga, but they have succeeded in avoiding the most transformative opportunity in the practice.

Other practitioners manage to bash their way through the practice without feeling themselves at all. Rather than using the practice to deepen their sensitivity towards their feeling body, they actually numb themselves as a way to "get through it." Or, they turn on the TV, play music, talk, etc. These are all ways to avoid the real work, the introspective encountering of the self through the practice. One is going through the motions physically, but they are not really practicing.

2. Use practice to feed and deepen *sankhara* patterns

This is also a regular occurrence. Those with self-deprecating and self-abusive tendencies can find very fertile soil in the Ashtanga practice to make these *sankhara* even deeper.

The model Ashtangi with the perfect physique and beautiful practice becomes an ideal that the conscious mind of the student attempts to embody, denying the reality of their own feeling body as they try to bash it into their vision of perfection.

The yoga selfie era of Facebook statuses and *Yoga Journal* covers has contributed much to this unfortunate phenomenon. As a result, eating disorders manifest or are worsened, knees and backs are forced until they break, and the rift between the conscious mind and the feeling body becomes wider and wider.

Or those with self-aggrandizing tendencies can also find fertile soil to deepen their patterns. The strength and energy generated by the practice are channeled into becoming even more manipulative and controlling. Once these types of people become teachers with other students looking up to them, the effects can become outright disastrous, for themselves and for the other lives that they succeed in damaging. There are too many stories of abusive and scandalized teachers and gurus. This is not an uncommon path to take either, unfortunately.

3. Quietly observe, and keep practicing

One can cultivate patience and objective observation. Whatever the feeling body is telling us, we listen. We try to listen as clearly as possible. And we accept what it has to say to us. And with that sensitivity, we continue our practice with awareness and allow the changes to manifest naturally.

Having a clear understanding of what we are really doing with the practice, combined with faith, focus, humility and patience, along with the support and guidance of a good teacher and a healthy tradition can allow us to gradually work through all the *sankhara* patterns that practice exposes us to.

This is difficult, it requires a real willingness to adapt and change. It requires humility and it requires surrender — to our tradition, to our teacher, and above all to our own feeling body. Those who do take this path become very grounded, balanced, functional and compassionate practitioners and teachers whose lives are greatly enhanced by what they do.

No one is perfect, and even with the best intentions, we all end up falling into category 1 or 2 from time to time. It is another reason that the support and feedback of a healthy practice community, a good teacher, and a lot of self-reflection are necessary. If we have these supports and this intention, and we persist, then we will succeed in practicing authentically and the practice will be a support to help our lives become the best that they can be.

ASHTANGA,
EMBODIMENT
& COMPLEX
SYSTEMS

PERCEIVING & BEING PERCEIVED

*The reciprocal relationship with
the non-human world*

— October 2015 —

GIVEN THE AMOUNT OF TIME in my life that I have spent hiking and hanging out in bear habitat, I consider myself lucky to have almost completely avoided any form of contact or encounter with bears. I've only once seen a bear while out walking, and that was a fleeting encounter as the bear ignored me and continued along its way—which is how the majority of human-bear encounters go.

I've done plenty of day hikes on my own, including many in bear habitat—but most of my backcountry hikes involving overnight camping have been with one or more other people.

A few days ago, I embarked on what was to be a five-day solo hike in Algonquin Park, Ontario—the first place I experienced backcountry hiking when I was a teenager and still my favorite place in the world to be immersed in nature. It was the third purely solo backcountry hike of my life. I've probably hiked through this area 15 times in my life, though the last time was in 2003.

Early October in this part of the world is ideal for hiking: The fall colors are in their glorious peak, the weather is crisp—but still mild enough to work up a sweat in the afternoon, it is generally dry, and the biting insects are non-existent—having perished in the onset of cooler nights in the preceding weeks.

I arrived at the access point to the Western Uplands trail around 1:30 p.m. after a 3-hour drive from the suburbs of Toronto where I was staying with my family. It was several hours later than I would have liked to arrive given the 12 km distance to the lake where I would spend my first night, and the limited daylight hours at this time of year. Still—I had enough time if I carried a good pace.

I put the finishing touches on my backpack—which as usual was far too heavy for comfort. In a group hike the shared supplies—such as tent, stove, fuel, cooking equipment, water filter, etc., can be split up amongst the group members. On a solo hike, it all goes on one person's back—along with the cold weather sleeping bag, extra clothing, thermarest pad, five days worth of food, and all the other necessary odds and ends to survive and have some relative comfort in the backcountry for a week.

It was a warm and sunny afternoon and as soon as I entered into the wonderland of colors and smells, all of my sense doors came to life and synchronized with my nervous system and inner being. I felt happy, calm and aligned on all levels. As humans, we place far too much importance on our relationships with each other and with our human-made devices. Our sense doors and nervous systems have evolved over millions of years to be in relationship with the non-human world. There is little wonder that most people feel unfulfilled in life, as they keep themselves isolated in a human-only world and attempt to satisfy their need for relationship in this very narrow realm.

In his excellent book *Becoming Animal*, David Abram suggests that the growing acceptance in popular culture of the connection between body and mind is not enough and that most of the therapists and healers exploring this connection have missed something very vital. He claims that to fully experience balance and wellbeing, we must also emphasize the connection between the human body-mind and the body-mind of the non-human world—the body-mind of the earth. To truly be balanced and whole, our senses need to be in relationship with the non-human world, as they have been "designed" this way by the coevolution of our species with all of the other non-human entities over millions of years. In essence, we are coupled to the non-human world to such a degree that it is a part of us and we are a part of it. Cutting off this vital aspect of our heritage and our being, as the modern city dweller does, is to cut off a part of what we are.

Maintaining a reciprocal and communicative relationship with all the non-human forms of life (and non-life) always has a profoundly balancing effect on the senses and nervous system, and on the deeper layers of our being—for those who choose to pay attention. In my opinion, those who are not able to have this kind of ongoing relationship with the non-human world have little chance at sustaining true clarity and harmony.

I feel that the major shortcoming of traditional perspectives on yoga and meditation is that they fail to address or recognize this vital aspect of being human. Just as the reductionist approach to science attempts to isolate a variable from its natural context in order to learn more about it, this approach to understanding the human psyche removes the human individual from the context of its manifold relationships with all that is "other." Liberation is sought by attempting to overcome or detach from the illusory or impermanent nature of these relationships to the physical earth and all of its non-human inhabitants. My own evolving perspective of spirituality is that the relationship between ourselves and the non-human world is so deep and ancient, that we need to practice in a way that recognizes these relationships as a part of who and what we are. We need to remain aware of and immersed in relationship with the rest of the planet earth, if we are to know ourselves completely.

Immersed in the manifold relationships with the non-human world, I never feel lonely or bored when I am alone in nature. In fact, I usually find that any concerns that have been weighing on me tend to lighten and become less significant once I step into a world that is dominated by that which is non-human. I thoroughly enjoyed the 4-hour hike to Maggie Lake, though the weight of my pack was bogging down my energy and awareness by the time I arrived.

Maggie Lake is large. There is a 6 km trail which circumambulates the lake and about 10 designated campsites scattered around its shores. I chose the second site which I came to. There was a large cleared area—perfect for a tent and some extra space on the soft pine needled floor for morning yoga if the weather allowed for it. There was a decent fire pit with some large flat logs surrounding it and someone had kindly left a neat stack of chopped wood. The site was only a few steps away from the rocky shore and clear waters of the lake.

I had not seen any other hikers on my walk in. Sound travels very well across a lake in the silence of the backcountry, and hearing no other sounds or signs of human beings, I guessed that I would probably be spending the night completely alone on this lake.

It was about 5:30 p.m. and the sun was already sinking low on the Western horizon over the lake. I figured I had about 60–90 minutes of daylight left. The beautiful and inviting campsite and lake would soon become completely dark—a form of darkness that is much denser than anything we can experience in human settlements. I had numerous things to accomplish before that happened and I began to feel a little stressed.

In order to prepare for the dark and cold night safely, I needed to set up my tent and lay out the things from my backpack in their appropriate places. I needed to find firewood and cut it, as the little bit that had been left at the campsite would not last long. I needed to set up my stove and cooking equipment, collect water, cook my food, eat my food, wash up my cooking equipment, filter water for drinking, repack my food and then hang all the food up in a tree to protect it from animals. This was quite a bit of work to accomplish in a short time, so I kept my focus strong and set into action.

I managed to get it all done, and in the last bit of fading light I roped my food bag over a high and strong-looking branch that I had located earlier when the light was better.

I was not completely satisfied with the location of the food pack. It is often difficult to find a perfect location—high enough that a bear cannot reach it from the ground, and far away enough from the trunk of the tree that a climbing bear could not reach over and grab it. The branch also needs to be strong enough to hold the food bag. This particular branch was a little low and a little close to the trunk. Still, I figured it would be good enough. I had never had an issue with animals getting food out of a tree at night and I had used many non-ideal branches in the past.

With the work finished, I was finally able to relax a bit and enjoy the darkness and solitude of the lake. I spent a few minutes sitting by the fire, and then wandered over to the lake to watch the final glow of daylight on the Western horizon fade and disappear. I noted that there were no other lights on the shores of the lake—no flickering campfires. I was indeed alone, probably the only human in at least a 10 km radius. It was a clear night and an incredible canopy of stars slowly emerged.

I spent some more time by the fire, feeling sleepy and vaguely disturbed in my body due to the tension of carrying my heavy pack over 12 km and the stressful rush to get everything finished upon arrival. I slowly relaxed and tried to read a little bit. I was too sleepy to focus on the writing, so I just sat quietly in meditation until I felt as if it was time to get into bed. I walked over to take one last look at the lake and open sky, in the now complete darkness of night.

The star canopy was incredible. I could not focus my gaze on it, it was a bit like an illusion where the more I looked, the more stars would appear and then seem to dance around, flicker and disappear. The sky was alive with an infinite number of points of light, all varying in brightness and seemingly moving around. I could relax my gaze and focus on the recognizable constellations which clearly stood out, but then when I tried to focus more the sky would seem to fill with more and more elusive points of brightness behind the constellations—a background of ever-increasing complexity. It had been a long time since I had seen a sky like this.

I walked back to the fire and put the last few things in their place for the night. I had a small machete for cutting wood which I was about to put under a plastic bag cover with my stove and water filter on an old tree stump. I reconsidered and then brought it to the tent with me. Just in case…

Though there are many documented cases of humans who have been killed or badly injured by bears—the probability of this happening is very low. One has a much greater likelihood of being killed or injured in a car accident on the road than of being killed or injured by a bear in the backcountry. Still—just as one takes reasonable precautions against car accidents, or protection (such as seat belts) in the event that one is in an accident—one also takes reasonable precautions to prevent bear encounters in the wilderness (such as treeing all the food after dark) and thinks about protection (such as a weapon) in the unlikely event that there is a bear encounter.

When I am camping with a group, I don't think about bears beyond taking these precautions. When I am camping alone, it is a different story. Alone, my thoughts and fears can run wild and on my previous solo trips the process of getting into my tent and lying quietly before sleep was always a very fearful one. I would imagine "what if…" and picture a bear coming into my campsite at night, perhaps with some interest in me as a meal. I would imagine what I would or could do—which generally would be very little. The feeling of helplessness and vulnerability that arose would trigger more fear reaction and the process would build until I consciously applied various techniques to put a stop to it. Still, I was never really completely comfortable in going to sleep at night when alone in the wilderness. The fear was always there, just below the surface, even if I had it under control. Encountering that fear was part of the process of hiking and camping alone.

Mountaineer Reinhold Messner, whom I consider to be a fascinating person and a great yogi, made similar statements. Of the many mind-boggling feats of mountaineering which he accomplished—a number of them were alone. He often stated in interviews that he climbed some of his most dangerous climbs alone simply to face his own fear. Being alone at night on the mountain was an almost unbearable fear for him, and the process of encountering that was a way to know himself better. Another very true statement he made was that when you are in a dangerous situation with another person, the fear is much less because you can share it. When you are alone in a similar situation, the fear is much greater as you can only experience it yourself and process it inside yourself.

I was happy to note that tonight seemed different for me. Maybe I was just so tired that I didn't have the energy to imagine a bear encounter. I did feel the familiar thoughts arising, but it was very easy to let them slide off and I felt quite comfortable and safe as I quickly drifted into sleep, warm and cozy in my winter sleeping bag. That was around 9 p.m.

At 12:30 I woke up sharply. A few times in my life I have been awakened with the awareness of a very real danger that I had to respond to. This was a similar experience. I woke up and was immediately very alert. The only way to describe what I felt was that I perceived a vector of energy running at a diagonal to the orientation of my body in the tent, its closest point perhaps five meters away from my head. The vector of energy ran directly to where my food was hanging in the tree, perhaps 15–20 meters away from my tent.

I sat up immediately and listened. Sure enough, there were some loud noises. Thumping and then some sticks snapping. I realized that something was near my food. There was no fear, just a heightened state of awareness and a calm lucidity. There were several different sounds. The heavy thumping, the snapping of sticks, and then another sound which was the very particular sound that a dead tree makes when you are trying to pull its roots out of the earth—a sort of earthy ripping sound.

There was little doubt that it was a bear. I tried to rationally deny it to myself, thinking that it could be some smaller mammal, but I quickly put my own doubts to rest as it was clear that the sounds I was hearing could only be made by a very large mammal, and a large mammal with some degree of dexterity—which ruled out every possibility except a bear.

I noted with some interest that I did not feel emotionally afraid. At an intellectual level, I was quite aware that this was a very bad situation and that the paranoid imaginations of my past were now actually happening: I was alone in the wilderness, in the dead of night, and a bear had voluntarily entered into my campsite and was aware of my presence there and clearly not afraid of me. "This…is…really happening." I acknowledged the reality of the situation to myself, but the emotional fear reaction that would come when I had imagined this situation in the past was notably absent.

Part of me wanted to react emotionally, as if it was the right thing to do, but the emotions were distant clouds. They could not touch me and I could not touch them. The center of my being and awareness was simply calm and collected focus. I reached for my headlamp and slipped it onto my head (without turning it on), grabbed and unsheathed my machete and held it in my right hand and quietly waited.

There is no standard procedure for a bear encounter. There are common threads of advice, but the advice can be different depending on whether it is a grizzly or a black bear as well as numerous other factors. In this region of Canada, it could only be a black bear. Black bears are generally considered to be less dangerous and potentially predatory towards humans than grizzly bears are—but black bears are also less predictable and there are certainly enough documented cases of black bears stalking and killing humans.

Bears tend to avoid humans in general. The vast majority of bear encounters happen because the bear is caught by surprise. Once the bear realizes that a human being is close by, it turns and leaves the area. This is the best-case scenario and the most common scenario.

The next scenario is that the bear realizes there is a human close by, but it does not leave or show fear—or the bear voluntarily enters into contact with humans. This increases the danger of the situation significantly and this was the situation that I found myself in at that moment. Bears are very intelligent and have keen senses. The bear could smell me and there is no doubt at all that the bear knew I was very close by, in my tent. This did not seem to faze the bear at all.

The only way the situation could become worse would be if the bear decided to investigate the possibility of making me into a meal. So far, I had no reason to believe this would happen.

"They" say that if a black bear approaches you or your camp, the first course of action should be to try to scare it off. Making a lot of noise, flashing lights, jumping around in order to look big are the commonly listed techniques. I could see this being potentially effective with a group of people, in the daylight. While guidelines can be good, blindly following them without analyzing the unique situation at hand can be troublesome.

I could have put my headlamp (which is particularly bright) on strobe, used my Fox 40 whistle, which I had also located and had in my other hand, and stepped out of my tent and shone the flashing light at the bear, blowing my whistle, yelling and waving my machete around. This might have been enough to send the bear running away into the night. It could also have made the bear feel threatened, and liable to attempt to defend its newly found food source from me.

Had I been with at least one other strong person, whom I felt confident would stay cool if the situation escalated further, I might have suggested we do just that. But I was alone and it seemed exceedingly foolish to try to scare the bear away and risk provocation.

I decided to sit and wait. The bear would either succeed in getting my food, have a good meal and leave, it would fail to get my food and leave, or it would either get my food or not, and then decide to investigate the tent and me. I figured the first possibility—that it would get my food and then leave was the most likely. The chances of it coming to the tent were very low, especially considering I had been careful to have no trace of food in the tent.

I devised a plan in the unlikely event that the bear did approach my tent. Once I heard it come close, I would begin to make a lot of noise. I would blow my whistle and yell. If that did not work and the bear attempted to come into the tent, I would move on to Plan B.

If the bear wanted to come into the tent and kill me, it could. A bear could slash or bite through the thin polyester walls of the tent in no time. I knew that I would have one big advantage, however: The bear would have to use its claws or its teeth to rip a hole in the tent before it could reach me. If I stayed cool and poised with my machete and my light, I would see exactly where its limb or face was going to come through the tent, and I would be able to take the first shot. The machete was brand new, the blade was sharp and about 2/3 the length of my forearm. If I struck well, the bear would be seriously injured before it had a chance to hit or bite me—especially if the strike was to its face. It would likely be enough to send the bear running off, bleeding and confused. I seriously hoped it would not come down to this, but it also gave me confidence to know that I had a plan of action which had a reasonable chance of success if it did come down to it.

I calmly waited. The noises went on for a long time. Eventually I heard another large thud and figured my food had hit the ground. The subsequent sounds of wrestling plastic confirmed this.

It had probably been close to an hour since I woke up and I had been sitting upright, half out of my sleeping bag with a machete in hand for the entire time. It was close to zero degrees and I was starting to get very cold as my upper body was exposed to the crisp night air with only a light layer of clothing on. I still felt little emotional fear and was increasingly confident that the bear would not approach the tent. I decided to lie back down and cover myself with the sleeping bag fully. I kept my headlamp on my head and laid the machete beside my sleeping bag, still out of its sheath. I kept both my ears off the pillow and continued to listen intently and wait.

Eventually the noise subsided. I figured the bear had departed. I was surprised to find that I felt very sleepy and eventually started to drift off. I awoke a short time later to more of the same noise. The bear had returned for more. I sighed and stayed in a lying position while the bear apparently went for another round of the same procedure. I actually drifted in and out of sleep while the bear continued to wrestle with the tree and my food. It probably went on for a total of three hours. Eventually, silence ensued and I went back into a deeper sleep.

I awoke to the first signs of dawn around 6:30 a.m. When sleeping outdoors, the subtle changes that immediately precede the onset of dawn can be tangibly felt and often lead to a natural awakening from sleep. Still tired, I went back to sleep. I was confident the bear had long since departed. Around 7:30 a.m., it felt fully light and I decided to venture out. As soon as I opened the tent door, I saw my food bag still hanging in the tree. I was quite surprised and happy but then quickly realized that the bag was empty. Walking over, I saw the detritus of my food and its wrappings spread around the ground. It looked a bit like a bomb had hit it, with tiny shards of plastic and little bits of rejected food everywhere. The hanging food bag (which was also my tent bag) had been pulled closer to the trunk of the tree, was looped over the branch a second time and had a gaping hole in the bottom of it.

I took stock of what was left of the food. The bear had been selective in what it ate. It almost completely avoided the dried foods which required a lot of cooking. These would have provided little nutrition for the bear if eaten raw, and the bear knew that. Unfortunately, some of the bags holding this kind of food were ripped open and the food spilled out over the ground. A few meals worth remained untouched. I began to pick up the pieces and salvage what I could.

I noted with some amusement that my Vega Sport Protein bars—all 5 of them—were the bear's favorite. There was not a single crumb left of any of the 5 bars, and all that remained of the wrappers looked as if they had been put through a paper shredder. This was a smart bear! Those bars were by far the most nutrient dense food that I had and would have been perfect for a black bear preparing for hibernation. The next favorite part of my food were all the other fresh and raw foods—dates, nuts, seeds, dried fruits—all of which had been completely opened and eaten, though a few crumbs of each still lay in the bottom of those bags.

Though I was sure the bear was long gone, making fire felt like the first thing that should happen. It was a cold morning—but the main reason for making fire was to re-establish myself as the reigning boss of the campsite. In the daylight and with a good fire burning, the territory was once again mine. Humans are diurnal animals and it is easier to feel confident and able to use our abilities to our advantage when it is daylight.

I tried to decide my next course of action. After rounding up the remnants of my food and deciding what was still usable, I had about 1.5–2 days worth of food left. To complete my hike I needed 3.5 more days.

During the night, I had felt there was little question that I would be heading back to the car first thing in the morning. Now, I felt a little more relaxed and open to other possibilities. There was no hurry. I felt hungry and still had my hot cereal and instant coffee, so I started to prepare both things and reflect on my next course of action.

I had three choices: I could try to continue my hike, and ration the food I had out—eating less, or increasing my daily walking distance so I could cover the distance in less time; I could try to shorten my route and spend one more day and night at another lake; or I could hike out the same way I came in and leave.

I didn't want to give up my hike. Four more days in the park would have been wonderful, and I had carried in enough food and fuel and clothing to do that. One perspective would be to look at my food loss as a "donation" to the forest, and continue on with what I had. I tried to think of different backcountry hikers that I knew or knew of, and I knew that some people would shrug the incident off and carry on.

On the other hand, I could take the perspective that what happened was a form of a warning and that the forest actually wanted me to leave. I could count myself lucky that the situation hadn't been worse, and leave with the good fortune I still had. Pushing on could be risking further and greater problems. If I distanced myself more than a day's walk from the car and another misfortune happened, it could be a very bad situation indeed. I knew the park was quite empty of other hikers and there would be no one to help me out even deeper in the park.

It was a beautiful morning, the sky was blue and the air so crisp and clean. The sun had risen and my spirits were high, in spite of what had happened. I did not want to leave this pristine place after only one night! I decided I would like to carry on and set about preparing to do so. After my breakfast I sat beside the fire and carefully stitched up my tent/food bag with a needle and thread. I reorganized and re-bagged my remaining food. I took my time and enjoyed the place.

After some time, I pulled out my map and tried to figure out the best options. If I quickened my pace so that I only spent two more nights, it would mean hiking 20 km a day, which felt like a bit much, especially given the shorter days of autumn. If I spent three nights and rationed my food out, it would mean eating very little. If I shortened my route and cut across to another lake that I had not planned for, I might not find an empty campsite. Besides—wherever I spent the next night, I knew that as soon as I made camp my thoughts would be predominantly with worry about another bear incident. It would not be a pleasant evening. I also noted that the bear had only left me with food that would require cooking. This meant I would need to use my stove every time I wanted to eat, regardless of the environmental conditions. Staying in the park was seemingly like less of a good idea. It was approaching noon and I needed to make a decision. It would be 4–5 hours' walk, whichever direction I was going in. I sat by the lake and noticed the sky was starting to change. Part of the horizon was acquiring a density which I knew was the beginning of an overcast sky. There was a good chance that within a few hours it would be completely overcast and raining. That sealed the deal. I decided to stay in camp a bit longer, eat some lunch and hike back to the car. My excursion was over.

It definitely felt too soon to leave the forest. The clarity and focus of mind that comes from the deepening of relationship with the non-human world and the removal of many of the human-made distractions is a real treasure that I only get to touch once in a while. To have to let go of it after only two days felt like a shame. Nonetheless, I was happy and I felt good. It had been a beautiful two days in the forest, at one of the best times of the year. The weather was perfect and I was lucky to have experienced what I did. To walk out in the current nice weather and a full belly would likely be better than pushing deeper into the park, to spend a night in the rain without being able to eat as much as I wanted to. I hiked out in a good mood.

I crossed paths with two groups of hikers on my way out. Both were heading to Maggie Lake. I related the incident to both groups and warned them. It was nice to note that both groups of people were more worried about me and my lack of food than they were about walking into a lake with a habituated bear hanging around. Both groups offered me food in spite of my assurance that I was not hungry. One of them literally forced me to take a few energy bars before they carried on their hike. People are very generous in the forest!

I learned a lot about bears. I used to think of them more as bumbling, brutish animals whose main advantage was in their size and strength—not in their intelligence. This bear was extremely intelligent. In reflection, I was impressed at how it executed the whole operation. It had clearly done this before. It knew exactly when to come—when my fire had died down to nothing and I had been in bed for several hours. It knew I would not dare to challenge it in the dark. It might have been watching me and planning since before dark. It knew how to get my food out of the bag in the tree, and then it knew which foods to eat and which to leave. It was not a bumbling foraging bear that randomly happened onto my campsite in the night—it was a well planned and executed theft by an intelligent and sentient being.

As humans, we often tend to objectify the non-human world to the degree that we forget that we are not only perceivers, but also perceived. All of nature perceives us. It all has intelligence—even the trees and rocks have a form of intelligence and can perceive us. This bear had immense perceptive abilities and it perceived and analyzed me in a lot of detail. I was an object, a factor in its quest for food before a long winter's hibernation and it made a number of correct calculations and actions to minimize my ability to keep my food out of its reach.

Another interesting thing was that my previous imaginings of a bear coming into my camp at night while I am camping alone were MUCH more frightening than when it actually happened. Looking back on the incident, I can honestly say that there was next to zero emotional fear while it was happening. Yet, all those previous times that I imagined it happening I would be gripped by an overpowering and visceral experience of fear.

I'm not sure if I will ever hike alone again. I love the experience of the solitude. When there are no other people, we absolutely have to be completely immersed in relationship with the non-human world. While one can experience this on a solo day hike, the longer one stays immersed alone in nature, the deeper this experience gets. It is wonderfully clearing and rejuvenating.

At the same time, I never want to experience what I just experienced again. Though I was able to remain fearless and clear-headed, and everything turned out OK (aside from losing my food and ending my hike early)—there is no doubt that being alone in such a situation vastly increases the risk factor, especially if the bear turns aggressive.

We'll see... time will tell.

ANSWERS TO QUESTIONS

❧ On the divide between "us" and "nature"

I have felt for a long time that the "protect nature" mentality was partly responsible for deepening the divide between "us" and "nature." Nature is not something we need to protect, it is something we need to be a part of. I've known numerous people who apply completely different rules of conduct when they are in a protected wilderness space vs. a space that is part of a human settlement.

It has been noted by several authors that animist and pre-agricultural cultures did not conceive of a distinction between themselves and "nature." "Nature" was a part of them and they were a part of it, there was no need to differentiate between the human world and the other world.

While we certainly cannot and should not revert to a pre-agricultural or animist type of civilization, we do need to consider that there are certain aspects of these cultures and civilizations which would serve us greatly, if we were able to somehow rediscover and instill them as we attempt to move forward as a collective group of cultures known as the human species.

If we are not to poison ourselves out of existence, then the sharp distinction between the human world and "nature" must be removed — at a conceptual level of collective consciousness.

The point I made in this essay is that just as removing the sharp distinction between body and mind is a step forward and towards a more authentic experience of the truth of our existence — so will removing the distinction between the body-mind of the human and the body-mind of "nature" be another big step towards individual and collective authenticity and wellness.

As for the fate of our species — and whether the above point can actually happen or not — I have my doubts. Sometimes being amongst like-minded people can give me the impression that things are changing for the better, but then stepping out into the seething mass of humanity at large reminds me that very few people will be willing or able to make the radical changes in mentality required for our species to change its course anytime soon.

I believe there is a vector of intelligence in the evolutionary path of our species, and of all other species, but I don't believe it will necessarily guarantee any particular result, nor is there any particular purpose.

Just as every cell in the human body eventually dies — but the human body continues to live on with new cells — so every species on the planet (including Homo sapiens) eventually becomes extinct, but the planet will continue to live on with new species.

Nonetheless, I feel it is my own duty as a human being to do the very best I can in order to live a life of authenticity in line with the truth that I perceive.

❧ On some interpretations of Patanjali's Sutras

I do take issue with some interpretations of Patanjali's Sutras: In my opinion, of the four types of "interfering thoughts," "Memory" and "Imagination"[1] are actually functional abilities that we are privileged to be endowed with. While some may consider them to be obstacles to "correct knowledge" and ultimately to liberation, I feel that without them we would quickly find ourselves in a lot of trouble.

Through the appropriate use of my faculty of memory, I can learn from my past, in order to make appropriate decisions about the present and future. If I use my memory to recall the experience of a previous bear encounter, I can use that memory to make appropriate decisions about any present or future situations that might also involve a bear encounter.

To that end, if my memory of a previous bear encounter informed me that the risks and dangers of that situation where the bear encounter occurred are greater than the benefits I gain from that situation, then I might make a wise choice by avoiding such future situations, or at least preparing differently for them.

Similarly, imagination can also be a very useful tool. If I am contemplating entering into a particular situation, I can use my knowledge of the various qualities and aspects of that situation to predict with some degree of probability, what may occur in that situation. This involves the use of imagination, which may then help me to decide whether to enter into that situation, or how to prepare for it appropriately if I do choose to enter into it.

I think the key is to use memory and imagination in a functional way, that helps us to best take care of ourselves and prepare for what we are going to encounter appropriately, while avoiding the dysfunctional reactive *samskara/sankara* patterns that both memory and imagination can bring up in us.

---

1. Sutras 1.5-1.6

"YOU STOP THERE."
[PART II]

Reflections on my second trip in Mysore with Sharath Jois

— February 2016 —

I RECENTLY COMPLETED MY SECOND three-month trip practicing with Sharath Jois at the KPJAYI in Mysore.

Last year I wrote "A New Chapter" and "You Stop There" about my first trip. These pieces expressed my perspective of the experience of starting over as a beginner with Sharath, after having had a daily Ashtanga practice for 12 years, having completed Fourth series with my previous teacher Rolf Naujokat, and having been a Mysore-style teacher myself for a number of years.

I had not been planning to write about this second trip in the same way. My impressions of practicing with Sharath remain much the same as I described last year and writing about it again seemed as if it would be both redundant and clichéd—two things which I strive to avoid.

It was a difficult trip for me, and a very personal one. I've been working with many inner struggles recently and this was the salient feature of my time in Mysore this year. Most of this is too personal to share publicly and initially seemed like another good excuse to not write about my trip.

Upon further reflection, I realize that the struggles and pain that everyone goes through are an important aspect of practice which is all too often ignored and hidden. Yoga websites, social media, and popular yoga culture are full of unrealistic and professionally staged photo and video shoots which depict us at our very best—glorifying the beauty of some advanced *asana* in a pristine natural setting or a temple and often accompanied by some "inspiring" cliché from one of the better known spiritual texts or teachers.

The reality is that our practices rarely look or feel like that. I have never practiced in front of a temple, and the only time I practice outdoors is when I am camping or there is no indoor space available. There are wonderful days where practice does feel light, free and blissful, but for the most part Ashtanga Vinyasa practice is difficult and often is a struggle. The images portrayed by these staged photo and video demos are not an accurate representation of the day-to-day experience of Ashtanga Vinyasa practice, and I feel that they promote unrealistic personal expectations and negative self-judgment in the minds of those who consume dozens of these images every day.

Even when the struggles and pains of practice and life are publicly acknowledged, they are often glorified and spiritualized as necessary sacrifices on the road to the reward of enlightenment. Superficial analogies are made to the battlefield of the *Bhagavad Gita* or other misinterpreted teachings where our pain becomes our noble cross that we have to bear on the path to personal salvation. I guess it is what keeps some people going, but it doesn't really work that way for me.

I do feel that there is some value in sharing the experience of the struggles which I encountered on this trip—at least those struggles pertaining to my *asana* practice. I had to relearn some important lessons.

At the end of my first trip to Mysore last year, Sharath had allowed me to practice up to *Dwi Pada Sirsasana*, which has always been a challenging posture for me. I wrote more about this in the essay titled "You Stop There."

Going back home to Bali at the end of last year, I felt no hurry to return to practicing Third and Fourth series, which were my main practices of the preceding 8 or 9 years. Practicing Intermediate series daily in Mysore and being asked to work more deeply on *Dwi Pada* had been beneficial and felt good. I was happy to continue with Intermediate series at home.

Practicing under Sharath's strict standards also made me realize that I would face another challenge on my subsequent trip: *Karandavasana*. While I could lower down and lift back up in *Karandavasana* to a standard that was acceptable to my previous teacher, I knew that it would not be sufficient to satisfy Sharath's idea of "perfection."

Dwi Pada Sirsasana and *Karandavasana* don't look very similar on the surface, but they share one very important feature. Both postures require a significant degree of lumbar flexion, posterior pelvic tilting and lengthening of the lower back and pelvic muscles connected to those movements. One could say that these two postures represent the extreme of "apanic" movement. This movement is very difficult for practitioners who have an anteriorly tilted pelvis and deep lumbar curve or lordosis—in other words, a "pranic" body structure.

It is interesting that both postures occur in Intermediate series. There are no postures in Third or Fourth series which require the same degree of *apanic* body movement, except perhaps *Bhuja Dandasana* at the end of Fourth series (which was also very challenging for me and I got stopped on for several months while learning that series with Rolf). All of the other leg behind the head variations involve one leg behind the head, which requires significantly less lumbar flexion than having two legs behind the head. All of the other arm balances (except *Sayanasana*) are done on the hands, not the forearms, which also requires less lumbar flexion.

Deepening my *Dwi Pada* to Sharath's standard was beneficial for my *pranic* body structure. Though I had already worked hard for many years to develop my body's ability to exist in the *apanic* state, deepening *Dwi Pada* had brought that movement to another level for me. It was also a very good preparation for improving my *Karandavasana*.

After experiencing the improvement in my *Dwi Pada*, I was determined and inspired to improve my *Karandavasana* before coming to Mysore this season. I continued to practice Intermediate series every day, and I put more attention on *Karandavasana*, attempting it three times in each practice session.

Many people focus on the fact that *Karandavasana* requires a lot of strength. The standard assumption is that those who cannot do it well are simply lacking in strength. For me, this was not the case — it was simply a mechanical problem arising from being 6 ft 3 tall and having an anterior pelvic tilt and lordosis.

My previous technique for lifting back up in *Karandavasana* would be to lean forward and let the face come even closer to the ground and then allow the rest of the body to lift back up to *Pincha Mayurasana*. While I did not rest my head on the ground, I would typically finish the lift up with my nose only about an inch from the ground. Fully extending my shoulders at the end of the lift up was not possible. My previous teacher had considered this good enough for me to move on, all those years ago.

I now realized this would not be good enough for Sharath, and that he would likely want full-shoulder extension when I lifted back up. I started to focus more on the shoulders in my practice of the posture. I found that when I attempted to extend the shoulders before lifting the rest of the body, I would not be able to lift the rest of my body up at all. Still, I knew that establishing the foundation of extending the shoulders was important, so I stopped worrying about coming up at all and tried to rebuild the posture based on better shoulder extension in the initial stages of lifting back up.

This proved to be quite frustrating, as there seemed to be no movement happening at all. After some time I began to use a strap above my elbows to help stabilize the shoulder girdle more and get a bit more leverage. This technique provided a glimmer of hope as I could see where the movement might start to come from, but it still seemed far away from actually happening.

I continued to do this diligently, three times per day in each practice session. Finally, after about six weeks it just happened—as most major breakthroughs do—and I found one day that after getting the initial lift in the shoulders, the rest of the body followed, and I was able to lift right back up and fully extend the shoulders into a perfect *Pincha Mayurasana*. I was able to do this quite reliably from that day onward, and I continued to practice it like that with the belt around my arms for several more weeks.

Once I felt confident with the aforementioned technique, I decided to get rid of the belt. I was shocked and disappointed to find that without the belt, I was back to square one. There was absolutely no movement happening. I was amazed that simply having a strap above the elbows would make such a difference and I felt that I had probably made a mistake by working exclusively with the belt. Though it had given me the experience of feeling what it was like to lift back up perfectly, it had not helped to develop the movement pattern in my body at all. It was a good reminder of why exclusive reliance on props is not very helpful.

I again began the diligent process of trying it 3 times per day, without feeling as if I was really getting anywhere. I would try 2 or 3 times without the belt, and then on my last attempt would use the belt and lift back up fully, just so I would not lose the body memory of the feeling.

This went on for a long time without much sign of progress. Eventually, I began to miss the experience of Third and Fourth series practice. I knew that I had to continue to practice Intermediate every day if there was any hope of improving *Karandavasana*, so I decided to try a different practice routine, where I would add Third or Fourth to the end of Intermediate.

I added a few postures of each advanced series per session and would alternate days, so that one day I practiced Intermediate and Third and the next day Intermediate and Fourth. This felt quite good and strengthening. I continued to practice Intermediate only on Sundays and Primary only on Fridays and on the other 4 days I eventually worked up to practicing two full series. This routine allowed me to maintain a daily practice of Intermediate and also get two days each of Third and Fourth.

It was part way through this process of adding back the advanced series that *Karandavasana* finally happened without the belt. This was probably about six months after leaving Mysore. It felt like quite an accomplishment to finally be able to achieve the one posture that is least suited to my body's natural structure. I also felt a sense of satisfaction that I would likely be able to go to Mysore without being held up in Intermediate series to work on another posture again.

Karandavasana came and went for a little while, but soon enough I could do it without the belt every day, and on most days I could do it on my first attempt. On the days when I could do it on the first try, I did not bother to repeat it and it started to become just another posture in my practice again, without so much extra emphasis.

I arrived in Mysore in November feeling very strong. I had had several months of practicing two series per day and everything felt aligned, balanced and open. Beginning practice in Mysore felt wonderful. As I noticed in my first trip, just being in that room took my practice to another level. I felt even more open, strong, and focused.

After the first week of Primary series, I attended led Intermediate to begin the second week of practice. Sharath gave me two new postures in that practice, acknowledging that my *Dwi Pada* was now good enough and taking me up to *Tittibhasana*.

A few days later in Mysore practice, I was part way through drop backs when Sharath looked over at me. "What did you do?" he asked.

"Tittibhasana," I replied.

"Pincha Mayurasana," he said.

"Now?" I asked.

"Yes, now."

I had already done several deep backbends and my spine was in a state of extension. Now I was supposed to just hop up into *Pincha Mayurasana*, out of sequence and under his analytical eyes. I managed to pull it off reasonably well. It was not my best *pincha* ever, and I could clearly feel that the backbending had taken away the usual stability I felt in *pincha*—but it was good enough.

"*Karandavasana*," he said.

Now I was unsure. My natural lordosis was deepened by the backbending, and I had clearly felt less stable than usual in *Pincha*. This would be a big handicap for attempting *Karandavasana*. I also had not done *Karandavasana* since before I arrived in Mysore, and Sharath was watching me.

I tried. It felt awkward and unstable lowering down and I was quickly losing hope of success. As I started to lift back up, my hands slid in towards each other as they usually did. Sharath groaned loudly, "Noooo." I made it about halfway up but then found my back was still too much in extension to complete the lift. I came down and looked at him.

"The hands are not correct," he said. He didn't seem to care so much that I hadn't lifted up, but chose to focus on the fact that my hands had slid in. I was surprised that he focused on the hands. While I realized that, ideally, my forearms should stay parallel to each other, I didn't think he would care too much about that detail as I had established all of the other aspects of the posture.

The next practice happened to be led Intermediate again. It would be my first time to attempt *Karandavasana* in the led class. I was able to follow his count moving into the posture, but by the time he had counted to five and gave the vinyasa to lift back up, I had already taken 12 breaths or so! I had never tried to lift back up after staying so long in the posture, and I was already quite tired as I was not yet acclimatized to the added strain of led Intermediate with Sharath. The result was that I could not lift back up again. I also noted that only a small percentage of the class were able to lift back up with Sharath's count.

I lay on my belly like everyone else and was about to get ready to go to the change room for finishing postures, when I noticed that he was taking his time to help several people lift back up. I also noticed that a few people were giving it a second attempt, so I thought I might as well try again. As soon as I had lowered down, Sharath's attention was on me. "Lift up," he commanded. As I started to lift up he again groaned, "No, no, the hands are not correct." I was still tired and felt intimidated and again was not able to complete the lift back up very well. "Try again," he said. At this point I had little hope, but gave it a third attempt. It was a little better than the second, but still not very good. "That's how ladies do it," he said. I looked up at him and he concluded, "All the ladies do it better than you. Now you go inside (to the change room for finishing)".

A few people actually messaged me after the class and told me not to take his comments personally and that he was just challenging me to do my best. I knew that was the case, and I actually took his poking fun at me as a compliment. He wouldn't have bothered to take the time to give me that attention if he didn't see some potential or a reason to.

I did feel challenged, though. I was pretty determined to make sure I didn't fail at *Karandavasana* in class again. The following class, which was again Mysore style, I was able to lift back up fairly well. My success didn't generate any reaction from Sharath. From that day onward, I was able to do the posture fairly reliably in Mysore class. However, at this point Sharath was ignoring me.

After a couple of weeks of practicing *Karandavasana* pretty well and being ignored, I decided that Sharath was likely waiting until I could do it without the hands moving in. So, I decided to start working on it a bit more at home.

I am a strong advocate of limiting *asana* practice to once per day. I often advise my regular students to follow this guideline strictly. If one has both the energy and the ambition, it can be tempting to do a little extra work on stuck areas in the afternoons or evenings. This rarely brings healthy results, especially if it is done regularly. It can be beneficial to perhaps have a few spontaneous exploratory sessions every now and then, especially if an opportunity to get a few tips from a more experienced practitioner arises, but doing extra training on top of an intensive daily Ashtanga practice is usually going to lead to problems.

I see the Ashtanga Vinyasa series as a system of bodywork which rebuilds the body and nervous system from the ground up. The sequencing of the series is very intelligently designed and take the body and nerves through a lengthy process of deep structural transformation. I personally believe that it is the most effective form of bodywork that is publicly available on the planet today.

Practicing the same sequence every day gives the body and nerves consistent repetitive inputs. Over time, the innate intelligence of the body begins to understand these inputs and eventually integrates those movement patterns into its permanent structural repertoire. In other words, the structure of the body itself changes in order to accommodate and integrate these repetitive movement patterns.

Any set of repetitive movement patterns will change the structure of the body. If one hunches over a computer or a mobile phone or a steering wheel all day, the body structure will change to reflect this. If one carries a heavy backpack over a mountain several times per month, the body structure will change to reflect this. If one grows up with abusive family members and is constantly recoiling in fear or shame, the body structure will eventually reflect this.

With the Ashtanga practice, the unique aspect of the system is that the new movements we learn and repeat each day are consistently arranging themselves around the internal form of *bandha* and deep and expansive breathing. The movements are therefore arranging themselves around the activation of the scaffolding of the innermost layers of structural tissue. If the postures are done with reasonably good alignment and conscious awareness, the structural changes that result will tend to bring the midline of the body into harmony with the field of gravity. Many long-term practitioners become taller and straighter as a result. Chronic tensions which arise from us being in a constant battle with gravity are automatically eradicated over time, as the body realigns.

This is truly a holistic process. It is also a particularly complex process. While each posture does "work on" specific sections of the body, it also simultaneously works on the body as a whole. Each Ashtanga series also works on the body as a whole, with the net effect of practicing all of the postures in the series being much greater and deeper than the sum of the effects of each individual posture.

In systems thinking, we can talk about "emergent properties" which arise from higher levels of organization but cannot be found in the parts of that system. A car, for example, has many emergent properties that cannot be found in any of the individual parts from which it is composed. A forest has emergent properties which cannot be found in each individual tree, animal, or rock. Similarly, an Ashtanga series, practiced in sequence with the connecting vinyasa and breathing has effects on the structure of the body which cannot be found from practicing any of the individual asanas in the series in isolation.

I think it logically follows from this that if the repetitive sequence of postures we are practicing is having a net effect on the structure of the body as a whole, it is a very complex process which even the most knowledgeable anatomy expert cannot possibly hope to completely understand. We should probably respect this complex process and not complicate it further with extra inputs. Practice the series in the morning; then take the rest of the day to allow the body to integrate those inputs before reapplying the process the following morning. Slowly but surely, the body changes. When it is done in this way, the changes are usually stable.

But, if we feel we are stuck on one posture, and then go home and later in the day apply some more repetitive practice of this posture (or hip openers or back openers or core strengtheners) out of the context of the sequence, then the inputs on the body become very different and the body now has to contend with a second set of unique and demanding inputs to integrate into its structure. Since these inputs have come without the usual context of the Ashtanga sequence, they may not necessarily even be in harmony with the first set of inputs that are coming from the sequence.

For example, one could experience being stuck at a posture that requires some degree of opening in the hips that is not currently possible. It might make perfect sense to then go home and spend 30 minutes in the afternoon doing extra exercises to stretch the hips. But it could very well be that the net emergent effect of that person's entire morning practice is currently to generate more opening in the thoracic spine during backbending. The body needs to compensate for the opening in the thoracic spine by tightening up somewhere else—i.e., the hips. So, by going home and then forcefully stretching the hips, one is actually sabotaging the intelligence of the body and the direction it is attempting to move in with the practice.

A tree can be shaped by an expert gardener—or even by natural environmental conditions—over time. The entire shape of the tree can be permanently and dramatically changed over a period of years by the cumulative micro effects of the daily inputs given by the gardener and environmental conditions. However, if the gardener attempts to force too much change in the shape of the tree too quickly with excessively strong manipulations and inputs, the tree will either break or wither and die.

Sustainable change takes time to integrate. Asking for too much change too quickly will never bring sustainable results; or, if it does, it will necessarily involve a period of fairly intense discomfort and instability before the results become healthy and sustainable.

This is why I strongly believe that one should not practice any strenuous *asana* beyond one's daily morning practice. The inputs of the Ashtanga sequence on the human body are very deep and powerful. It is wise to treat them with respect and give them the space they need to settle in and be integrated.

In complete contradiction to the above explanation, I decided to start working on *Karandavasana* at home. Why did I disregard my own views on doing extra practice at home? It's a good question, and an important question. I never would have done this had I not been in Mysore. There was definitely an element of wanting to perform and to prove something. Sharath had challenged me and had done so publicly. I wanted to meet his challenge, and I had a limited period of time during which I could do this. I also felt that having practiced the advanced series for nearly 10 years and having just gone through a phase of practicing two series per day that my current practice in Mysore of Intermediate series only up to *Karandavasana* was fairly easy and non-strenuous. My practice was only one hour long and finished by 5:30 a.m. It seemed relatively harmless to attempt a little more later in the day at home.

I was certainly wary about the prospect of practicing *Karandavasana* at home without the context of the sequence. For the shoulders to support the movement safely, they require a significant amount of warm up and need to be well aligned. If any problems arose from this extra practice, I figured they would come from too much strain on an improperly prepared shoulder girdle.

I attempted it at around 11 a.m., before lunch and still a little bit warm from my morning practice. I would do a few simple shoulder openers and then go straight into attempting *Karandavasana*. I was happy to find that there was no strain at all on the shoulders and that I could do it quite well. I started with 3–5 repetitions of the posture, and over the next few days worked my way up to 8–9 repetitions, usually done in sets of 3, with a bit of a shoulder release in between sets.

I found that I actually felt very good after doing this. I would feel more open in the chest and shoulders and feel taller and straighter, which I always interpret as a sign of "correct practice." I would normally do this extra little home practice 4 days a week, from Monday to Thursday, and then give it a rest on the other three days. Though there was no significant change in my *Karandavasana*, after a few weeks I did start to manage to keep the hands a little more apart after 4 or 5 of the repetitions at home.

In the shala, my performance of *Karandavasana* did not improve. In fact, it seemed to be getting a little more difficult as time went on. I could still do it in the shala, and usually on my first attempt, but it was sloppier and the hands would come in more than in my home practice of the posture.

I didn't have much hope of being able to achieve *Karandavasana* without the hands coming in before the three-month trip was over. I resigned myself to being stuck on the posture for the remainder of the trip. Several people mentioned to me that Sharath would likely move me on within a few weeks, and that the way I was practicing *Karandavasana* was definitely good enough — he just wanted to make sure I had to work a little bit harder before getting moved forward in the series. Whether this was true or not, I realized that the posture could be improved and I did want to be able to practice it without the hands coming in, so I continued with my home regime.

Part way through my second month of practice at the shala, things started to get more difficult. I noted the same thing on my first trip: The first month felt very open, light and easy, while in the second month and third month things started to tighten up and practice became more challenging. All of the other postures in my practice began to feel a little stiffer and the flow seemed to be less natural. Practice became a bit of a struggle overall, though I could still do everything reasonably well.

Around this time, I also started to notice a strange effect after my home *Karandavasana* sessions. After finishing my 8 or 9 repetitions, I would stand up and feel a bit of cramping at the bottom of my sitting bones. It felt like the insertion point of my hamstrings was quite a strong sensation. It would only last a few seconds, and I would simply do a standing forward bend and then everything would feel fine. I assumed it was the hamstrings and I found it very peculiar. I wondered how it was that *Karandavasana* was creating a strain on the hamstring, since my hamstrings are open and strong and the effect of *Karandavasana* on the hamstrings should be fairly negligible. In hindsight, this was the first warning sign of something going wrong and I should have paid a lot more attention to it.

The sense of struggle in my practice carried on for the next few weeks of my second month. *Karandavasana* was becoming more difficult as well. It seemed to take more effort to lift up and it felt sloppier. I also started to feel more tired during the day, and began taking naps, which I had not been doing in the first month.

In the second half of the second month, there was one day where Sharath seemed to be giving everyone new postures. I was having a particularly difficult time that day. It was hotter than usual and I felt quite low in energy and stiffer than usual. As I came to *Karandavasana*, I wondered if I would be able to do it at all. I was looking forward to being in the finishing room. I did manage to do it, and as I straightened back into *Pincha Mayurasana* after lifting up, I heard Sharath say, "You did?" I jumped back into *Chaturanga* and then heard him say, "You did Karandavasana?"

I looked at him and said, "Yes, I did."

"Show me again," he replied. I groaned to myself. I was so sweaty and exhausted, I was not sure I could do it a second time. I tried. As I had feared, I was not able to lift back up. When I looked up, Sharath had already walked away silently. I chuckled to myself and thought, "blew my chance"…

After that day, I was not able to lift up in *Karandavasana* at all. My ability to do the posture vanished completely. Each day in the shala, my attempts to lift up would get worse and worse. For a few days, I was only able to lift part way up. Then, I could barely even get my legs off my arms at all. Finally, it came to the point where I actually could not even start to lift up. My brain would give the command to lift up, and the muscles simply would not respond. I would just slide off my arms and shake my head in bewilderment. It felt like a mental block as much as a physical one. Though I never bothered looking up to see if I was being watched, those who were practicing near me told me that Sharath was watching me intently each time I attempted to do it. After a week or two of this, he came over one day to backbend me at the end of my practice and shot me a disappointed look that said it all. My only response was to laugh sarcastically and shrug. No words were necessary.

Losing the ability to lift up should have been my second warning sign that something was going wrong and I was perhaps overdoing things by practicing at home. This sign was much clearer than the little moments of cramping below my sitting bone, yet I also ignored this warning sign. I became frustrated and actually started putting more effort into the home practice, sometimes attempting it more than 10 times per day, even though I was no longer able to lift up at home either. It began to feel as if I was beating a dead horse, and yet, I kept beating it.

I know from experience in the practice that big breakthroughs are often preceded by a period of time where things seem to hit rock bottom. Sometimes things have to come apart before they can be rebuilt in a better way. I theorized that this could be what was happening to me now. My assumption was that losing the ability to lift up at all in *Karandavasana* was hitting rock bottom. I was wrong.

During the final week of the second month, I began to feel really unstable in my practice. There was a strong sense of resistance and avoidance and I could feel what I can only describe as a quivering, shaking feeling deep in my nerves. While my inner focus and composure were still there, the deepest root of my physical stability seemed to feel strongly threatened. I began to feel other elements of my practice which were second nature to me also slipping away. Jumping into *Bakasana* became sloppier; during one led Primary series class, I could barely even lift up and jump back between each posture. The whole practice felt clunky and seemed to take me back about 15 years to what my first year of practice felt like. It was humbling, to say the least.

Finally, the hitting of rock bottom happened: During one Mysore practice, after completing *Bakasana* I jumped through for *Bharadvajasana* and suddenly felt what seemed like a bolt of lightning shoot through my left leg. It was probably one of the most intense pains I have ever felt in my life and my leg went partially numb. I practically went into a state of shock.

I have had experiences before where something really gets tweaked in the practice, and then by carefully continuing the practice, it disappears just as quickly as it came. This was much stronger than any "tweak" I had ever felt before, though. I very carefully put my body into *Bharadvajasana*, which I could do, but the entire body was still quivering in shock. When I tried to jump back, the electric pain shot through my left leg again. I gingerly stepped through and did the other side of *Bharadvajasana*. I repeated the process for *Ardha Matsyendrasana* and it was very clear that this tweak was not going to release. I could not even fathom attempting *Eka Pada Sirsasana*, so I just sat there for a minute, unsure of what to do. The intensity of the room swirled around me and I had a very lucid feeling like suddenly being jerked violently out of a dream.

I decided to end the practice. I walked over to the stage and told Sharath that something had happened to my leg and I needed to stop practice. He looked at me and then quickly nodded and said, "Okay, don't do backbending." I went into the change room with the intention of doing the full finishing sequence, but the pain was so strong that I could not even lift my body into *Sarvangasana* or *Sirsasana*. I struggled to place my body into *Yoga Mudra* and then lay down to rest. Getting up and rolling up my mat was excruciating and I was unsure I would even be able to walk out. Thankfully, I did manage to do that.

I was concerned, but figured that it would be something that I could release with a few days of Primary series practice. There were three more days left in the week and I managed to do a very painful Primary series on those days, though certain postures were not possible at all. It did not seem to get any better.

It was a very strange pain, and unlike anything I had experienced before. There was no pain in the spine or back, and the spinal movements themselves seemed to be unrestricted. Anything that required the same kind of abdominal and pelvic strength or flexion that *Karandavasana* requires would send a shooting pain through my left outer thigh and all the way down to my foot. Certain types of forward folding, with the legs in different rotations also elicited the same pain. Other types of forward folding were fine. It depended on the rotation of the hips and the degree of strength required. It was very clear to me that this pain was caused by my excessive *Karandavasana* regime, as any postures which resembled the movements of *Karandavasana* triggered the pain most strongly.

Backbending was the only movement that did not elicit any pain and actually felt more open than usual. I decided to return to Intermediate series practice, though anything beyond the twists would not be possible. With some trepidation I came to led Intermediate practice the following Monday. It went okay (though still very painful) up to the backbends and twists. As we came to *Eka Pada Sirsasana*, I decided to stop and got ready to leave for finishing postures. Sharath was well aware of me and watching from the stage. He encouraged me to attempt *Eka Pada*. I was surprised to find that I could do the right side. For the left side, he told me to at least attempt it as much as I could, which was not very much. He stood near me for the next few postures and guided me with some suggestions for modifications, making sure I stayed up to *Karandavasana*.

It felt empowering to complete the practice, and I found the leg was actually somewhat better afterwards. Stretching it to the degree that was possible seemed to help a bit. I still had some hope that the problem would resolve itself sooner than later.

I felt a deep sense of surrender as we began Mysore practice that week. For the preceding two months, I had felt quite a bit of performance pressure around *Karandavasana*. Now that my practice was in smoldering ruins, and I knew there was no chance of doing *Karandavasana* at all and that several other postures in my practice had to be modified or avoided, there was actually some sense of relief. Though my practice was very painful and unpleasant, that sense of surrender to my circumstances also created a sort of relaxation and letting go. I developed a new routine which involved skipping the left side of *Eka Pada*, *Dwi Pada* and *Yoga Nidrasana*. I could do *Tittibhasana* and *Pincha Mayurasana*. For *Karandavasana*, I would lift up and cross my legs but could not lower down, as even the lowering movement would start to trigger the pain.

It was a challenge to be in this state. It was very humbling, and a good experience to go through. Sharath's attitude towards me also changed. He became more outwardly kind and less pressuring. Though each day was an immense struggle, moving slowly and carefully and bearing the pain that many of the movements elicited, I did see that slowly but surely most of the movements were gradually returning. Each day and each week I would feel a little more open, and could go a little further into certain movements, or use the internal strength a little more without triggering the bolts of pain. The practice became about finding that fine line of generating enough movement to stimulate creative healing but not so much that would cause aggravation of the symptoms.

Facing the intense physical discomfort and the emotional vulnerability of having to go through this process in public was a very deep form of practice. In many ways, it was about dropping back into the real purpose of the practice. Instead of obsessing about the external appearance of one particular posture, I was able to drop back into the internal process of working with my reactions to my own inner experiences.

My third month in Mysore was a difficult process of slow recovery from the injury caused by my own excessive ambitions. As I was also struggling with other aspects of my Mysore experience and my experience of life in general, I was eagerly looking forward to the end of my trip. I longed to return to my home in the humid and quiet rice fields of Bali, where I could practice alone and in the dark before teaching with only the sounds of crickets and frogs to accompany me as I limped through my practice and continued to encounter my own pain. I had completely let go of all ambition to "move on" past *Karandavasana* and was ready for the trip to end.

A couple of weeks later, I had healed to the extent that lowering into *Karandavasana* became possible again. Lifting back up still seemed light years away. In my second to last led Intermediate class, I attempted *Karandavasana* as usual and then rolled up my mat to go to the change room for finishing. As I started walking, Sharath turned towards me and said, "Show me." I actually laughed out loud sarcastically. He then turned back to whomever he was helping. I just stood there for a minute, and wanted to tell him, "No." What was the point? *Karandavasana* was not going to come again for a long time. He remained focused on someone else, so I sighed and put my mat back down and gave it a second attempt. I was shocked to find that I actually was able to lift halfway back up. I felt a deep focus and strength that I had not felt since the beginning of the trip.

For one brief moment, everything came together again inside me. Sharath didn't say anything and I then went to the change room for finishing.

The next day in Mysore class, I prepared for backbending after my attempt at *Karandavasana* and Sharath again called to me from the stage and told me to repeat it. I failed again, and he attempted to give me some helpful instructions, which were things I already knew but that my body just could not execute in its current state. I still had no hope of lifting back up again anytime soon. I was expecting it to be at least a few more months.

I then continued to attempt *Karandavasana* twice per practice session, as it seemed like that was what Sharath expected now. I could feel that he now wanted to move me past the posture but could not justify doing so until I could lift up again. I, however, was quite content to wait until the next trip!

In the following led Intermediate class, which was my last one of the season, he again asked me to "show him" after I started to walk towards the change room. The same thing happened as in the previous week's class; I was able to lift up part way and felt that glimmer of what it used to feel like, but was not successful in lifting up fully.

On Thursday of that final week, which was my second to last Mysore practice of the season, I lowered down into *Karandavasana* as usual. Somehow, I then lifted back up. It was shocking. I didn't feel as if I had really tried to do it, and I had had no ambition or expectation to do so. Yet, somehow my body came up. I was so surprised that I actually started trembling. I unfolded my legs and extended my shoulders straight. It was sloppy and certainly no better than it had been in the beginning of the trip, but I had done it. I jumped back to *Chaturanga* from *pincha* and immediately heard Sharath's voice from the stage—"Mayurasana."

I looked up towards him, just to make sure it was not a coincidence and that he actually was talking to me. He gave me the biggest smile I have ever seen on him, and nodded and gestured with the *Mayurasana* arm position.

It was an intense moment. Suddenly, all the pain and the dark tunnel that my practice and life had been for the past while, dissolved into a moment of lightness. It was as if a thick fog had suddenly lifted. I smiled back at him and nodded and attempted *Mayurasana*. He immediately informed me that it was not correct and critiqued several aspects of how I did the posture.

The following day I was able to do *Karandavasana* again. Even though my body still had a long way to go to heal completely, it was an unexpected and somehow fitting way to end the trip.

Having been home in Bali for two weeks now, I am still working through the injury. I managed to put my left leg behind my head and to do *Supta Kurmasana* for the first time since the injury in my practice this week. Still, there is a lot of pain to work through and I anticipate it will be another 2–4 months before I am pain free. Interestingly, *Karandavasana* has returned to feeling quite smooth and feels like one of the least effortful parts of my practice at the moment.

This trip to Mysore was a very important one. In many ways I feel it was a calibration of my relationship with Sharath. I think we both learned a lot about how to deal with each other, and my next trip will be much better as a result.

The interesting question that still stands out to me is why I chose to disregard my own understanding of how to practice? Why did I allow myself to succumb to the ambition of excessive practice in order to perform?

I would never have chosen to do that anywhere else, whether at home or if I was practicing in another shala. Was it that the environment of Mysore brought out some unhealthy inner tendency of mine which I had not yet completely resolved? And, was it my time to face that tendency again?

Sharath pushed me hard on both of my trips, for reasons that only he can know. One thing that is clear to me, however, is that Sharath would not have approved of my extra practice of *Karandavasana* at home. He also strongly advocates not practicing *asana* more than once per day. If I had asked him what I should do to improve my *Karandavasana*, he definitely would not have told me to go and do what I did.

I know this, and I knew it then, so I certainly take most of the credit and responsibility for my own actions. I will certainly learn from my mistake, and this will serve me well on future trips to Mysore as I get into more advanced practice there.

I share this story for various reasons. I feel it is important to publicly express and share the darker side of practice as well as the dangers of "incorrect practice." As social media and pop culture increasingly promote *asana* practice as an image contest and a fashion show, the dangers of harming oneself by getting caught up in this trend increase.

Even though I was not attempting to create the perfect *Karandavasana* so that I could post it on Facebook, YouTube, or the cover of a magazine, the fact is that I was still trying to create a perfect *Karandavasana* at least partly for image-related reasons. This is what led to my excessive practice which led to my injury.

The most interesting thing is that I intellectually understood all of this very well before this experience. Even though I have watched numerous fellow practitioners and students injure themselves in a similar way, it seems I had to finally experience it for myself in my own body to fully comprehend the truth of it.

ANSWERS TO QUESTIONS

❧ On the nature of the injury in this trip in Mysore

My symptoms closely match those of piriformis syndrome, but not exactly. There is certainly nerve compression, but it is not the sciatic nerve. The areas of the leg that experience pain and numbness correspond closely to the dermatone innervation of SI.

As *Karandavasana* demands more lumbar and hip flexion than any other posture in the Ashtanga system, I figure that by doing it so repetitively, I induced a shift in the lower lumbar and sacral vertebrae which compressed the nerve roots coming out of L5 and S1.

At the same time, the strength required to perform the posture probably drove the left periformis into spasm. Those cramps I felt at the bottom of my sitting bone which I mentioned above were likely the beginning of this.

I did consult an anatomy expert on these two theories, and his question to me was "Did you always put the right leg first in lotus?" This works the left periformis much more strongly than the right one, and it is why the left side got injured. As part of my current remedial work at home, I am doing *Karandavasana* with the left leg in lotus first half of the time, in order to help balance things out. I will likely continue alternating sides in the posture from now on (except in Mysore, of course).

As I mentioned in this essay, and as my anatomy expert friend also suggested, it is difficult to put a diagnostic label on something like this, due to the complexity of the situation. I tend to view the body as more of a whole, and I don't think this situation can be reduced to a simple diagnosis of an injured part. Simply going back to moderate practice, and also balancing out the sides seems to be slowly healing it.

ASHTANGA,
EMBODIMENT
& COMPLEX
SYSTEMS

STARTING THIRD SERIES [AGAIN]

Reflections on an eleven-year relationship

— April 2016 —

I FIRST BEGAN TO PRACTICE Third series of the Ashtanga Vinyasa system in early 2005, shortly after relocating to Whitehorse in the Yukon Territory of Northern Canada. I had learned Primary and Intermediate series from Mark Darby in Montréal the year before, and following a period of travel and then settling in a very remote and isolated corner of the world, I was far away from anyone who could offer me guidance in my Ashtanga practice. I've always enjoyed self practice, and having had four years of experience in the Iyengar yoga system (including being trained as an Iyengar teacher) before starting Ashtanga practice with Darby, I was happy and confident to be isolated and on my own with this new system of practice.

I arrived in the Yukon in September 2004 and settled in for my first winter in the north, with eighteen plus hours of darkness per day and temperatures as low as -40 degrees Celsius. I spent the winter house-sitting for a friend of a friend who lived a few kilometers north of town. My only transportation was my feet, and I would take a biweekly trek into town to teach a yoga class, purchase some supplies, and then trudge back up the long hill through the snow and biting cold wind. I had no internet connection and had little else to do besides walk the dog in the forest around the house, read books, cook food, and focus on my daily practices of Ashtanga yoga, Pranayama and Vipassana meditation. It was a special time and I have fond memories of that winter, in spite of its hardships.

Though I had only been practicing Primary and Intermediate series for a little over a year, and they certainly both needed more work, I grew curious about Third series. I had already experienced a significant amount of structural transformation from Primary and Intermediate series, and now that those changes seemed like they were starting to settle and take root in my body and being, I grew eager for more intensity and change.

Matthew Sweeney's first edition of his *Aṣṭāṅga Yoga as It Is* book was the only publicly available resource for the advanced series at that time, so I ordered it, and a few weeks later it arrived in my frozen mailbox, all the way from Australia, in the other corner of the world.

With enthusiasm and vitality, I immediately began to experiment with the postures of Third series at the end of my Intermediate series practice each morning. I would add several postures of Third series each week and I quickly bit off more than my body and nervous system could effectively digest. Within two months, I had taught myself all of the postures of Third series, and practiced it four days per week.

The structural changes and discomfort which I experienced over that winter can only be described as "extreme" and "intense." My upper body responded with massive shifts, and my rib cage and shoulder girdle literally changed shape from the inside out. I felt things move that just shouldn't move in a human body. I can still vividly remember a two-week period, when every time I moved from upward dog to downward dog, the entire right side of my rib cage would slide out of its articulation with some other set of bones. This particular sensation was not painful, but it was almost sickening to feel a part of my body that should not really move actually slide out of place and then return back again. I kept practicing and eventually this effect stopped happening.

I would use my pranayama and meditation practices later in the day to "recover" from the overwhelming intensity of the effects of a hastily learned Third series on my body and nerves. It was fortunate that I didn't have much else to do in my life at that time, because it would have been challenging to remain functional within a relationship or to do any more than the minimal amount of teaching work that I was doing at the time.

I discovered another important principle during these months, which is that daily, long-term Ashtanga Vinyasa yoga practice is not necessarily compatible with other forms of body work. I had met someone in Whitehorse who was a beginning Ashtanga practitioner and a Rolfer. I had experienced the 10 session series of Rolfing about five years earlier, and held this practice in high regard. This Rolfer and I agreed to do an exchange, where I would give her a private Ashtanga class in exchange for a Rolfing session once per week.

In the first Rolfing session, I described to her what I was doing in my practice and the tension and discomfort that I was experiencing in my upper body, due to all the shifting and changing. I also described the very strange and disturbing sensation of the right side of my rib cage literally sliding out of its usual articulation with some of the other bones. She had me lay face down on the table and said, "Let's see what is happening." She started by feeling my rib cage, applying gentle pressure, and suddenly my rib cage did the sliding thing. She gave a little yell, and literally reeled back several steps. "Oh my God!" she exclaimed. "What was that?"

I laughed and said, "That is what I was describing. I was hoping you could tell me what it is."

"Wow, are you okay? I don't even want to touch you now," was her response.

I convinced her that the rib cage sliding actually did not hurt at all, and that I wanted her to see what she could do. With some trepidation, she started again. By the end of the one-hour session, I felt great relief. The tension in my upper body seemed to have completely vanished and I felt an immense sense of freedom. She told me that she felt my energy was expanding outwards uncontrollably, and that she had attempted to instill a sense of "the container." I thanked her profusely and we agreed to meet again the next week.

Within a few days, the pain and tension in my upper body had all returned. The following week, the Rolfer released the tension again. This cycle repeated itself a few times. Eventually, I realized what was happening. Third series was asking my body to change. Because I had learned the series so quickly, the changes were dramatic, and they were very destabilizing. The pain and tension were a result of the body attempting to accommodate all of the rapid and dramatic structural changes. The Rolfer was doing her best to stabilize my body again, which would always release the pain and tension. However, by stabilizing my body, she was bringing it back towards its old structure — the one that Third series was attempting to change. So, there was a tug of war going on. Third series was asking my body to do one thing, and the Rolfer was asking my body to do something else.

Once I realized this, I explained it to her and told her that I needed to just trust my practice and to allow all of the effects of the practice to work themselves through my body without any other intervention. Fortunately, my 29-year-old body was strong and forgiving, and my faith in the method of practice and in myself saw me through. A few months later I came out the other side with a somewhat stable Third series practice and Third series body.

Around the same time that I felt my body begin to stabilize, the daylight began to rapidly increase and the weather slowly followed the lead of the change in daylight and began to warm up. I then experienced my first spring and summer in the north, culminating in a complete absence of darkness during the peak months, and I began to enjoy the fruits of my long and difficult winter of self-directed transformation. I felt as if I had a new body—and in many ways, I did. I felt straighter, taller, and more naturally in tune with the field of gravity. In particular, I noticed much more ease in my seated meditation practice, which I did for two hours a day. It became effortless to hold my spine in alignment with gravity and to keep my shoulders and chest open and relaxed in relation to the spine for the entire period of sitting.

I diligently practiced Third series as my main practice (4 days per week) for the following three years, all without consulting a teacher. By this time, I had established my own yoga school in the Yukon and began to feel a calling to go back out into the wider world—Yukoners often refer to anywhere that is not in the Yukon as "the outside"—and connect to the greater global Ashtanga community.

When I was living in Montréal, a few trusted people recommended Richard Freeman to me, and this had stuck in the back of my mind. I now felt a strong calling to go and see Richard, and I applied for his month-long teacher intensive in Boulder, Colorado. I was accepted, and went to practice there in 2007.

At that point, I probably had a fairly respectable looking Third series practice, by anyone's standards. However, I was not entirely familiar with the standard pedagogical methods of the Ashtanga community, and wondered what the reaction/reception would be when I wandered into a new place and rolled out a self-taught Third series. I did mention in my application for the course how I had learned my practice, including that I had taught myself Third series.

The Mysore-style classes at Richard's studio were not very traditional. Though practitioners were expected to follow the traditional series, not everyone did, and I never saw anyone being told which postures to practice or not to practice. People came in and practiced whatever they felt like practicing, and this was generally accepted by the teachers. It was a comfortable situation for me to walk into at that stage of my own practice journey.

I practiced Primary, and then Intermediate series in my first two days at the studio. Having not been questioned by any of the teachers, I decided to try Third series the next day, which happened to be a Mysore class that Richard was teaching. Richard took a significant amount of interest in what I was doing, gave me a few corrections on vinyasa and alignment, and basically gave my Third series practice his approval. I continued to work on Third series under the guidance of Richard and the other teachers at his studio for the remainder of my time there.

I thoroughly enjoyed the month that I spent in Boulder, and subsequently returned two more times in the following year to participate in Richard's "advanced intensive" courses. I enjoyed practicing amongst other like-minded individuals again, and Richard seemed to attract the types of practitioners to whom I could relate and connect. Richard himself is a very inspiring practitioner and teacher.

As enjoyable as my time there was, I don't think I learned very much about my *asana* practice, or how to use the Mysore method of practice appropriately as either a student or a teacher. It felt nice to receive verification that I had basically taught myself Third series correctly, and for the strong points in my practice to be acknowledged. I also appreciated that the alignment principles which I had come to understand through my own practice were in line with what Richard was teaching. Richard's eloquent verbalization of the alignment principles helped to crystallize my intuitive understanding of *bandha*. However, by not being given any restrictions or pressure around the limitations in my practice, or my method of learning it, there was very little stimulation for evolution and transformation in my practice.

At this stage, in 2007, I also felt drawn to go and practice at the KPJAYI. I had actually been to the old AYRI in Lakshmipuram in 2000 when I was still a student of Iyengar yoga. I met SKPJ, who allowed me to watch a Mysore-style class. I was unimpressed with what I saw at that time, and hadn't felt any desire to return, even after I adopted the Ashtanga practice in 2003. Now, I had regained my interest and was starting to consider another visit to Mysore. When I mentioned this to a fellow student at Richard's course, she mentioned to me that if I was traveling to India, I should go and practice with Rolf Naujokat in Goa. She felt that Rolf and I would get along very well. This recommendation resonated strongly with me, and I made plans to go and practice with Rolf in Goa that same year.

When I arrived at Rolf's shala in Goa on my first day, he informed me that I should practice "only Primary, and no adjustments." I enjoyed practicing Primary series in the energy of the room very much, and Rolf came over to help me with catching my legs in the final backbend. He then asked me about my regular practice. I told him I was starting Fourth series. "Oh, great!" he exclaimed. "Who taught you all those postures?"

I was unsure how to answer his question. I knew it would likely not go over well if I told him I had taught myself Third series. Things here felt a little stricter and more controlled than they did at Richard's studio. "Richard Freeman taught me." I lied.

"Oh, Richard taught you all those postures? Great! Tomorrow practice Intermediate, and then let's see."

In my Intermediate series practice the following day, Rolf and his wife Marci noticed several weak spots, including *Dwi Pada Sirsasana* and *Karandavasana*, as well as a few other things. They both adjusted me quite strongly in several postures and gave me a particularly hard time. The next day, Rolf asked me to practice Intermediate series for the remainder of the week. The strong adjustments continued, and Marci was particularly aggressive towards me. She kept asking me questions about my practice in a way that felt like an interrogation.

It was an intense experience, and very different from the easy-going and positive energy I had felt at Richard's studio. On the one hand, I felt a strong focus and increased depth in my Intermediate series practice, due to the adjustments and strong pressure they were putting on me. At the same time, I felt intimidated and picked on by their comments and questionings. The combination of the intensity of the *asana* practice and the relations with them brought me to my edge — that place where real self-encountering occurs.

On the third or fourth day of practice, as we were preparing for the opening prayer, Rolf called me into a separate room. With kind, but firm energy, he asked for more details about how I had learned Third series. He specifically asked if Richard had taught me the postures "one by one." I told him the truth, which was that I had basically taught myself Third series and that Richard had then helped me with it and approved of it. Rolf's response was very clear: "No, no, no. This is not the correct method as I learned it. You need to learn each posture one by one from a qualified teacher. This is how my teacher taught me." He also pointed out the three or four places in my Intermediate series that needed improving. He told me that they wanted me to practice only Intermediate series with them, and that if I didn't like it, they would be happy to give me a refund and I could go somewhere else.

My answer was also clear. "I'd like to practice with you," I said. "I really enjoy being here and will practice whatever you feel is appropriate."

Rolf's eyes lit up. "Good!" he exclaimed. "We also like you very much. You have very focused energy. We are only a little bit mean to you because we like you and you have the capability to improve your asanas."

Once that was cleared up, practicing with Rolf and Marci became a little smoother. On the one hand, I was disappointed to have an entire series taken away from me, but on the other hand, I could feel much more depth developing in my practice of Intermediate series. It was quite an epiphany in terms of my understanding of how this method of teaching works most effectively. By being shown where my limitations were, and being forced to stop and encounter them, I was required to put my attention, awareness and effort in the places I had previously avoided or glossed over. This pressure was the stimulus for evolution and transformation in my practice and in myself.

After about a month, I had improved my Intermediate series to the degree that Rolf had wanted to see. He congratulated me each time I attained the form that he wanted to see in *Dwi Pada*, *Karandavasana* and *tic tocs*. One morning, as we entered my second month of practice, he told me: "Now, your Intermediate is very strong, much better. Now, we start Third series. Today, you try *Visvamitrasana* after headstands."

I was still not overly familiar with the "correct method" of being given postures one by one, so I assumed that his instructions meant that I should just start practicing all of my Third series postures. At the end of Intermediate, I began practicing Third series, and was on the third or fourth posture when Rolf looked over and exclaimed, "No!, I told you *Visvamitrasana*, not all those other ones!" He told me to go back and redo *Visvamitrasana*. After watching me practice it, he said, "Very good, now do backbending and next week *Vasisthasana*."

I was again disappointed to find that starting Third series with Rolf did not mean I could just go ahead and do my Third series practice, but that it meant practicing ONE posture from Third series and then waiting again. However, in the subsequent days, I noticed that I was really focusing on *Visvamitrasana*, and attempting to make it as perfect as I could. There was a new-found feeling of stability and depth in the posture.

Rolf then began a trend which would continue for the subsequent seven years that I would practice with him. Every Monday, he would give me one new posture. Each time I practiced that new posture, it was in some ways like experiencing it for the first time. After having focused on deepening the posture which preceded it for a week, and then placing all my awareness and attention on practicing that one new posture as well as I could for the following week, the result was a significant deepening of my entire Third series practice.

At the end of that first trip in Goa, Rolf had taught me up to *Urdhva Kukkutasana C*. On my final day, as we said goodbye, he told me, "Now you know how it works here with me. If anyone says they did Third series in Goa with Rolf, they will have a really strong practice." I assured him that I enjoyed it very much and would be back the next season. I had lost all interest in going to the KPJAYI. I knew that Rolf was my teacher.

Going back home, I immediately returned to my old routine of practicing Primary and Intermediate series once per week each, and Third series on the other four days of the week. It was interesting to note that the postures of Third series which I had relearned with Rolf that year felt much better and more stable than the rest of the series.

Over the following two winters, in trips of three or four months each time, I completed Third series with Rolf. Each time I returned to Goa, I would drop my usual full Third series practice and pick up where I had left off the previous season with Rolf. The routine did not change. Every Monday I would get the next posture. I never asked, and he never forgot. Once I had reached *Viparita Salabhasana*, he split my practice so that I was only practicing Third series each day, without Intermediate series as a warm-up. Once I had completed Third series with him, he told me: "Next year, same procedure for Fourth series. If you can do them, I will teach each posture one by one. If you can't do them, then you have to wait."

I had never practiced Fourth series before, so the subsequent four years became the first time that my personal practice at home actually matched the practice I was doing in Goa with Rolf. Due to the years of preparation I had done, I could do most of Fourth series postures on my first try when Rolf gave them to me; however, there were a few postures which were difficult, and he had me stop on those postures for periods ranging from several weeks to several months. After four more seasons, in trips of four or five months each, I completed Fourth series with Rolf. I then had a personal practice of Primary, Intermediate and Third series one day per week each, and Fourth series three days per week.

Rolf's teaching method changed quite a bit between my first season with him in 2007 and my final season with him in 2014. Over the years, he grew to accept and assimilate Marci's ideas of how to modify some of the postures and the changes she made to the Ashtanga system itself. By the end of my seven-year period of learning with Rolf, none of the other students were being taught the traditional postures in the traditional way, and Rolf and Marci had developed their own unique interpretation of the Ashtanga system.

With me, however, Rolf maintained the same traditional method that he had learned himself from SKPJ for all seven years that I practiced with him. I feel extremely fortunate to have learned the entirety of both the advanced series from Rolf in this way, and I believe he enjoyed teaching me as much as I enjoyed learning from him.

My understanding of how the Mysore method of practice works most effectively was shaped during this formative period of learning with Rolf. Several important aspects of the pedagogy of this method became clear to me, especially during the first few seasons that I practiced with Rolf.

There are practitioners who have enough motivation, strength, and understanding of the practice and of their own bodies and nervous systems to teach themselves new postures. One can even teach oneself an entire advanced series, as I did. I don't necessarily feel that this is a bad thing to do, especially if there are no qualified teachers available to learn from.

However, self-teaching can result in more mistakes, creating unnecessary pain and discomfort. This is especially true for an immature practitioner, as I was when I taught myself Third series in my first winter in the Yukon. I taught myself Third series far too quickly. I was enthusiastic, and underestimated the deep reaching structural effects that daily practice of this series would have on my body.

An experienced and mature teacher who understands how the series works on the human body would never allow a student to move through the series so quickly, even if the student could do all of the postures. When Rolf taught me Fourth series, he sometimes slowed the pace down even more, sometimes waiting two weeks before giving me the next posture. "You do that one fine," he once said, after not giving me the next posture in the series one week. "But we'll just wait another week so you have more time to digest it."

This concept of "digesting" postures is an important one. The first few times one performs a new posture, its effects on the body are more superficial. One can often feel new areas of the body and nerves being affected by the posture, but this is just an initial taste. It is a first meeting and exchange between the body and the energetic and structural dynamics of the posture. The body does not yet feel the need to integrate those elements deeper into its permanent structural framework.

Over the subsequent weeks, as the posture is repeated each day, the effects of the posture work their way much deeper into the body and nerves. The body starts to understand that this posture and its effects are now part of its movement repertoire, and the body must then shift its structure accordingly in order to accommodate these new patterns. The tensegrity[1] patterns of the entire body need to change, and the fascia and bones themselves sometimes have to change their position in relation to each other during this process. These deeper effects will not play out until the posture has been repeated numerous times—usually for several weeks

---

1. Tension and integrity - *tensegrity*, a balance of tension members

or months — on a daily basis.

We can think of the body as a very complex hierarchy of systems. There is a dynamic arrangement and communication between the musculoskeletal, nervous, breathing, digestive, immune, endocrine, and other systems. Within each of these systems, there are also subsystems which are interacting and coordinating with each other. Within each subsystem, there are further levels of sub-subsystems, etc. We can make the picture even more complex by also adding in the "non-physical" components of a being, such as emotions, thoughts, beliefs, etc. These also organize themselves into patterns which also influence the physical systems. These systems and elements of the being all communicate and coordinate with each other in an ongoing dynamic exchange, making compensations and compromises so that the being as a whole always maintains the optimal level of functionality and ability to maintain itself as a discrete entity in the world.

The habitual behaviors in which an organism engages in its relationships with the world will also influence how the different systems and subsystems of the organism functionally arrange themselves. A person who has spent fifteen years climbing mountains on a regular basis will have a very different type of inner balance and stability which defines their "self" than a person who has spent fifteen years living in a city and working at an office every day.

If the office worker suddenly decides one day to climb Mt. Everest, and attempts to do so, all of the systems of his body would have to very quickly find novel ways to try to support this new and extreme behavior of the organism. Almost certainly, it would be too overwhelming, and the result would likely be severe physical and mental debility or death.

However, if the office worker started by taking a few short hikes on the weekends, progressed to some easy multi-day backpacking trips, eventually moving on to hiking up hills and smaller mountains, and so on, it is quite possible that this person could eventually climb Mt. Everest in a way that would actually benefit his overall being. By giving the systems of the body time to calibrate and adjust to the smaller and more graduated behavioral changes over a period of years, these activities can be successfully integrated into that person's being, and the final step to actually climbing Mt. Everest could then also be safely incorporated into that person's being.

Similarly, if the long-term mountain climber and adventurer suddenly quit all forms of this type of activity, moved to the city and took up a job as an office worker, this person, too, would likely experience overwhelming changes within his physical and mental being. All of his physical and mental systems would have to rearrange themselves drastically to accommodate the extreme change in lifestyle and sensory experience, and he would also likely experience physical and mental unwellness due to this sudden and extreme change in behavior.

The asanas we practice also affect the way our systems and subsystems arrange themselves and relate to each other. It should be clear from the analogy above that smaller steps in learning new asanas is going to be much smoother for the body to digest and integrate in a healthy and balanced way than suddenly adding a large number of difficult and advanced asanas.

Rolf also told me that SKPJ once said that you need to perform a posture 1000 times in order to master it. My interpretation of this statement is that this is how long it takes for the body to fully digest and completely assimilate a posture into its permanent structural and movement repertoire. If one practices a posture five to six days per week, this adds up to about three and a half years to get 1000 repetitions of that posture. If we think about our practice, the postures which we have been practicing daily for over three and a half years do tend to feel very natural and innate, while the ones we find difficult are usually those that we have learned more recently.

The process of complete digestion cannot be rushed. Attempting to learn too many new postures too quickly will overwhelm the body, and it will not be able to digest and incorporate them effectively. The result will be structural chaos and instability, which comes along with quite a bit of pain and discomfort, as I experienced in that winter in the Yukon. A strong person may be able to persevere and come out the other side with benefit, but it seems reasonable that we should try to avoid unnecessary pain and discomfort.

One more analogy would be to compare the human body to an ecosystem. Ecosystems are also composed of many interacting subsystems in a complex pattern of arrangements. Any change in one part of the ecosystem will affect the balance of the system as a whole. Furthermore, these resulting changes in the ecosystem will not necessarily be immediately apparent. For example, if we add a new species to an ecosystem, the immediate effect on the ecosystem as a whole might seem minimal. After some weeks or months, however, we may notice that other species which were already present in that ecosystem have begun to either decline or thrive, due to the addition of the new species. If we then observe the ecosystem after an even longer period, say months or years, we may find that there are secondary and tertiary effects, as the species which began to thrive or decline will then affect other species and elements in the system which are dependent on them, and so forth. It may take years before the ecosystem reaches its final state of equilibrium to accommodate the cascade of effects resulting from the addition of one new species.

A healthy ecosystem will likely be able to integrate the addition of one new species (or environmental condition, etc.) with minimal chaos. As it "digests" the new component, gradual changes will characterize the process of integration. Over months and years, the ecosystem will rearrange itself and a new balance will be struck. The ecosystem has been altered, but it was able to function relatively well, as a whole, during this integration period.

Now, imagine if we suddenly added five or ten new species or environmental conditions all at once. The result would likely be much more dramatic and probably much more detrimental to the basic functionality of the ecosystem as a whole. While the system would eventually find a new balance over time, the process would not be gentle, and we would likely witness great chaos and suffering in the ecosystem while the very complex set of new dynamics attempt to sort themselves out.

Again, the analogy to adding asanas to our daily practice should be clear. I feel that all of the preceding discussion lends itself to support the idea that it is ideal for us to learn each new posture one by one from a qualified teacher. A qualified teacher is one who has already learned and digested the postures and series that we are working on, and they therefore understand, through their own experience, how these postures work on the systems of the human body, both in the short term and longer term. They can then give us appropriate guidance as to when to wait and "digest" versus when to move forward and add new postures.

There are some "older generation" Ashtanga teachers who are very lenient in giving out postures. Even if a student has not effectively integrated the preceding postures in the series, these teachers will continue to add on more postures to a student's practice, seemingly indiscriminately. Some of these teachers were taught this way by SKPJ in the early days, and claim that this is the "original" way of teaching this method.

SKPJ refined his methods quite a bit over the years that he taught. One of the most notable aspects of this refinement was that he slowed down the pace at which he taught postures to students, and that he demanded increasing perfection in the asanas before moving students on in the series. Sharath has continued with this trend even more. Some of the older teachers will claim that this was simply a way to manage and deal with the rapidly increasing numbers of students. I suspect it is more likely that SKPJ and Sharath witnessed the negative and detrimental effects that learning the series too quickly had on some of those first students, and realized that learning the series more slowly was more appropriate. The term "research" in the old AYRI name was quite appropriate, I think.

If a practitioner is self-taught, or has learned a particular series from one of the more lenient teachers (both cases apply to me in my first five years of practice), I think it is very healthy and beneficial to practice with a teacher who has stricter standards and is not afraid to stop students in the places they still need to work. As I described in my experience with Rolf (and later with Sharath), being stopped provided the stimulus for more transformation and development to happen in my practice. Stopping students creates an awareness and a healthy pressure which stimulates more focus and energy to flow into the weakest areas of practice. It is a psychological "trick," but it is a very important part of the method. I have experienced the benefits of this myself as a student, and by applying it as a teacher I have also witnessed its effectiveness.

Being asked to "master" each particular posture before moving on in the series develops patience and self-encountering. We all have postures and movements we dislike and instinctively try to avoid. It requires great effort and attention to consciously go against our instincts and encounter these experiences every single morning. This is the field where authentic and deep personal transformation occurs. If we are required to "master" a particular aspect of a posture or vinyasa before we are given the next posture, then we have no choice but to apply the attention, awareness and effort necessary to make that happen. This is often where we truly encounter the most stuck areas of our bodies and beings, and it is how the practice changes us as people. Time and time again, I have noticed in myself and in my students, that if we are not required to master something before moving onward in the series, then we will never bother to maintain the level of effort and attention necessary to create that mastery. Once we have been moved on past a posture, it naturally loses importance and prominence in our awareness.

Another important reason for "mastering" a posture before learning the next one is for physical integrity and safety. Each posture (or set of postures) in the system serves as a preparation for something more difficult which is to come later. If we don't fully develop and integrate the movement patterns which are required with the current postures, then when we come to more difficult postures which are based on those same movement patterns, we will be in trouble.

One early example of this comes in the *Marichasana* series. Many newer practitioners struggle with binding in these four postures, especially in *Marichasana D*. Some practitioners will require months or even years of persistent work to successfully bind in all four postures. I have noticed that many teachers are lenient, and eventually move students on in the series before they can successfully bind in all four *Marichasanas*.

Without developing the ability to bind in all of the *Marichasanas*, *Supta Kurmasana* and *Garbha Pindasana* will be impossible in most cases, as these two postures rely on the movement patterns developed in the *Marichasanas*. Students who are still struggling with the *Marichasanas* and then move on and also begin to struggle with *Supta Kurmasana* and *Garbha Pindasana* end up putting too much pressure on their bodies.

Struggling with *Marichasana D* alone might be a sustainable degree of challenge for the body to go through each day. If the student stops there and finishes the practice, the body will eventually develop the movement patterns necessary to bind in *Marichasana D*, without experiencing too much discomfort or excessive pressure. However, if the student attempts to practice *Marichasana D*, along with several other postures further along in the series which also require deep movement of both the hip and rotator cuff, then it often ends up being too much struggle for the body to go through each day. The result can be a lot of pain and a significant increase in the risk of injury.

Over my years of teaching, I have noticed that the students who have been taught all of Primary series very quickly, and yet are still struggling with many of the postures in the series, are invariably the ones who report having knee, hamstring and shoulder injuries in their first six months of practice. These students are often grateful when I scale their practice back to half of Primary series or less.

In 2013, I came across an article which inspired me to go to the KPJAYI and practice with Sharath Jois. This inspiration stuck with me, so in 2014 I applied and was accepted. Six months after completing Fourth series with Rolf I found myself in Mysore where I was required to drop my advanced practice and start again from the beginning. In 2007, when I began practice with Rolf, I had to drop one full series from my personal practice. In 2014, when I began practice with Sharath, I had to drop three full series from my personal practice. Fortunately, I understood that this is required of everyone on their first trip to Mysore, so I was prepared to do this.

I enjoyed refocusing on Primary series, and then on Intermediate series with Sharath. I did experience some frustration and self-encountering, but overall it was a very beneficial process for me, and it strengthened and verified my understanding of the system which I have expounded on in this essay.

Returning home after this first trip with Sharath in early 2015, I was faced with a rather large gulf between the practice which I had been doing with Sharath in Mysore (at that time up to *Dwi Pada Sirsasana*) compared to my previous personal practice which I had learned from Rolf over seven years.

After my first trip with Rolf in 2007, I quickly returned to my old personal practice; but this time I felt in no hurry to immediately return to my previous personal practice of the advanced series. I had enjoyed returning to Intermediate series and refocusing on the postures which could be deepened, and it had been many years since I had practiced Intermediate series daily. I also knew that I would continue to practice Intermediate with Sharath again the following year. This time, going back home, I initially maintained a daily practice of Intermediate series only for several months.

After a few months at home, I began to miss the practice of the two advanced series, and felt a natural desire to add them back into my practice. This presented a dilemma: It had now been about six months since I had dropped the two advanced series (at the beginning of my trip to Mysore). It seemed as if it would be a bit much to just jump back into full advanced practice after a six-month gap of not practicing these two series. I realized that adding the advanced postures back gradually would likely be a healthier and smoother process. I also felt as if I still wanted to maintain a daily practice of Intermediate series until my subsequent trip with Sharath, which was only a few more months away.

My solution was to start gradually adding Third or Fourth series postures to the end of Intermediate series four days per week in my daily practice. On two of the days, I would add Third series postures to the end of Intermediate and on the other two days, I would add Fourth series postures to the end of Intermediate.

I added between one and three advanced postures on most of the days that I practiced like this. The first day of practicing each new advanced posture (after a gap of six months of non-practice) usually felt a little shaky, yet it was also very interesting to see how familiar they felt in my body. By the second or third repetition of the new postures, they felt completely stable, and in many cases they felt even deeper than they had been before my trip to Mysore with Sharath. Dropping those advanced postures for six months and refocusing on the basics had not diminished my ability to practice them—in many cases it actually improved my ability to practice them. This was a very interesting result to observe!

I treated the experiment as if I was practicing the advanced postures for the first time. I only added new postures from Third or Fourth series if the ones I had already added felt completely stable and open, and the practice as a whole felt stable and nourishing. Because I already had a ten-year relationship with Third series, it all came back very quickly. I was able to add two to three postures from this series just about every time I did the practice, and it was not very long before I was practicing two full series—all of Intermediate and all of Third—on the two days per week that I did this practice.

Fourth series took a bit longer. I had only completed Fourth series a little over one year earlier, and my relationship with it was far less stable than my relationship with Third series. My body had not fully digested Fourth series before I went to Sharath for the first time. The first part of the series (which I had a longer relationship with—up to five years), came back more quickly than the second half. There were several points in the adding back of Fourth series where I did stop myself and waited for a few days or weeks, when the overall effect of the series on my body and nerves seemed to require a little more time to stabilize. It was several weeks or a month after I completed Third series that I also completed all of Fourth series and was practicing full Intermediate and full Fourth series two days per week.

In the beginning of this process, I was unsure if practicing two full series per day would be sustainable for me, especially when followed by three or four hours of teaching each day. But by adding the advanced series back gradually, it turned out to be fine. It felt very stable and very strengthening. I enjoyed it quite a bit.

Soon enough, it was time to return to Mysore, and drop the advanced series yet again. There was more work to do in Intermediate with Sharath in my second trip.

Returning home after my second trip in Mysore (which was just two and a half months before the time of writing this), I was faced with a similar situation as I had been in the previous year. This time, the situation was complicated by the fact that I had been injured in Mysore, and was still in quite a bit of pain. I was still unable to practice a few of the postures in

Intermediate series due to the injury, so adding back the advanced series was not even a consideration at this stage.

It took about two months at home to reach the point where I was practicing full Intermediate without needing to modify anything, and for the pain from the injury to have completely dissipated. At this point it had once again been nearly six months since I had dropped the advanced series from my practice, and so I again began the same procedure off gradually adding back Third or Fourth to the end of Intermediate, four days per week.

This process began three weeks ago, and I am now up to seven or eight postures from each of Third and Fourth series at the time of writing this essay. Once again, I am treating it as if I am practicing them for the first time. The injury I sustained in Mysore had quite a deep effect on my body. Though I am no longer experiencing pain, I do still feel structural effects, and a lot has changed in my body as a result. Because of this, I feel I am experiencing the effects of Third and Fourth series in yet another unique way. I am witnessing their effects on the body from a new perspective — perhaps from a healing one.

Three weeks ago, when I decided to start adding the advanced series back, I was unsure if I was ready. Though I was pain-free in my Intermediate series practice, I felt quite tired, heavy and stiff overall. It seemed counterintuitive to start making my practice longer and more intense in this situation. Yet, something told me to try, and so I did. In the first week, I added just two or three postures of each advanced series. It was amazing to feel the overall shift in the energy and the experience of my entire practice. Adding these new postures created a significant sense of space in my pelvic area and injected a new flow of vitality into my body and my practice. It felt as if everything came back to life. It is clear that I made the right decision. I look forward to continuing the process over the next couple of months.

ANSWERS TO QUESTIONS

❧ On "All [Ashtanga] methods are good" and "All paths lead to the same goal"

I don't personally subscribe to the idea that "all methods are good" and "all paths lead to the same goal." Some methods and paths are more effective and healthier than others, and I think all practitioners should examine wisely and make healthy judgments about which methods to pursue.

I disagree with the characterization of the approach of teaching students many postures which their bodies are not ready for as being "liberating," which seems to be fashionable nowadays. I could fill an entire book of case studies which I have observed or been directly involved in, where this approach has caused serious injury. I also discussed this point in this essay, though I did not mention specific cases. I find it hard to see what is "liberating" about meniscus surgery, spinal damage and hamstring tears which result from attempting to practice postures that are beyond the body's current capacity.

It is these kinds of teaching methods, and resulting injuries, which give Ashtanga a bad reputation as being "unsafe" in the yoga world.

To be more specific, *Baddha Konasana* is a fairly advanced posture for a beginner with little experience in yoga or movement training. I do, in fact, know of injuries in the knees, groin, and spine that have been sustained when a person who is not ready to attempt *Baddha Konasana* has been asked to perform it — and even worse, been pushed deeper into it by a teacher. However, if one completes all the postures which come before *Baddha Konasana* in Primary series sufficiently, then *Baddha Konasana* will come fairly easily for that person and the posture will serve its purpose for its particular placement in the series.

Regarding Intermediate series backbends, I have worked directly with several practitioners who have been injured by attempting these postures prematurely.

Two incidents stand out in my mind: The first was when, years ago, I had an assistant who was "authorized to teach by a senior teacher" cover my Mysore classes while I was away for a few months. This was before I realized what that senior teacher's teaching approach was like. When I returned, I was shocked to find that many beginners had been aggressively moved into Intermediate series, well before they had developed any of the prerequisites. To make a long story short, out of 20 or so students in my class, five or six of them had sustained knee injuries and several had sustained back injuries while I was away. Two of the knee injuries came from being asked to practice *Bhekasana*. I then had to attempt to rehabilitate these unfortunate people, and some of the knee injuries were still lingering years later.

Another incident which is prominent in my memory was when a student came to practice with me for a month and told me that he had sustained a back injury because his previous teacher had him working on *Kapotasana*, and was trying to adjust him deeper into it. When I saw his practice, I was shocked that any teacher would even consider having him start to work on *Kapotasana*, let alone the well-respected older generation teacher that he came from. He was not even close to being able to stand up and drop back from *Urdhva Danurasana*. I scaled him back and focused on bringing strength and stability in *Urdhva Danurasana* with him, and within one month his practice and backbending had stabilized significantly and his back felt better.

As I mentioned earlier, I could fill an entire book with case studies like this. My opinion is formed out of these numerous experiences.

I have observed a lot of Ashtanga practices over the past 13 years. At this point, I can predict with about 80 percent accuracy which branch of Ashtanga teaching a student has been trained in when I see their practice for the first time. Sometimes, I can predict the specific teacher they have come from. Those who are trained in the modern method, by Sharath or the teachers whom Sharath has personally trained, usually have a very stable, grounded, mature and well-integrated personal practice. Those who come from the more liberal (or as some put it, "liberating") branch of Ashtanga usually have a sloppy, disembodied, impatient and immature practice. Of course, there are exceptions to these general trends—but the trends are very clear to me in the large sampling of practices that I have observed.

One big problem I see is that some teachers carry the attitude that those who take up Ashtanga practice should attempt to learn as many postures as they can. The goal is quantity over quality. Some people may never need to learn all of Primary series. Half Primary may be enough to support them in a healthy way to live a better life. Practicing half of Primary series in a well-integrated, aware and patient manner is going to confer much greater health and wellbeing than practicing Intermediate or advanced series with a disembodied, impatient and acquisitive attitude.

ASHTANGA,
EMBODIMENT
& COMPLEX
SYSTEMS

BECOMING ANIMAL

*Using Ashtanga Vinyasa Yoga and Meditation
as embodiment practices for the cultivation
of organic intelligence*

— July 2016 —

A PRACTITIONER IN MY MYSORE program recently asked me: "If one side of a posture is more open than the other, and I feel I can keep going deeper in the more open side, should I hold back to try to even it out with the less open side?"

My response drew from what I feel is one of the most beautiful aspects of the Ashtanga Vinyasa practice. What follows is an expanded version of my response to this question:

Don't attempt to consciously direct the organic intelligence of the body. There is a deep intelligence in the sequencing of the postures and vinyasas. They are designed to restructure the body in a particular way over many years of daily practice. The body also has its own innate, organic intelligence. The intelligence of the body interacts with the intelligence of the practice in a complex way, which even the most knowledgeable anatomy expert cannot even begin to see clearly.

The tensegrity patterns which hold the body in its stable structural state exist within a vast and complex web which has its own inherent intelligence.

As the practice influences the body and the tensegrity patterns of its structural state, all kinds of complex shifts, changes and evolution in those patterns are taking place. What we observe on the surface may sometimes seem illogical or counterintuitive—such as one side of the body becoming more open than the other side, or some types of transient pain. But, if we could see what is happening beneath the hood, in the myriad of complex inner patterns which we cannot directly perceive, what is happening may make perfect sense. The temporary outer expression of the body is simply a passing phenomenon which is a by-product of a much vaster internal process. The organic, instinctive intelligence of the body knows very well what it is doing. It is often better not to impose our conscious ideas about the restructuring process onto the body, because our conscious ideas are based on very limited information—the outer expression which we see on the surface.

Trust the innate intelligence of the body to direct that deeper internal process in the best way possible. It is more relaxing that way. Sit back and surrender to something that does not actually require conscious manipulation. Do all of the postures and vinyasas of your practice every day, in order, with sensitivity and awareness. Whatever the body happens to be allowing on that particular day, go into it. Allow it to happen. Don't hold back. Whatever the body happens to be resisting on that particular day—encounter it, but don't force it. Respect the resistance. Come up to the edge of it and feel it, but don't push too hard against it. Flow through the practice in this way and just sit back and watch as the magic unfolds within, and the patterns of tension and release continue to shift, change, and evolve over time as the structure of the body shifts, changes and evolves over time. It is a beautiful journey.

I've maintained a daily practice of the first four Ashtanga series, without any alteration to the modern sequencing for 13 years. The description above represents my current perception of how the system works most effectively and healthily on the human body, based on my own personal experience as well as the experience of observing hundreds of students who have practiced with me. The concept of "surrender" to a greater intelligence than that which we can directly perceive is a key theme in the above description.

I believe that "surrender" is an inherent property of a healthy human mind. The human mind has a powerful capacity to conceptualize, and to attempt to control its inner and outer environments. This is a wonderful capability, and we can and should use it when it is appropriate. It is also important to understand that relaxation cannot occur without surrender, or a relinquishing of control. If we are always attempting to control and manipulate ourselves and our surroundings, we will exist in a constant state of stress. This is a pathological condition. Stress is unhealthy to any organism. Some tension is necessary for life to exist, and some degree of conscious conceptualization and manipulation will increase our quality of life, but a dynamic balance between a state of tension (or stress) and relaxation (or surrender) is likely to be the most functional and healthy. This balance is another form of *bandha*.

Spiritual and religious systems also cite the concept of "surrender" as being an essential ingredient in the path to liberation and freedom. In other pieces I have written, I have discussed how this surrender often takes the form of giving one's personal power away—to a god, to a guru, to a dharma, to a concept, to an imagined and unattainable ideal, etc. In these contexts, surrender becomes a subtle but powerful way for people to be subjugated and controlled and essentially to mistrust themselves. I feel that modern religion and spirituality emerged and became rooted in human cultures by capitalizing on the inherent need and characteristic of the human mind to "surrender," and feeding it lofty abstract concepts such as gods, gurus, heavens and ideals of liberation to which it should surrender.

It is no coincidence that modern forms of religion and spirituality came into existence around the same time that agriculture did (about 10,000 years ago), and the modern human population began its path of unchecked expansion and growth. The need to organize greater numbers of people into increasingly cooperative networks based on increasingly unnatural and specialized tasks (i.e., modern human society) required a common ideology, a common myth, a common shared story that we could all agree on and be bound together by. Religion and spirituality evolved to fulfill this crucial role and requirement for modern, organized human society to work.

Religious and spiritual concepts which claim to be of divine origin, and are therefore essentially unchallengeable by mortal and imperfect humans fulfill this role perfectly. Early modern humans agreed that in order to attain freedom, heaven, salvation, or eternal peace, they had to surrender themselves to the demands of the higher powers—the gods, the gurus, the concepts, the liberation ideals—which governed the universe. This proved to be very effective and allowed human society to continue to cooperate and expand its numbers and its power to the point we have reached today, where we live in a dream bubble of our own making and have very little relationship to our organic, animal roots as members of the interconnected web of species on the planet earth.

This worked to increase the numbers of our species in the early phases of the agricultural revolution—and increasing numbers of copies of genes is the currency of success as far as biological evolution goes. However, having transcended some of the laws of biological evolution at this stage in our species' journey, we have come to a point of deep crisis, and our very survival is likely at stake, unless we are able to radically shift our worldview and our reality.

If surrender is an inherent trait of a healthy human mind, then it must have already existed in the human mind before the emergence of agriculture and modern religion and spirituality 10,000 years ago. It is likely that the new abstract religious concepts to which humans learned to surrender subverted the traditional ways that human beings utilized the mind's ability to surrender for the millions of years that the Homo genus existed before the comparatively recent advent of agriculture and modern religion and spirituality.

My current feeling is that when human beings existed in hunter-gatherer clans prior to 10,000 years ago, the mind's surrender would have been to the innate biological intelligence of its own organism. Though the state of consciousness of pre-agricultural humans cannot be definitively understood, I feel it is possible to speculate based on the anthropological observations we have of the few hunter-gatherer societies which have survived in the modern world, as well as introspective observation of the way my own consciousness behaves in different environments and lifestyles that I have engaged in throughout my life.

In pre-agricultural times, humans likely spent much of their existence in an embodied organic animal state of intelligence. This would have been a very beautiful form of self-awareness and self-understanding, which placed great confidence in the human sense of instinct and intuitive understanding. This state of consciousness and self-awareness is very different compared to that which our rational and analytic dominated minds tend to exist in today.

To survive in the forest, without the network of support of a modern human society, the sensory and perceptual systems of these humans must have been highly developed. The variety and degree of intelligent skills that each and every human being would have developed and mastered over a course of a lifetime would have been enormous. Those who were not able to do this would not have survived. The embodied state would have been a prominent feature of this existence. Consciousness would have generally stayed within the framework of the physical, biological organism, and this likely led to a very deep sense of trust—or surrender—to that innate organic intelligence. I imagine it was a very complete and whole way of living, and the existential crises and feelings of disconnect that so many people experience in the modern world likely did not exist for those human beings. There was probably not much need for lofty spiritual aspirations, because an embodied life that directly perceived its place within an interconnected web of species was likely full and complete in nearly every way.

Modern humans currently face a serious crisis as a species where we are literally poisoning the planet that we are a part of, and which we rely on for survival. It is quite possible that in the not-too-distant future, the planet earth may no longer be hospitable for human life and Homo sapiens will become extinct. I believe that the fundamental reason we are allowing this to happen is that over the past 10,000 years, we have moved from a reality and a self-awareness which is based on intuitive, instinctive, organic intelligence to a reality and existence which is entirely an abstract construct of the human mind. Our sense of self and awareness is now based on the ideas and suggestions of these imagined and artificially constructed concepts, rather than the organic physical reality of our bodies and the rest of the planet which we are a part of.

In a recent TED talk, author and historian Yuval Harari gives a very lucid description of the difference between objective, physical reality and the imagined fictional reality that humans have created, and which we now almost entirely exist in. The objective, physical reality of trees, rivers, wind, rocks, animals, and our own organic intuitive intelligence is our biological heritage. It is the reality that humans existed almost exclusively in for the millions of years before the agricultural revolution. Over the past 10,000 years, and especially in very recent times, that objective physical reality has been almost entirely replaced by an imagined, fictional reality created by the human mind. Money, countries, cultures, corporations, laws, religions, heavens, hells, and gods have no basis in physical reality. Yet, we base nearly all of our lifestyle habits, behaviors and decisions on these fictional entities which the human mind has created. As Yuval Harari says in his talk, these imagined entities are now the most powerful forces in the world, even though they are not real. It is no coincidence that the rise of power of these creations of human imagination has occurred at the same time that the objective reality of lakes, rivers, trees and animals has become neglected, abused and destroyed.

Not only has the objective reality of these other physical entities of the planet earth been forgotten and neglected, but the objective physical reality of our own instinctive, organic, intuitive human intelligence has also been neglected and abandoned. How many people today can say that they truly live in a way that most of their decisions, behaviors and actions draw from an ability to perceive and understand what is going on within their own organism at the level of embodied experience? I think very few people can honestly say that they live this way. Most decisions, actions and behaviors are based on the fabricated ideologies and expectations that come from society, culture, family, job, religion, scriptures and idols.

Where does the modern human being place its faith and its capacity for surrender? Is it in abstract, fictional concepts, or is it in the intuitive organic intelligence of our own bodies and beings? I think the answer to this question sums up the vast majority of what is wrong in the world today, both in terms of intrapersonal wellbeing, and in terms of our collective problems as a species.

If we turn to spiritual practices as part of the solution, then we need to be sure that we are not using them to perpetuate the problem. As I stated earlier in this essay, I feel that modern spirituality and religion arose as a part of this process of abstraction and the manufacturing of a fictional reality. Any spiritual practice which asks us to give our power away by surrendering to a fictional idea is not going to help in the current crisis that we face. Nearly all the religions and practices that exist today fall into this category.

What will help are practices which help us to rediscover and deepen our relationship with ourselves by cultivating, and ultimately surrendering to, the intuitive, organic intelligence of our own bodies and beings. This increases self-trust, self-confidence and a sense of wholeness. We need to stop giving our faith and trust away to ideas and ideals, and start cultivating and placing our faith in our organic intelligence. We need to stop surrendering to the whims of gods, jobs, countries, cultures and money and start surrendering more to the power and intelligence that lies within the nerves and flesh of this animal human body. By reconnecting to and developing reverence for our own objective, physical nature, we will naturally reconnect to and develop reverence for the objective reality of trees, rivers, rocks and animals. The path back home to nature begins through our own bodies.

This leads me back to the description of the process of Ashtanga Vinyasa practice that I began this essay with. I have maintained a 16-year daily practice of two of the most powerful embodiment techniques available on this planet today—Ashtanga Vinyasa yoga and Vipassana meditation. Both of these techniques are also connected to extensive dogmas and ideologies which are products of the human mind. By saying that, I do not mean that the philosophy surrounding these techniques is worthless. Certainly, some of the ideas of fictional reality that human beings have created are positive and helpful.

Yet, after 16 years of open-minded practice and experimentation, I have found that the real reason these techniques work for me is not due to the fictional ideologies that they are connected with, but because I use them as a way to embody my consciousness and to develop the capacity of my organic intelligence.

Whether I am sitting still in meditation and experiencing the subtle ebb and flow of sensation throughout every part of my body and being, or whether I am flowing with my body and breath in a profusely sweaty sequence of advanced asanas and vinyasas, the essence of what I am doing is the same. When I practice either of these techniques, I am practicing the letting go of my rational, analytic mind, and letting go of the governance of human-made ideas over my being, and I am dropping deeper into and surrendering to the organic intelligence and the felt physical reality of my human body and its sensations and feelings. Many people consider asana to be something that is designed for training the body and meditation to be something for training the mind. For me, they are just different aspects of one and the same thing. They are both somatic, body-oriented practices which are extremely effective at cultivating and deepening the sensitivity of our intuitive and instinctive intelligence.

In both of these techniques, there are steps in learning which require rational and analytic understanding. In Vipassana meditation, we must learn how to apply our focus to different parts of the body, how to scan, feel and move on, what to place importance on or not place importance on, etc. In the Ashtanga Vinyasa technique, we need to learn how to move the breath inside the body, how to sequence the asanas and vinyasas, how to position the body correctly according to basic principles of alignment, etc. Yet, these are all very superficial aspects of the techniques. They are only meant to be a doorway which opens up into a much deeper experience of embodiment and a state of consciousness which flows intuitively and instinctively.

In a mature Vipassana meditation practice, there is very little conscious directing of the awareness. Once one has learned how to move the awareness through the body and feel the somatic experience of sensation everywhere, the conscious directing mind can step back and allow the intuitive aspects of the process take over. In many of my meditation sittings, I drop into a dreamlike state, where I am continuing to scan and feel my body, but the conscious mind actually becomes suspended and the subconscious dreams, visions and images become my predominant mental experience. This is a feeling of the self at an extremely deep organic level — the subtlest layers of somatic tissue sensation with the corresponding mental images and patterns which arise spontaneously from that felt awareness, with no overlaying of conscious ideals or ideologies. What plays out in those states is very healing, clarifying and restorative. Deep and sometimes detrimental patterns of the psyche are disrupted and reconfigured. Much of what the mind requires from actual sleep and dreaming is accomplished in these sittings, and the need for sleep and dreaming is significantly reduced.

In a mature Ashtanga practice, there should also be minimal conscious direction. Once one has learned the correct vinyasa sequencing, and the correct breathing and alignment principles, all that remains to do is to shut the analytical mind off and to flow through the practice instinctively and intuitively. This is where the real magic takes place. When one's mind simply flows with the movement of the breath and the physical body—especially the subtler internal movements connected to *bandha*—one can feel the dynamic intelligence of the organic body itself take over. The body understands intuitively how to move or not to move. It understands how to expand and slow down the breath, how to slide deeper into a position, and when to back off and not push against some form of resistance. Some mature practitioners speak of experiencing a state where "some other force" is moving their body and breath through the practice. This force is certainly connected to *bandha*, but the essence of that force is the organic, intuitive animal intelligence. It feels very good to surrender to this intelligence in practice. When the conscious, analytical mind overlays its ideas and ideals onto the practice and subverts the organic intelligence, the problems of lack of self-trust, self-confidence and self-acceptance occur. This also becomes a breeding ground for injury.

Conscious analytical and objective analysis of breathing or alignment techniques may sometimes be beneficial and necessary, especially in the beginning stages of practice. But, in a mature practice which is used as a technique of embodiment and cultivation of organic intelligence, this conscious analysis should constitute only a very small percentage of how the energy and attention is directed. The analytical, objectifying practice is a much more superficial level of practice than the practice which flows from a purely intuitive and instinctive state of being.

When one is able to practice in this intuitive way, self-practice in isolation often becomes preferable to practicing in a group or under the direction of a teacher. I am sometimes asked if I am okay with practicing alone for most of the year, and without the guidance of a teacher, or whether I am able to go as deep into my practice and progress on my own as I am with a teacher. The truth is that nearly all of my deepest, most beautiful, and powerful practices occur in that very intimate space when I am alone, with myself in the dark early morning hours. It is easiest to slip into the purely embodied state when one is not concerned about being watched by others, or about integrating instruction from others. When we are alone, and in the dark, we are forced to feel ourselves more.

It is good to visit a teacher from time to time, and if one is fortunate enough to live close to a good teacher, it can be good to practice most of the time in the teacher's shala. However, all mature practitioners should strive to be as independent as possible in their practice. Relying on a teacher to "take you deeper" is a giving away of one's power. It makes one reliant on the power of the teacher, and it undermines one's ability to surrender to and develop confidence in one's own intuitive organic intelligence.

A good teacher knows this fact very well. A good teacher can see when a practitioner is able to access their own organic intelligence, and therefore requires very little input or external direction in their practice. Giving input or adjustment where it is not necessary will disrupt the student's internal process. As a teacher myself, I find that as my experience and maturity grow I place more and more importance on allowing the practitioners' own internal journey to unfold within the container of the shala room, with as little input from myself as possible. The best moments in teaching for me are when I can step back and scan a full room of twenty or more practitioners, and feel as if there is no one that I need to attend to in that moment. The only sound is that of everyone's breathing, and everyone is immersed in their own internal journey. This is where the magic of group practice really happens; when everyone is practicing in the intuitive animal state of organic consciousness.

When a student requires assistance to attain a particularly difficult asana, or if they are stuck in some inefficient movement pattern, I will certainly help them. I might help them every day for weeks or months at a time. But, as soon as I get the sense that this person has the capability to find their own way into it, then I start to leave them alone and just watch. It is fascinating to see the animal intelligence take over at this stage. Everyone has their own unique way of finding their way into something new. This is also why I feel it is important not to impose strong and rigid micro alignment ideals onto people. For me, the most fulfilling moments as a teacher are not when I physically or verbally help someone to attain something, but when I watch them learn how to attain it themselves, without my help.

It is not only through physical yoga and meditation that we can access and cultivate the organic intelligence of the human body and nervous system. As I stated earlier in this essay, our hunter-gatherer ancestors probably existed in this state nearly all of the time. Their life and their sensory relationship with the more than human world of animals, rivers, wind, rocks and trees would have been completely inseparable. They were part of this greater whole, and living in the world absolutely required living in an embodied state.

Any activity which requires us to be both physically active and sensitive can help us to cultivate and deepen this organic intelligence and to deepen our trust in it. Hiking is one of my favorite ways to do this. Long before I discovered yoga or meditation, I used to spend a lot of time hiking with a good friend. We enjoyed going out to the forest late at night, and to walk along the forest trails without the use of any light to guide us. We would use other abilities aside from our vision to feel the forest and navigate through it without stumbling or falling. It is a skill which develops very easily and quickly, once one surrenders to the innate capabilities of the human body. Sometimes one of us would break into a spontaneous run, and the other would attempt to keep up and follow, somehow navigating all of the hidden obstacles, and making lightning fast bodily decisions as each rock, tree, twist or turn suddenly presented itself. Things would happen much too quickly for the analytical conscious mind to make decisions. It was purely the organic instinctive body intelligence which would lead the way.

I was reminded of this wonderful kind of experience a couple of weeks ago as I was descending through the forest trail after climbing Gunung Abang here in Bali. The trail is narrow and steep, and full of large rocks, tree roots and erosion ditches. I had been walking down fairly slowly, carefully scanning the ground and placing my feet in the appropriate places. After reaching a particularly steep section, the stress of continuing to move slowly and carefully seemed to be too much, so I broke into a bit of a run, and then just kept going. I picked up speed and suddenly my body was flying down the trail, with that familiar experience of having to make lightning fast decisions as each rock, tree, ditch or turn in the trail presented itself. There was a great sense of freedom in letting go of the stress of calculating each and every movement, and just surrendering into the instinctive organic reactions of the body to guide the way as I sped down. Even though any wrong move at that speed could have led to serious injury, my confidence in and surrender to the organic intelligence of my body made me certain that I would be fine. It was a far more uplifting and liberating way to experience the descent.

When watching a master musician perform, one can get the sense that the same thing is happening. Things are happening far too quickly for the performer to be calculating or analyzing the notes or strokes or various techniques that they are applying. If one watches and listens with an open mind, one can literally feel the embodied state of the performer as they drop into their own organic intelligence and allow the body and sound to flow spontaneously.

I love to watch the bats around my house at sunrise and sunset. They move with such lightning speed and precision as they catapult themselves around, catching insects to eat and avoiding obstacles. Occasionally, they will fly into my open house and effortlessly zoom around, seeking their prey, and avoiding all the walls, pillars, roof, floor (and me!) Sometimes one will fly straight at me, and I will instinctively duck down, even though I know there is no chance of it hitting me. The amazing thing is that bats do not use sight at all. They feel their environment through echolocation—emitting high frequency sounds, and then navigating with their sensitive ears, according to the pattern of those sound waves bouncing off the objects around them. When I watch them, it absolutely blows my mind to witness the stunning organic intelligence and precision that nature has endowed these creatures with.

We humans too, have these kinds of capabilities. We have simply forgotten how to use them for the most part. I believe we can also develop and refine them to a very high degree. Watching an advanced and embodied Ashtanga practitioner flow through their practice is much like watching a graceful animal move through its environment. The quality is the same, because both are moving from a place of organic, embodied intelligence, and not from conscious manipulation. While physical or sensorial activities such as hiking (or any kind of sport) or music can aid us in accessing the embodied organic intelligence more readily, I believe that embodied yoga and meditation stand out as being particularly effective in cultivating this layer of our human nature.

In Ashtanga Vinyasa asana practice, the technique of moving the body and breath with vinyasa allows us to access the deepest and subtlest layer of somatic movement, which is that of *bandha*. *Bandha* will not be readily accessed by most other forms of embodied activity, such as hiking, sports, playing music, etc. Accessing the physical state of *bandha* in body and breath takes us to a much deeper place of embodiment and organic intelligence, and hence awakens perhaps as yet untapped layers of the human potential in this realm. Similarly, in meditation techniques which focus on embodiment, if we can sit still in a well-aligned posture where *bandha* is present, and we train the mind to feel the subtlest sensations in the deepest layers of organic tissue, we also access untapped layers of the human potential. Many people tend to focus on the idea of these techniques leading us to altered states of consciousness. I prefer to think of them as leading us to much deeper states of embodiment and a very effective deepening of our organic intelligence.

These techniques will not automatically accomplish this for everyone. Intention must be there. Those who practice yoga and/or meditation from a place of dogma, and who constantly impose these ideologies onto their actual practice, will only end up objectifying and vilifying their physical body and their organic intelligence. Those who view the body as something that is "lower" or an "obstacle" that needs to be overcome through rigorous practice will certainly not become more embodied or sensitive through their practices. These practitioners usually end up creating more dissonance in their relationship with their own bodies and mistrust or even disdain for their organic intelligence. They often display a lack of self-trust, a lack of self-love, and a lack of true self-understanding. When they discuss their practices, it will always be in the language of dogma and striving, and never in the language of felt, personal experience. I see many devout yoga and meditation practitioners who dutifully and devotedly recite their prayers and mantras before and after their practices, yet when I observe their actual practice, I see no sensitivity, trust or faith in themselves, in their body, or to the actual technique they are practicing.

The practice becomes a way to further mistrust the body and to give their power away to an idea. These same practitioners will usually display very little sensitivity in their daily lives. Rather than using the practices to increase somatic sensitivity and awareness, the practices are used to distance themselves from their own organic experience, while they overlay the ideas of the dogma they are following onto the body.

Whether or not one finds meaning in the philosophies and dogmas connected to the practices, I feel the most important thing is to approach the practices with an intention to become more embodied, and with an intention to surrender to the instinctive organic intelligence that lies within the physical tissues and nerves. This ultimately leads to self-trust, self-love and an embracing of the organic animal intelligence of our human heritage. If the practices are to help make us "whole," then we need to bring this long neglected and forgotten aspect of being human back into our way of being. Once we learn to love and trust ourselves as the animals that we are, we can then relearn how to love and respect the rest of the planet earth, which we are inseparably a part of, and which we rely on for our own survival and longevity as a species.

Returning to the wholeness of a hunter-gatherer existence is not feasible for the human race. We have forsaken our roots long ago, and there is no turning back now. And there have been many beautiful and wonderful ideas that have developed in the past 10,000 years of human culture which we cannot and should not forsake. I think the issue facing us now, is to understand that we have strayed too far from our roots, to the degree that wholeness and longevity are no longer possible in the state we currently exist, both as a species as a whole in our current position on the planet, and as individuals in the state of consciousness that our modern, manufactured reality has promoted. What is required is a radical shift in perception, and I believe that shift must involve reincorporating our organic, animal intelligence back into our way of living and being. I view effective embodiment practices such as Ashtanga Vinyasa yoga and Vipassana meditation as being excellent tools to aid in this process, if we choose to use them in this way.

ANSWERS TO QUESTIONS

❧ On the "future of humanity"

As I mentioned above, we have forsaken our roots to the degree that we cannot possibly go back to our former way of existence now. The carrying capacity of the planet for a population of Homo sapiens hunter gatherers is probably not more than a few hundred thousand. That would require about seven billion of us to voluntarily commit suicide in order to make that viable. Obviously, this is not an option. The only way to go now is forward.

I also don't feel that everything that human beings have created in the past ten thousand years is harmful or should be discarded. The world wide web, in particular, is an incredible tool for sharing information, knowledge and ideas. Unfortunately, most people use it as a way to become further disconnected from all that is organic and embodied. In my mind, it is fathomable to have the best of both — to honor, embrace and live through our intuitive animal nature, and to become reintegrated into a healthy network of systems of species on this planet; and at the same time to continue to use our gifts of rational intelligence and creativity to make our lives (and the lives of other species) better and more enjoyable.

Attaining this balance would require a massive overhaul of everything that we currently know — lifestyles, belief systems, worldviews, etc. It would require cooperation, creativity, and innovation from all of the most influential levels of human societies around the world. The pantheists, the responsible atheists such as Dawkins, Harris, and Hitchens, the open-minded scientists such as David Eagleman, the late Carl Sagan and Lyn Margulis, the deep ecologists such as the late Arne Naess, the organizations such as David Abram's Alliance for Wild Ethics, and the non-dogmatic, independent mystics, who seek the fullest expression of the human experience without any other agenda, are the ones that we need to listen to most in our moving forward.

While I feel that attaining this new balance is within the realm of fathomable possibility, I honestly doubt that the human species can pull it off. There is just too much ignorance, delusion and attachment to belief systems. Taking a walk through the cities and rural areas of some of the most densely populated parts of the planet makes this clear. Because I am alive at this time, I find meaning in living the best life that I possibly can, in line with the aspects of truth that I perceive and feel. I also feel it is important to share my ideas and perceptions for those who would like to listen, and perhaps apply them in whatever way possible.

❧ On Vipassana meditation

The essence of the Vipassana technique is brilliant—increasing the sensitivity of somatic awareness, and cultivating non-reaction to that felt somatic experience. And, when that technique is stripped of its dogma and worldview, it works extremely well for me in the way that I described in this essay.

The problem is that the dogma and worldview connected to the Vipassana technique prevent "surrendering to the adaptive unconscious." The underlying dogma of Vipassana is that the unconscious reactions of the adaptive unconscious are just that—blind reaction. And, in this worldview, that is seen as the primary source of suffering. Nearly all Vipassana practitioners that I know do end up vilifying and objectifying the body—and the adaptive unconscious—for this reason. They create a deep inner struggle as they grapple with their "sankharas"—which they see as something that needs to be eradicated, when it actually is a very healthy intelligence of the adaptive unconscious. They may display equanimity, poise and focus—but this struggle creates a very subtle but deep lack of self-love and self-trust, which you can observe in their speech and subtler actions. There can be no surrender to the self—to the adaptive unconscious—because it is seen as illusory, impermanent, and a source of suffering. Surrender therefore has to be placed on abstract and imagined concepts—such as the Buddha, Dhamma and Sangha. I carried this worldview for over 10 years, and the most liberating experience I had was when I allowed that worldview to crumble. What I have described in this essay is the new worldview that has begun to form itself out of the ashes of the old one.

That said, I do recommend going to the retreats in order to learn the technique. Immersing oneself in the technique in that particular way is very effective. I think that some dogma is necessary in order to pass on a structured technique of any kind. In learning something, we do need to accept that the dogma within the learning structure may not fit us perfectly. I feel that the important thing is for each person to eventually "make the practice their own" by applying their own logic and intuition to it. The danger lies in when people fail to do this, and accept all of the aspects of a teaching unquestioningly.

During my Vipassana retreats, I made many deviations from the group mentality and prescribed behavioral codes, in order to make the technique and retreat environment workable for me. This, including doing my asana practice each morning. In centers where one has one's own private room, it is possible. I am grateful to the organization for providing such a learning environment. I sat over 20 retreats in a 12-year period, but have not been back to sit a retreat in two and half years now. I am not sure what the future holds for me in that respect. I am happy with using the technique on my own as part of my daily life, and as part of my own worldview right now.

❧ On long sittings in Vipassana meditation

Amongst those who sit these kinds of retreats frequently over many years, many practitioners eventually develop very debilitating bodily pain and joint and tissue damage which paradoxically prevents them from being able to sit comfortably at all later in life.

I do still sit. It is certainly possible to sit intensive meditation retreats regularly, and not suffer this kind of physical damage. However, this requires that one is able to evaluate the effect of applying the ideology on themselves with critical discernment.

Sitting for 10–12 hours a day for 10, 20, 30 or even more days in a row will compress the joints of the body. I have sat over 20 of these kinds of retreats over the last 16 years, the longest being for 60 days, and many being for 30 or 45 days. Due to my long-term asana practice, I feel I can sit with "near perfect" alignment in a way that minimizes the compression and strain on the joints. Yet, my conclusion after all this practice is that it is impossible to completely avoid unhealthy compression in the joints in this kind of retreat.

However, if one is attuned to the effects of this kind of sitting on one's physical body, and is listening to what the sensations are telling them, it is possible to make appropriate decisions to alleviate this joint compression so that it does not cause any kind of pathological damage to the body.

For me, that means doing my asana practice every morning while sitting a retreat, sitting with healthy alignment, and also getting up and taking a walk at regular intervals during the day. By applying all of these things, I have never experienced any physical problems from sitting, nor do I expect to, in the future.

In other long-term meditators who have suffered physical damage, I observe the following: A) They do not practice asana or any other kind of physical activity that strengthens the body and relieves joint compression—neither long term nor in the retreat itself; B) They have a very poor sitting posture which exacerbates the joint compression; C) Most importantly, they do not actively evaluate the ongoing effects of the practice on their body and being.

The reason for all of the above is that rather than paying attention to the effects of the practice on their body and being, they accept and attempt to apply the ideology in an extreme way that borders on blind faith. They sit for as long as possible and as continuously as possible, without the appropriate balancing physical precautions and relievers. The pain that they experience which signals impending pathology in their bodies is interpreted through the narrow lens of the ideology as just another part of the technique and another way to practice equanimity towards their sensations.

The result is long-term damage that is irreversible.

I see this as such a paradox because in my experience the sensation-based nature of Vipassana practice has been a way to become very intimately aware of deeper aspects of myself at a sensation based level. It has made me more sensitive to what is and what isn't good for me and to make better decisions for myself based on that.

Yet for some people it doesn't have that effect. Even though they become more aware of the physical sensations, those sensations are used as a tool to objectify and even vilify the body. On one level the awareness of sensation and ability to remain non-reactive is increasing, but on another level the ability to listen to what the sensations are actually telling them is being increasingly repressed.

So, it is not the practice itself which is bad—and that is why I still do it. It is the way the practice is applied, with blind devotion to an ideology without individual discernment and discrimination, which is bad.

This is an echo of the theme I have been trying to expound: That each teaching can only be beneficial if we are able to apply it with discernment and discrimination. We need to attempt to follow the instructions of the teacher and the teaching in earnestness, but at the same time, we need to be critically evaluating and interpreting its effects on our body, spirit and mind. This may eventually mean rejecting, adapting or modifying parts of the teaching and the technique.

In my opinion, this is the mark of a very mature practitioner and a true seeker of deeper understanding of the self. I would also refer to this as "making the practice your own."

FURTHER REFLECTIONS

*On organic intelligence, animism,
Gaia & relationship with
the non-human*

— September 2016 —

I**T WAS CLEAR AND CRISP ON** Saturday morning—a bit of a rarity in this year's dry season—and perfect for a visit to Gunung Abang, the third-highest mountain in Bali. I had already hiked up Abang three times this year, and like any place that I visit regularly, I felt as if I had begun to develop a relationship with it.

I arrived at the trailhead around 7 a.m., and the clear weather held for the duration of the hike. The mountain had been shrouded in mist and cloud on each of the other occasions that I had visited, so it was a very different experience this time to walk up with the morning light shining brightly through the thick forest. I found myself noticing and experiencing many different things, as if it was a brand new place at times.

Unfortunately, the weather wasn't the only thing that was different about Abang this time. One of the things that I enjoy most about this hike is the lush and dense forest. The trail used to be fairly narrow, and the vegetation closed in tightly against it in many parts of the hike. The trail was also quite eroded in many places and full of large rocks and roots, which made the hike technically challenging. All of these factors would stimulate a more participatory sensory engagement with my environment, which would lead to a feeling of a much fuller relationship with the forest and with the land. Feeling this kind of relationship with my environment is the essence and purpose of hiking for me.

As I began my hike on Saturday morning, I immediately noticed that the trail had been leveled out. The erosion ditches were gone, and it also seemed much wider than before. My first thought was, "Wow, trail maintenance in Bali! That's impressive." It seemed odd to me. I've never encountered more than a small handful of people on this trail, and as I walked on it became apparent that a lot of work had gone into flattening and widening the trail. Soon, the trail grew to be at least 4–5 times as wide as I remember it being. There was a notable absence of the big rocks and tree roots that I remember. Massive amounts of vegetation had been cleared on either side, and the trail was now very flat, uniform and in many places neat "steps" had been cut into the dirt.

While I still enjoyed the morning, I increasingly noticed that I felt much less connected to the forest than I preferred to be. The forest seemed so far away from me, on either side of the now massive trail. It was more difficult to feel the forest, and I had to make a conscious effort to do so. I made rapid progress on the ascent, and I began to feel that a lot of the meandering twists and turns had been removed from the trail. I started to feel as if I was on something like a paved highway. Whoever had revamped the trail had taken the same approach that someone building a highway for automobiles would take. Instead of respectfully integrating the trail into the surrounding environment, a large and direct swath was cut through the landscape, with convenience, speed and ease of access being the main concerns. "Whoever planned this is certainly not an ecologist," I thought, as I imagined how much erosion was going to take place during the next rainy season on this wide, exposed and flattened swath of dirt.

I then began to wonder if this had perhaps been done for a large religious procession. Why would such extensive and unnecessary changes be made to the trail for a small handful of hikers? There are three small temples on the hike—two on the way up, and one at the top. They are all seemingly insignificant temples. The one at the top was a decaying old bamboo structure, along with a very old looking and crumbling stone archway, which had fallen into disrepair. I doubted there would be any major procession for such a minor temple.

I reached the top in record time, even though I had walked quite slowly and stopped to take a lot of pictures. This confirmed my suspicions that the trail had been altered to become much shorter and more direct. It served the function of a highway. I still managed to enjoy the walk, for the most part, in spite of the changes to the trail.

I am currently reading a book called *Animate Earth* by Stephan Harding, who is a colleague of David Abram. In the book, Harding writes about Abram's eloquent descriptions of the reciprocal relationship between a human and its environment. The environment is not simply a static, soulless object for us to perceive, measure, manipulate and dominate, as most modern worldviews assume it to be. The environment is alive and participatory, and it perceives and responds to us as much as we perceive and respond to it. Animals, plants, and even the inorganic parts of the environment all have an ability to perceive, and they respond to us. The relationship moves in both directions, hence the land and the environment must be engaged with in a respectful relationship, just as we would with another human being. All animist and indigenous cultures have held this fact at the heart of their worldviews.

To understand that our environment (meaning everything that is not us, including all of the animals, plants and inorganic parts) is alive; that it has intention, intelligence and preference; that it perceives us as much as we perceive it; and that it is ultimately a whole which we (homo sapiens) are just a small part of, and ultimately inseparable from, could be considered to be a form of animism. This type of understanding occurs outside of the realm of the rational, analytic and objectifying understanding that science and most of modern human society is based on. It arises from the subjective feeling and intuitive aspects of the human experience—or our organic, intuitive, animal intelligence.

What I enjoy most about hiking or immersing myself in natural places is the cultivation of this kind of feeling based and reciprocal relationship with the forest and with the earth. A good friend of mine and I used to give names to the specific trees, rocks or places that we would frequently encounter on our walks. We would speak of the trees or places we intended to visit on each of our hikes. To us, these trees, rocks and places were actual entities which we had reciprocal relationships with, and visiting them was not unlike visiting a human friend. They would respond to us as much as we responded to them.

One of our favorite tree friends was a massive old oak tree, which resided on the top of a hill along one of our usual routes. We aptly named it "the tree on the hill." It was a well known being to us, and we frequently paused and spent some time under its large branches when we passed by. One day, some years after I had moved away, my friend wrote to me and reported, "the tree on the hill died this year. It didn't get any leaves this spring. Later, some people came and cut it down. When I walked up the other day, there were just a bunch of sawed up logs where it was supposed to be." I recall feeling a great sadness upon reading those words. An old friend had passed away. I imagined what it would have been like to walk up the hill and to encounter a pile of sawed up logs instead of being greeted by the tree. A very strong and unpleasant visceral feeling arose deep inside me. My friend also reflected that he had felt extremely disturbed when the tree on the hill died. It seemed to be a representative statement of the gradual decline of that section of the forest, which we had witnessed over the years as the surrounding human settlement encroached deeper into it.

I often feel as if I directly perceive how a specific forest or environment "feels." Is it happy and thriving, or unhappy and wounded? How does that feeling relate to the forest's impression of me and to its reaction to my presence within it? These perceptions don't come from analytical observation and evaluation. They come as direct feelings and intuitions, as if the forest as a whole is speaking them to me.

As an extreme example of this, in my early 20s I worked in the silviculture industry in Northern Canada during the summer months for a few years. My job was to plant trees—reforestation—in areas which had been clearcut by logging companies or burned by forest fires. When working in a freshly clearcut area, where the stumps, branches and remnants of the trees were still lying around not yet dead, but in the final stages of dying, I always felt as if I was walking through the scene of a horrific mass murder or genocide, with the bodies of the dying victims strewn everywhere. I could feel the pain and anguish of the remnants of the forest, and all of her living and non-living entities. I sometimes felt the forest was very angry, and that my presence offended it deeply. There were some days in places like these where everything would go wrong. Every five minutes, something would appear out of nowhere and trip me up until I fell flat on my face. Or I would step on a jagged branch of a dead tree, and it would jump out of the ground and whack or scratch me deeply. One day, after being tripped or scratched for the hundredth time or more, I yelled out to the wind in exasperation: "It's not my fault! I didn't do this to you!" The forest didn't care. It was hurt, angry and lashing out in whatever way it could.

Other times, when I am in healthy and thriving forests or environments, I feel an immense loving energy emanating from my surroundings. I feel completely accepted and integrated into the environment, as if it will take care of me and no harm could possibly come to me. In the Yukon region of Northern Canada, where I used to live, people usually carry bear spray, which is meant to be a last resort defense in bear attacks, with them when they hike. I never felt the need to carry bear spray, even though I was often strongly criticized and called foolish. When confronted about this, I would smile and state that I go hiking with the intention of loving my environment, and that the environment recognizes this and loves me back.

I have a friend in the Yukon who is extremely adept at listening to the non-human world. One day, I was having tea at her house and she related a story to me about the construction going on in the lot beside her property. She told me that the contractor of the construction project had approached her and inquired about the potential removal of some trees that were on her property, close to the lot where the construction was taking place. The contractor had said that the trees were in the way of some equipment that they needed to use, and he proposed to cut them down and then replace them with new trees once the construction was completed. Since the trees were on her property, he would need her permission to do this. She told me that she had replied to him that she would ask the trees if they were willing to be cut down, and then let him know the following day. She said that when she went out later to ask the trees, the clear message coming from the trees was "no." She reported this to the contractor the following day. "How did he respond to that?", I asked. She said that he began to argue and attempted to bargain with her. She told me that she finally cut him off by sharply saying, "Look! The trees said 'no,' it isn't my decision. End of discussion."

On my hike on Saturday, I definitely felt like the forest was moderately wounded. The previous times that I had done this hike, the forest had always reached out to me and embraced me. Today, it remained aloof, and a bit sullen. Walking in the middle of this newly widened trail, with the large swaths of vegetation removed from either side, I felt like the forest chose to ignore me. When I approached the edges of the trail, to take a picture, or to touch something, or to look more closely at something, the forest would come around and respond to me. But I clearly had to make an effort to engage with it for that to happen. The forest was sulking a bit, and it was not a natural-flowing relationship as it had previously been.

When I reached the summit of Gunung Abang, I understood what had happened. I was correct in my guess that the desecration of the forest was for religious purposes. The small clearing at the summit was completely unrecognizable. It had been dramatically landscaped. All of the big old trees that I remembered as residing there had been cut down. The vegetation was all cleared away. The entire shape of the clearing had changed. The entire area was bare exposed dirt, with a shiny new concrete temple complex built in the middle of it. It looked like a construction site. It was a construction site. It was very disturbing, and I again experienced a strong and unpleasant visceral feeling. Even though the removal of the trees made for a more open clearing, and the views all around were more expansive than they were before, I did not enjoy being on the summit at all.

The last hike that I did before this one, which was in the dense forest of Gunung Batukaru, also contained temples and stone idols. Yet, these man-made structures all felt completely integrated with their environment. In fact, there were a few man-made things that I hadn't even noticed until I descended by the same route and passed by them a second time. They were so well integrated with the forest that they remained hidden to the casual glance.

When telling a friend about this later, he asked, "Did it seem Hindu or animist?"

"Definitely animist," I replied. The stone carvings actually felt alive to me, as if some force had breathed soul and life into them and the forest had also accepted and integrated them as a part of it. I distinctly remember two small stone wild cats, which sat on the ground, nestled into the trees and undergrowth on either side of the beginning of the trail. They did not stand out to the eye, but once I stopped and looked at them more closely, they came to life. They were fierce, and snarled menacingly at me, as if to warn me about entering the forest. I sneered and growled right back at them, as if to say, "Ha! I am not afraid. Don't worry, I belong here." They relented, and I walked through happily.

Saturday's experience was the exact opposite. Whoever built the new temple on the top of Gunung Abang, and paved a highway through the forest in order to do it, had absolutely no relationship with the land or sensitivity to the feelings of the land. There was no life or relationship in the man-made modifications, only soullessness. The temple, and the highway through the forest were not built for the forest, or within a relationship with the forest. They were built for something that exists only in the realm of abstract and disembodied human thought and fantasy. This is the way of the world today. Whether we worship capitalism and money, or abstract and disembodied gods, or an unfeeling and objectifying science, we are turning away from our authentically felt and reciprocal relationship with the rest of the planet earth—with the living entity called Gaia—which we are inherently a part of. The rest of the planet—Gaia—knows that we are doing this. It is intelligent. It has feelings. It perceives our actions. And it is not very happy.

Our relationship with the earth is the essence of our existence, it is a defining feature of who and what we are. We are whole when we are lovingly and respectfully integrated into the form and life of Gaia. We speak to Gaia, and Gaia speaks to us. When we stop listening to her and we stop participating in the relationship with her, Gaia becomes ill and displeased.

I wrote about one of my previous descents from the summit of Gunung Abang in the essay titled "Becoming Animal." I described how I broke into a run on the way down, and allowed my body to make instinctive and intuitive movements from a place of organic animal intelligence. On Saturday, I realized that this organic intelligence does not arise entirely from within me. I realized that organic intelligence arises out of my reciprocal relationship with my environment. It is an emergent property of that relationship, which cannot be experienced in isolation of that relationship.

Descending from the summit of Abang on Saturday, I broke into a run a few times, but felt much less steady or confident than I did in my previous descent, which I wrote about in "Becoming Animal." On Saturday, as I ran, the slope felt too uniform. It was just bare dirt. There were no "obstacles." No rocks for my feet to find. No tree trunks or branches for my hands to find. On my previous descent, the "obstacles"—and specifically my relationship with them—stimulated and cultivated my organic intelligence. Nearing a sharp bend in the trail, my hand would instinctively grab a narrow tree trunk, and I would use it to swing around and make the turn in mid-air. Or, perhaps the tree trunk had called out to my hand, "Here, turn now! Let me help you!" Nearing a big rock, my foot would instinctively step on it and use it as a springboard to propel myself up into the air and over another obstacle, such as a ditch or another rock. Or, perhaps the rock had called out to my foot, "Here, I will give you a lift!" Nearing a sharp drop off, my hand would instinctively grab a hanging branch, and use that to slow down my momentum, so I could navigate the drop more carefully. Or, perhaps the branch had called out to me, "Hey, slow down now! Be careful. I will help." None of this was possible on Saturday. The flat and leveled surface of dirt, with its unnatural carved steps, did not allow for any of these spontaneous relationships with my environment. Every time I broke into a run, I soon felt as if I was uncontrollably picking up speed on a sheer descent, with nothing to moderate or modulate it, and I would have to force myself to slow down and walk again.

Within the human body, each organ, or muscle, or specific population of cells or microorganisms is a discrete and distinct entity of its own. It has characteristics which make it distinguishable from the other parts of the human body. At the same time, it is also a part of the greater human body. Its integrated role in the functioning of the whole human being is as much a part of the essence and definition of what it is, as are the characteristics which allow it to be distinguished as a discrete and separate entity. Remove a heart from the human body, and it will cease to be a heart. It will quickly stop beating, die and decay into detritus. To be a heart, is to be a healthy and integrated part of a human being.

Similarly, human beings are also discrete entities of their own. Each human is different and distinguishable from other humans, and each human is different and distinguishable from other animals, plants, rocks, and the rest of the planet earth. Yet, each human, and the collective population of humans as a group, is also part of a greater whole—that of the living entity that has been called Gaia, or the self-regulating organism which is the planet earth. Just as a heart cannot be removed from its relationship to the human body and expect to continue its existence as a heart, a human being cannot be removed from its relationship to Gaia, and expect to continue its existence as a human being.

There has been a lot of talk about colonizing Mars in the news recently. This fascinates me. When I imagine what it would be like to live on Mars—if it were possible—I feel it would be a hell. It may be possible to manufacture artificial life support systems which would allow humans to survive on Mars for some period of time—just as it is possible to set up controlled laboratory conditions where a heart can be kept alive and beating outside of a human body for some period of time. Yet, there is no doubt in my mind that such an experiment would eventually fail, and those humans who made it to Mars would die a terrible death through a combination of physical complications and psychological insanity. The human organism simply isn't designed to function and survive outside of the greater whole of Gaia — the planet earth. Our role on this planet — within Gaia — is a part of the definition of what and who we are. We cannot exist outside of that definition.

The spiritual implications of this are vast. Science asks us to surrender to objective reasoning, and to reduce anything in the realm of feeling or intuition to subjective speculation. Capitalism asks us to surrender to money and unfettered growth. Monotheistic religions ask us to surrender to an abstract and disembodied God, and to a heaven that lies beyond this planet, which we will be rewarded with at the time of death. Our physical experience on this planet is reduced to being a testing ground for our ethical virtues and our worthiness of ultimately escaping to a better place at the time of death. Eastern renunciate religions ask us to remove ourselves from the attachments that relationships bring, in order to know the self. The Eastern ascetic attempts to cut himself off from relationship as much as possible in order to escape its samsaric clutches, and to enter into solitary and isolated contemplation. The planet earth and all of the relationships and connections we have with it, are reduced to being viewed as illusory, a cause of suffering, and ultimately meant to be transcended.

With these types of worldviews prevailing in 7.3 billion powerful and technologically equipped human beings today, it is no wonder that Gaia is wounded, and crying in pain. None of these worldviews recognize that our inherent nature is that of being in intimate and reciprocal relationship with the greater whole of this beautiful, living planet. None of these worldviews recognize that our relationship with Gaia is a fundamental and defining feature of our existence as humans. It may very well be that the only hope to re-establish the health, happiness and vitality of Gaia, is to revive the worldview and spirituality of animism: To re-engage in our reciprocal sensory relationships with the non-human world, to re-learn how to listen to the non-human world, and to rediscover that this relationship with a greater whole is a defining feature of what it means to be human.

To be human is to be in relationship with the non-human, and to play a balanced role as a part of the greater whole of Gaia. We co-evolved in intimate, intricate, and reciprocal relationship with all the other parts and components and the whole of Gaia over millions of years. To know the self, can only mean to know the role of the self within its manifold connections to the rest of Gaia. To imagine that a human being could find truth and liberation by transcending its relationship with Gaia is as ridiculous a notion as imagining that a human heart could find truth and liberation by transcending its relationship with the human organism.

In the previous essay, I wrote about surrendering to the self, and to the intuitive organic intelligence of the self. Comparing the experience of my two different descents down Gunung Abang—one on the old trail, and one on the new trail—helped me to come to the beautiful realization that the organic animal intelligence of the self can only arise out of the reciprocal and participatory relationship of the self with the rest of the environment. To surrender to the self and to surrender to the organic intelligence of the self means by definition to surrender to Gaia and to our relationship with her.

Fortunately, Gaia—the living, self-regulating organism which our entire planet is—is much greater than us. We are only a small part of it. One day the human species will be no more, and of all their gods and idols will die along with them. But Gaia will live on. Gaia doesn't need us. Nature doesn't need us. Life doesn't need us. We are replaceable, and we will eventually be replaced. Other forms of life will evolve out of our dust and our detritus, and they will grow over our monuments and our ideas, until all traces of the human species are buried under the ashes of time. Gaia will survive and thrive, long after we are gone. This fact gives me great comfort.

SUKHA

— April 2017 —

BANDHA ARISES NATURALLY WITHIN AN Ashtanga practitioner when the qualities of *sukha* (softness, lightness, ease) and *sthira* (firmness, stability, strength) are both established and cultivated within the context of a dynamic relationship with one another.

The commonly held belief that *mula bandha* arises from consciously squeezing the pelvic floor (or other muscles in that area) is incorrect, in my opinion and experience. I attempt to teach the essence of how to find a more relaxed and natural experience of *mula bandha* during my immersion and pranayama courses.

In response to a question during my recently completed immersion course, I explained that the "sthira" aspect of *bandha* arises from establishing a full and conscious contact with the earth — not from gripping or clenching anything. Whichever parts of our bodies are touching the ground must engage in a deliberate relationship with the ground. This contact must be firm, full, and sensitive. "Mula" is often translated as meaning "root." Establishing a deep connection to the ground, with our bodies, is the essence of rooting.

Once this rooting is established, and the energy of the earth begins to flow up and into the body, we must then find "sukha" in order for the energy of the earth to spread, percolate and distribute itself everywhere. We simply need to "get out of the way" of that rising energy whose natural tendency is to spread and expand. This requires a softening, a release of tension, and an allowing for relaxed expansion to occur. Any form of clenching or gripping will inhibit this relaxed expansion from taking place.

When helping students with backbending, I notice that the vast majority of practitioners are most blocked in the hip and pelvic extension aspect of backbending. I feel that this is often at least partly due to a forceful misapplication of the concept of *mula bandha*.

THE GEOMETRY OF BANDHA

—April 2017—

BANDHA NATURALLY EMERGES WITHIN a person when the two polarities of the spectrum of any given aspect of our existence are in relative balance and communication with one another. If we stand in the middle of a high mountain ridge, we can clearly see what lies on either side of the ridge. Similarly, in the balanced state of *bandha* we can easily feel the qualities of either end of the spectrum of our potential experience. From this vantage point, we have maximum freedom and spaciousness in our perspective and in our energy flow. From the middle ground, we can move in either direction at will, and hence have the greatest range of options available to us.

The following photograph of *Trikonasana B* (which was not staged and was taken during a regular practice session) illustrates the physical dynamics of *mula* and *uddiyana bandha* nicely. This is one of my favorite postures for feeling the dynamics of *bandha* at work.

Mula bandha arises when the opposing forces around the pelvis are in a dynamic balance with one another. In *Trikonasana B*, the pelvis and the spine are oriented parallel to the ground. The legs do the work to pull the pelvic bones backwards, away from the camera, along the axis of the earth. The right hand and the deeper muscles of the torso work to pull the spine and torso in the opposite direction, culminating in the crown of the head reaching towards the camera, along the axis of the earth.

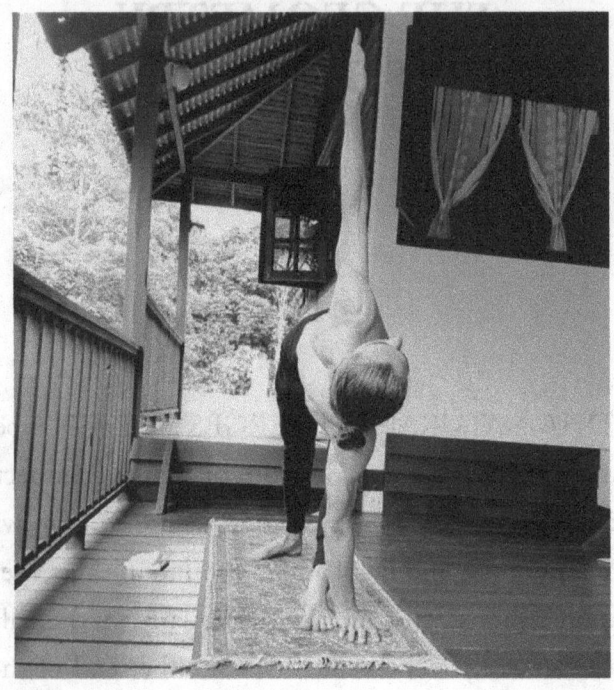

If you look carefully at the above picture, you can see that the crown of my head and my pelvic bones are well aligned and connected with each other, are moving in opposite directions and the movement of this force is parallel to the axis of the earth. There is maximum length and space through the midline of my body. This is *mula bandha*.

The internal feeling that arises in this state is one of traction and suction through the midline. The pelvic floor comes online without any conscious effort or squeezing, and feels as if it is naturally being "suctioned" towards the crown of my head. This frees up energy to flow through the center of my body, along what is also known as the *sushumna nadi*. This energy flow can be tangibly felt, especially when the breath is slow, deep and full, which serves to brighten and deepen the subtler internal sensations.

An important point to understand is that the tone in the pelvic floor is a natural result of the geometry of the posture. There is no conscious engaging or squeezing of the muscle, and doing so would actually inhibit or block the free flow of energy and breath.

Uddiyana bandha manifests when there is a dynamic balance between the opposing forces around the core of the upper body. If you pay attention to my arms in the aforementioned picture, you can see how this is achieved. The arms are working perpendicular to the axis of the earth, along the axis of gravity—so *uddiyana* is manifesting in the opposite plane that *mula* is manifesting, if we consider the reality of the body in two dimensions.

My right and left arms are well aligned with one another, are working along the axis of gravity, and are moving in opposite directions. The right hand is making a full and firm contact with the ground, and the rebounding/reactionary force of the ground is being transmitted up my right arm, through the core of my upper body, and into the left arm, which is reaching up towards the sky. The energy between my right hand and my left hand flows freely and without blockage. This is more difficult to attain than the flow of energy in *mula bandha*, as it does require an ability to release tension in the shoulders and upper back, which is typically where the flow of energy between the arms would get blocked.

The release of tension is the key concept to understand in both *mula* and *uddiyana bandha*. In *Trikonasana B*, I see many people using force and strain to attempt to crank the upper arm and shoulder backwards, instead of simply letting it relax and naturally lengthen along the axis of gravity. Once we are able to tune in to the flow of energy along the axis of gravity, and apply the downwards pressure into the earth with the bottom hand, the rest of the work is simply about letting go and creating space to allow the energy to move through. This ultimately feels relaxing and… spacious.

The net result of *uddiyana bandha* is that we have maximum expansion and spreading of energy in the upper body, perpendicular to the axis of expansion and spreading that *mula bandha* generates.

Mula and *uddiyana bandha* ultimately work to create space and expansion in opposite planes in our two-dimensional model of the body. They are both attained through correct geometry and harnessing of the natural forces that arise between our bodies, our breath and the earth. They work together reciprocally (*mula* will enhance *uddiyana* and *uddiyana* will enhance *mula*), and they ultimately communicate with each other via the medium of the flow of relaxed and deep breathing. When *mula* and *uddiyana* are both in place, the body is free of all unnecessary tension (whatever is NOT necessary to hold the posture or state of being), the nerves relax, the breath naturally slows down and expands, and we are at the peak of our physical, mental and energetic potential as living organic beings on this planet.

SOME THOUGHTS ON ALIGNMENT

— April 2017 —

IN A TALK BY MR. LEHMAN[1], he describes one important reason that I don't obsess over what I call "micro-alignment" Principles in teaching yoga. There are some branches of yoga, as well as some outspoken teachers within the Ashtanga fold, who strongly insist on very rigid and dogmatic postural alignment. Some of these teachers tout their training in fields such as physiotherapy, kinesiology, etc., as giving them greater authority to dictate how the traditional postures should or shouldn't be performed. They generally take a "one size fits all" approach to postural alignment, believing that there is a right way and a wrong way, and that everybody must conform to what they have decided is the right way.

I had the misfortune of working with one of these teachers for a number of years, and it was neither a healthy nor pleasant experience. I experienced deep physical trauma from being forced into rigid and unnatural alignment patterns. And I was much less subject to her dictates than most of the other students were.

As a teacher, I observe the practices of other students who come from

---

1. https://youtu.be/cnLxcEMdjVk

extensive training with these types of teachers, and the tendency I see is that they don't have any less pain than other students. In fact, in many cases they have more pain than others, and their movements tend to be rigid, stressed and lacking in freedom or fluidity. Their approach to the practice tends to be intellectual, rather than intuitive or embodied. They tend to have very little confidence in their own practices or their own bodies, often because these teachers have spent a lot of time pointing what is wrong with their bodies. Mistrust is a key feature in their practice experience, and probably also in their experience of life.

We humans come in all different shapes and sizes. One of the most beautiful things about the Ashtanga practice is witnessing how people of different body shapes and sizes, strengths and weaknesses, can all find their own unique way to move through the standard postures and vinyasas of the Ashtanga series. My goal as a teacher tends to see how I can stimulate and inspire people to have enough confidence in themselves to find their own way through the postures and movements using the tools that they naturally have, rather than pointing out what is wrong with, or what they have to change about their bodies.

When I do adjust alignment, it tends to be an attempt to bring them into a deeper experience of one of the *bandha*s, or to change very inefficient movement patterns. I don't necessarily see them as "corrections," but more as a suggestion to try a different way of moving. When a student complains about pain, I will sometimes make more extensive adjustments in alignment, but as Mr. Lehman states in the video, this is often more to break up a chronic pattern that has become stuck, rather than judge any particular pattern as being absolutely right or wrong.

We will tend to feel most healthy when we are practicing, and moving through life in general, with a sense of embodiment, self—confidence and freedom to be who we are and to honor the instinctive and innate patterns of our own unique and natural body structure.

A SYSTEMS-THINKING PERSPECTIVE

On the resolution of pain in Ashtanga Yoga Practice

— May 2017 —

> *I've been studying low back pain for the last 50 years of my life and if anyone says they know where low back pain comes from, they're full of shit.* —Alf Nachemson

I COMPLETELY AGREE WITH THE message of this video[1]. After watching it, I felt compelled to write more about my interpretation of pain, injury, pathology and healing, especially in the context of the Ashtanga Yoga practice.

The structurally transformative process which arises from correct, long-term application of the Ashtanga Yoga System of practice necessarily involves some experience of discomfort. Many practitioners don't understand the inevitability of these unpleasant phases of the Ashtanga experience. Rather than accepting and patiently working through the discomfort using the method of practice, some practitioners immediately seek help from outside modalities in an attempt to eliminate the pain or discom-

---

1. https://www.youtube.com/watch?v=u3EK9h4JQlo (Mar 1, 2017)

fort as quickly as possible. Fortunately, the treatment they seek is usually not as dramatic as surgery, but the surgical tourism industry in countries like India does serve a number of Ashtangis who want a quick and easy diagnosis and treatment solution for their knee pain.

When a student reports pain to me, my general advice almost always falls along the lines of "Continue to practice. Back off somewhat, perhaps we'll need to temporarily modify your practice, don't push into the pain, but continue to practice." Depending on the characteristics of the individual situation, I'll probably have some more specific advice to go along with that, but in general terms that about covers it. With continued careful practice, if the pain doesn't get worse, or it moves around to other areas of the body, or it spreads out, or it slowly improves, then I generally feel confident to tell the practitioner that they don't need to do anything else. They shouldn't seek other forms of manual therapy, nor do they need to consult a doctor and have medical scans. With continued intelligent and aware practice, it should work itself out and resolve itself.

The pain which arises out of daily, long-term Ashtanga practice often represents a deeper reorganizing and recalibrating of the tension and structural patterns of the bones, tissues and fascia. This reorganization is actually a sign of correct practice and is a desirable result. Those who don't want significant internal transformation shouldn't practice this system of yoga.

Tension is an inherent property of a healthy human being, and of any stable structure in the universe. Tension is a necessary condition for life itself. Disorder and chaos are the path of least resistance (and least tension) in the universe. For a complex structure (whether it is a molecule, a human being, a society, or a solar system) to remain stable and not degenerate into chaos and disorder, some organized force — involving tension — is an essential property of the system. Complete elimination of tension is therefore not the goal of our practice. A human being that is free of all tension is a human being that has experienced death and disintegration.

The component parts of the dead human being are free to disintegrate into chaos and disorder until they are absorbed by other stable structural systems. Death is the only true state of freedom from tension.

The goal of our practice is to reorganize and recalibrate the tension patterns in our body-mind system so that we can have a more functional and stable relationship with the environment which we live in and are a part of. The state of *bandha* could be considered as the optimal state of tension for the human being. When opposing forces are balanced in *bandha*, the tension moves to the deepest "structural" layers of the body, such as the pelvic floor and the key supportive muscles for all of the joints, which are "designed" to hold us steady and stable in relationship to the earth and its field of gravity. In *bandha*, the tension is largely removed from the sleeve muscles, which are "designed" to be free and ready to respond to the need for movement. Hence the state of *bandha* is a dynamic balance between the forces of tension and release (or, bondage and freedom). This creates healthy and functional tensegrity patterning within the human structure. For me, this functional repatterning is the goal of asana practice.

We can think of ourselves as having two temporally distinct, but interconnected postural states. One of these states is the transient postural state which we happen to occupy at any given moment in time, throughout our daily lives. This is a relatively superficial and temporary postural state, and largely reflects a relatively temporary and superficial action (or inaction) of the muscles and tissues of our body. It is also reflective of our emotional state at that given moment. The other postural state which we can consider is the long-term postural tendency, which reflects the deeper structural habits and patterns that we have adopted over our entire lives. This postural tendency is a cumulative result of the habits we generate through each of our transient postural states throughout our lives, along with the genetic tendencies which we are predisposed to from birth. This long-term postural tendency could be thought of as a deeper and more crystallized (though not impossible to change) state of tension patterning within the human system.

Postural states reflect tensegrity patterns which organize the forces of tension and release within the body-mind structure. The momentary transient and the long-term postural states influence and inform each other in a reciprocal relationship. Each momentary transient postural state provides an input into the human system which influences the more crystallized form of the long-term postural tendency. If the transient state is similar in nature to the long-term tendency, then the input of the transient state will strengthen and support the structure of the long-term tendency. If, however, the transient state contains aspects which are different in nature from the long-term tendency, then the input of the transient state will tend to induce a shift or change in the tensegrity patterning of the long-term tendency. The causal relationship between the two types of postural state also flows the other way. The patterning of the long-term tendency will also influence and inform how we hold ourselves in each momentary transient state.

In my view, the role of asana vinyasa practice is to use conscious awareness in the transient postural states of each asana and vinyasa that we occupy during our daily practice, so that these transient postural states provide tensegrity patterning inputs which are healthier and more functional in nature than the patterning of our long-term postural tendency. When this happens, the transient states of each asana and vinyasa of our practice encourage and induce a shift and transformation towards a healthier and more functional posture in the long term structural tendency.

When we do this day after day, using muscular strength, flexibility and awareness to provide the same repetitive tensegrity patterning inputs of the particular Ashtanga series that we are working on, the tensegrity patterns of the deeper structures of the human system, which reflect the longer-term postural tendencies, eventually must shift and change in order to support the new transient movement patterns which we are regularly engaging in.

If we practice each posture and vinyasa with some degree of the balanced energetic state of *bandha* in place, then over time, our long-term postural tendency will also tend to reflect the properties of *bandha* more naturally and readily. In a state of *bandha* we are in a more harmonious and functional relationship with the field of gravity. For example, when we stand in *samasthiti* with *bandha* in place, we tend to stand somewhat taller and more effectively spatially organized than we would if we were simply standing around, unaware of our posture. Practitioners who apply *bandha* well in each of the transient momentary postures (asanas and vinyasas) of their daily practice will actually grow taller over time. I have experienced this myself. My natural resting posture is now at least several centimeters taller than it was before I started daily yoga practice. I have also observed this happen in some long-term students of mine.

This process of shifting and changing the long-term structural tensegrity patterns of the body through asana practice is where the transformational pain arises, which many long-term practitioners experience from time to time. The long-term effects of shifting the deeper tensegrity patterns are healthy and beneficial, but the short-term experience of getting from here to there can be uncomfortable. Imagine what has to change deep within the structural organization patterns of your body for you to grow taller. It is unlikely that this would happen without some pain or discomfort along the way.

Continued practice through these periods of discomfort is the best (and often the only) way to resolve this discomfort. By continuing to provide the inputs of the transient postural states of our daily practice, we encourage the patterning of the long-term structural tendency to continue to evolve, until it eventually reaches a new stable conformation. There is an "intelligence" and functionality in the pain we are experiencing in this transition period. If we halt the process by stopping practice, or confuse the process by adding other, different inputs (such as resequencing the asanas, bodywork, manual therapy, surgery, etc.), then the process gets sabotaged and in some cases this can make the pain worse, or simply transfer it to other parts of the body-mind system. If, however, we continue to provide the familiar inputs of our daily practice, the evolution in our long-term postural tendency will continue to move with the intelligence of these familiar inputs of the Ashtanga series. Eventually, the longer-term postural tendency will settle into a new, stable conformation. Once this new stable conformation is reached, the transformational pain generally subsides naturally. Sometimes the pain subsides gradually, getting a little bit weaker each day as the body continues to shift and stabilize into its new structural state. Sometimes the pain disappears instantaneously, perhaps during some movement in our practice or perhaps while we are at rest later in the day.

Whether the pain dissipates gradually or instantaneously, it is continued practice (i.e., continuing to provide the same transient structural inputs which have induced the shift) which will bring about this resolution. This advice can be counterintuitive to what many practitioners (and the general population) tend to believe. Upon experiencing pain most people tend to feel that they should A) stop practice for a while and B) consult a physician.

A physician will almost always prescribe rest and recommend avoiding yoga practice until things get better. For the reasons I have already mentioned, this will not likely provide effective long-term resolution. A modern physician may also order X-rays and scans, which may confirm disc degeneration, herniation, or ligament, tendon or cartilage tears. As Alf Nachemson stated, a significant percentage of the "normal" population also have some or all of these "pathologies," yet they don't have any significant pain symptoms. Some degree of structural "pathology" is actually "normal." Yet, if an Ashtanga practitioner (or anyone, whether they are a practitioner or not) who is in pain receives the news that their scans have confirmed some structural pathology, then the person will necessarily create a network of physical and psychological labels and restrictions around their pain. They will likely limit and restrict their practice and general life movements based on intellectual theories, rather than on phenomenological experience. The movements which they do allow themselves to perform will be done with fear and trepidation, with the anxiety of making their fragile condition worse. This mentality and set of physical restrictions will not promote healing in most cases.

Ashtanga is a systems-oriented type of practice. It is therefore important to try to understand its effects from a systems-oriented perspective. The systems perspective of nature and the universe has begun to develop and evolve relatively recently. It is slowly gaining traction in the scientific community, and I believe that it is an accurate and realistic way to understand life and the universe. It trumps the reductionist methodology which has been the pervading feature of both Western and Eastern approaches to understanding reality for most of the past several thousand years.

Event Oriented Thinking
Thinks in straight lines

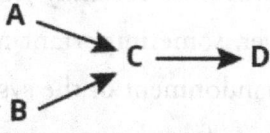

In event oriented thinking everything can be explained by causal chains of events. From this perspective the **root causes** are the events starting the chains of cause and effect, such as A and B.

Systems Thinking
Thinks in loop structure

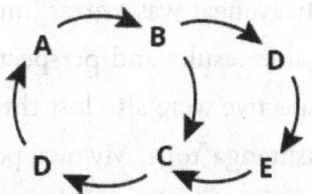

In systems thinking a system's behavior emerges from the structure of its feedback loops. **Root causes** are not individual nodes. They are the forces emerging from particular feedback loops.
http://www.thwink.org

Reductionism attempts to understand something by breaking it down into its component parts and then examining the properties of those parts. It looks to the properties of the parts as being the root causes for the properties of the whole. This is what Western science has done for hundreds of years, and this is also what Eastern religions and philosophies, such as Buddhism, do. While both Western science and Buddhist philosophy have yielded accurate, valuable and useful perspectives on reality, they have not effectively explained everything that we experience.

Reductionism is also frequently used to analyze and understand asana practice and its effects on the human system. One of the most well-known asana reductionists was B.K.S. Iyengar. Mr. Iyengar took the Ashtanga system, which he learned from Krishnamacharya, and analytically broke it down into its component parts. He took the asanas out of their systematic relationships with one another through the vinyasa system, and turned each asana into a system of its own. He then took each individual asana, and broke it down into its component parts of the actions of each individual muscle, bone, etc. He then noted the effects on each individual body part in each individual asana, and how these effects contributed to the overall functioning and health of the human being. Not surprisingly, Mr. Iyengar's work became of great interest to the modern medical community, which operates on the same reductionist paradigm.

Mr. Iyengar was a great innovator, and his work certainly yielded some valuable results and perspective. However, some important results and perspective were also lost through his abandonment of the systems view of Ashtanga Yoga. My own personal journey, from being trained as an Iyengar practitioner and teacher to becoming an Ashtanga practitioner and teacher, is that the systems perspective and experience of Ashtanga practice is deeper, richer, and more encompassing than the reductionist Iyengar technique. I value my experience with Iyengar Yoga. I am glad that I had it for four years in the beginning of my yoga journey, but there is a reason that I have been a daily Ashtanga practitioner for the subsequent 14 years. People sometimes tell me that they are drawn to me as a teacher because I have an "Iyengar background" and they want that focus on alignment.

My response to them is that the two systems are actually incompatible, and cannot be practiced together. I don't use any alignment principles, props, or techniques from my Iyengar training in my Ashtanga practice and teaching. Alignment is certainly a feature of the Ashtanga system, but it is a very different perspective on alignment. In the Ashtanga practice, alignment is integrated into a systems perspective and experience.

Returning to pain and pathology, an example of a reductionist approach to pain experienced by an asana practitioner might be to obtain medical scans or use other diagnostic methods to find some pathology in one particular muscle, joint, ligament, etc. Upon discovering (or theorizing) some localized pathology, the experience of pain in asana practice would be understood to be directly caused by that pathology. The treatment would then be to remove that pathology—either through surgery, or less dramatically, through some form of deep tissue release or targeted manual therapy. There would also likely be a number of significant changes made to the person's asana practice, based on the diagnosis of pathology in some body part.

Another reductionist approach in asana could be exemplified by a teacher telling a student "Your knee pain is caused by your tight hips," and to then prescribe a set of supplementary "hip opening" exercises to be done in conjunction with the regular asana practice. I've seen numerous practitioners who believe that "opening the hips more" or "opening the shoulders more" will be the cure to all of the issues which they face in their practice. I am frequently asked by students who are struggling with some particular asana "which body part" is stiff or stuck or needs to open more, and is therefore responsible for their inability to perform the asana.

A more Eastern-influenced form of reductionism would be to characterize all aspects of bodily pain, tension, or "blockage" as being psychological in origin. In this view, the mind is seen as being the root cause of all bodily experience and any pain in the body is reduced to some dysfunction or blockage in the psychological realm. The poor student is then left to haplessly believe that their bodily torment is due to some mental issue which they have no real way of addressing.

The key theme in all of the above examples is the reduction of the holistic experience of the state of a person's body-mind to a single root cause, and then to assume that the holistic state of the person's body-mind can be "fixed" by simply changing or fixing that one root cause. This is the essence of reductionism.

A human being is an extremely complex system. There are 11 organ systems in the human body (skeletal, muscle, nervous, integumentary, endocrine, circulatory, lymphatic, digestive, respiratory, urinary, reproductive), as well as various layers of "non-physical" experience, such as the cognitive, emotional, energetic, etc. All of these systems and layers of a human being are interconnected and coordinated in an unfathomably complex network of dynamic relationships and feedback loops.

When this human body-mind system places itself into the transient postural states of a particular asana or vinyasa, there will be an effect of all of these physical, and non-physical systems of the human being, as well as in the network of connections and relationships between all of these systems. The overall effect is a shift in the entirety of the state of the human being. This shift in the whole being is known as an "emergent property" and it cannot be explained by looking at the properties of any of the component body-mind parts, or by looking at how the asana affects any of those single component parts. Emergent properties of a dynamic and complex system literally "emerge" out of the complex dynamics of the relationships between all of the component parts. The key point to understand is that the emergent characteristics of the whole are a result of the properties and dynamics of the relationships between the parts. The emergent characteristics of the whole are not features of the parts themselves. These emergent features can only be understood by looking at the system as a dynamic whole.

A single Ashtanga series, from *Ekam* position of *Surya Namaskar A* up to *Utpluthi*, should also be thought of as a system. Practicing any of the Ashtanga series in their entirety will give certain effects, features and results, which cannot be found or explained by looking at the characteristics of any of the individual asanas in that series. They cannot even be explained by looking at all of the individual asanas in the series. The effects that one experiences by practicing a particular Ashtanga series are emergent properties which emerge out of the relationships between all of the asanas and vinyasas in the series taken together and they can only be understood by perceiving the series as a complex and dynamic system which is a whole in itself.

A system can vary in its relative stability. When the dynamic relationships between the parts of a system are changing or shifting significantly — such as when the long-term postural tendency is undergoing significant shifting — the system can be said to be unstable and in a state of transition. Whatever emergent features — such as pain — the system is experiencing at that time should be thought of as properties of the whole system, not properties of any of the parts of the system. The pain is a property which emerges out of the restructuring of the relationships and feedback loops between the parts of the system, as the system transitions from one structural state to another structural state. The pain is not a symptom of any one root cause or "dysfunction" of any component part of the system.

I suggest that in many cases of pain or discomfort experienced through long-term Ashtanga practice, adopting this perspective is the most accurate way of understanding and dealing with what is taking place. The system of the Ashtanga series is exerting an effect which is causing a shift or change in the tensegrity dynamics of the relationships between the parts of the system of the whole human being. The pain is something that emerges out of the shifting of this complex and dynamic set of relationships. The pain is not a property of any one part of the system and should not be attempted to be addressed through a perspective of linear causation.

This brings us back to the quote from Alf Nachemson which I put at the beginning of this piece. No matter how learned one may be in anatomy and physiology, I don't think that anyone can conclusively say that they understand exactly where a person's pain is coming from — especially in this type of situation. This is because the pain is not due to any one root pathology in any one part of the body. The pain is simply a reflection of the shifting relationship dynamics between all the parts of the whole human system. How these patterns are structured, and how they are changing, is far too complex for any human mind to completely understand.

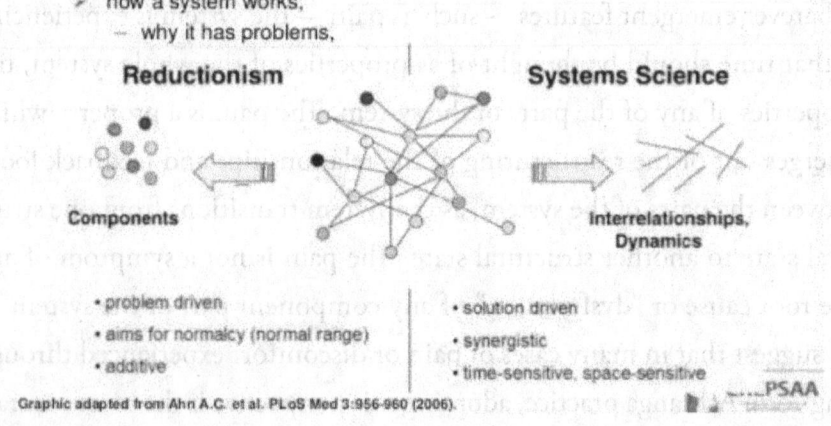

The resolution to the pain necessarily involves retaining a systems perspective. In cases of "transformational pain," the system of the Ashtanga series should continue to be practiced with as little modification to the dynamics of the system as possible. This way, the inputs that the practice is exerting on the human system remain consistent, and the intelligent reorganization process which the practice is inducing retains some stability. The human body-mind system will eventually imbibe and embody the transient daily inputs of the Ashtanga series in the more stable long-term postural state which it is moving towards. Continued intelligent movement will resolve the pain. Restriction and reductionist oriented intervention probably will not.

In my 18 years of daily yoga practice (14 of which have been Ashtanga), I've gone through many periods of pain, which have lasted anywhere from a few days to the better part of a year. Some of this pain has been severe, and accompanied by serious mobility restrictions. In most cases, these periods of pain were a by-product of a deeper restructuring/recalibration of my body's relationship to gravity, as I have described in this essay. Most of the time, the pain could be localized to a general area of the body, but usually not to a specific structure (i.e., a particular muscle, tendon, bone, joint, etc.). My approach to dealing with these periods has always been the same: Pull back to a more basic version of my daily practice. Often this would mean a less advanced series, or even a partial series. I would practice as much of the series as felt energetically sustainable, even if it was still accompanied by pain or discomfort. Often, my decision on which series to use "therapeutically" or how much of the series to practice was intuitive. I find that decisions based on systems thinking often feel more intuitive, because they require a different form of cognitive understanding than the more analytical reductionist approach which we are habituated to in most modern societies around the world. Generally, if I had to modify more than one or two postures or vinyasas in that series which I had chosen to practice, I would stop my practice at that point and go into the finishing sequence. Using this method, day by day and week by week, I would always see a gradual improvement. Improvement is defined as an increase in mobility and a decrease in pain and (equally importantly) an increase in a sense of confidence and mental/energetic stability and vitality. This could also be simplified by saying improvement is defined as a movement towards stabilization in both body and mind. As my condition improved, I would add postures and series back to my practice until I arrived back at my standard normal practice again. Some days, it might be just one inch more of space in one particular posture that could be taken without inducing pain, but if I paid attention, there were always some signs of improvement and usually on a daily basis. The pain would often move around, shifting to different places in my body, spreading out, until eventually it would disappear completely. Other times, it would happen more dramatically. I have had experiences where very serious pain completely vanished from the body instantaneously, after performing a particular posture or movement in the course of my practice that day. Whether the "recovery" was gradual or sudden, the technique was the same: careful, aware and embodied movement, to whatever degree of capacity I had at the time, encouraged and actively led to the eventual resolution of the pain.

One particularly interesting experience came during my first few months of my Ashtanga practice in 2004. I had a lot of energy and enthusiasm at that time in my life, and I was practicing with an older-style teacher who generally didn't stop practitioners at the asanas they couldn't yet perform fully. Due to my Iyengar background, I could already do many of the postures, so within a few months of beginning Ashtanga practice, I was doing all of Primary and all of Intermediate series as a 3.5-hour daily practice. Needless to say, I was in a significant amount of pain and experiencing dramatic structural changes. I watched the coming and going of different pains and the resulting structural shifts in my body with great interest and curiosity.

When I had begun practicing Iyengar yoga some four or five years prior to that, I learned how to practice dropping back from a standing position into a backbend on a beach in Northern Goa. I wasn't ready for that movement, but after watching a flexible girl in our class do it, I wanted to try. My teacher obliged and encouraged me to try. Through sheer will power, I managed to arch back and land successfully in a backbend. It was exhilarating and empowering. Two days later, when our class was "working on" backbends again, I wanted to try dropping back again. I managed to succeed, and this time my teacher came over and pulled me back up to a standing position. We went on to practice standing postures, and I felt a pain in between two vertebrae of my lumbar spine. The pain grew stronger over the course of that day and ended up staying with me for the rest of my four-month stay in Goa that year. It also brought up a lot of negative emotions. Eventually it resolved itself completely.

During the first few months of my Ashtanga experience in 2004, my nemesis became *Kapotasana*. It was very difficult for me to catch my heels, and every day when I was about to arch back into *Kapotasana*, my teacher would appear in front of me and pull my hands directly to my heels from the air. It was always terrifying, but once it was done it felt exhilarating. It happened every day. My teacher could be on the other side of the room as I was preparing, but as soon as I started to arch back, he would magically appear in front of me and pull my hands to my heels. The transformative effects of the practice on my entire being during that time were profound, and that one particular daily experience of *Kapotasana* seemed to be at the heart of everything that was going on. Sometimes, I would sit in meditation later in the day, and spend an hour with my eyes closed, meditating on my experience of *Kapotasana*. Over and over again, I would replay in my mind, in my nerves, and in my body what it felt like to have one hand, then the other hand on my heels, my elbows down and then…boom… that rush. Like a tape looped on repeat, over and over again. It was all part of the deeper integration of the experience into every layer of my being and the transformative process that was taking place.

Eventually, I started to feel some minor back pain between the same vertebrae that I had hurt years before in my Iyengar beach drop-back experience. Day by day, the back pain grew worse. I began to re-experience the same emotions which I had felt when I hurt my back in Goa, and I grew increasingly fearful and anxious when I prepared for *Kapotasana* each day. Still, the energetic rush that ensued after being pulled into *Kapotasana* made it all okay. One morning, I woke up and my back was very sore. It felt exactly as it had after the injury in Goa, and I also felt very depressed. "Great," I thought. "I've arrived back here. At least four months of back pain…" I forced myself to go to class and practice, but I made a strong and solemn determination that I wouldn't perform *Kapotasana* for some days. "When he comes over, I'll tell him I can't…"

I kept an eye on my teacher as I practiced the postures leading up to *Kapotasana*. Sure enough, when the time came he appeared in front of me. "No, no, not today," I said firmly. "Just go. Breathe," he replied. "No, my back, it really hurts…", I said. "Go!" he commanded impatiently. I sighed and started to arch. I felt the familiar pain between my vertebrae and he went to grab my first hand to pull it to my heel. I panicked and managed to yell out, "No!" I resisted his pull and tried to come back up. "Shut up and breathe, don't cry," he hissed from above me. He kept pulling and I panicked even more and started flailing around until I had wormed my way out of the posture and out of his grasp and collapsed in a heap on the ground. It was such a scene that everyone in the room had stopped practicing to look over and see what was going on. My teacher stood over me, shaking his head disappointingly. Another teacher who was practicing close to me called over, "He needs to squeeze his legs more so that he doesn't get back pain." My teacher looked up and responded loudly so that everyone could hear, "Huh! There's nothing wrong with his legs or his back, he's just got a WEAK MIND today, that's all."

His technique worked. From my collapsed and disempowered state of body and mind on the ground, I suddenly felt a rush of anger and energy surge through me. How dare he call me weak-minded! I'll show him! I quickly got back up and muttered, "All right, I'll do it!" He smiled amusingly and stepped back to watch me. I took the preparatory position and unhesitatingly started to arch back into *Kapotasana*. Instead of fear and trepidation, I felt a strong sense of pride and confidence. There was no back pain and I reached back and caught my heel with my first hand without help for the first time ever. My teacher then stepped in and gave me a tiny bit of help on the second hand. I put my elbows down. "See?" He said from above, "Now what was all that crying and fussing for?" The pain between my vertebrae had completely vanished and it never returned.

The above example is dramatic, and I certainly don't recommend or apply these kinds of methods in general. Nonetheless, it shows how quickly and suddenly the tensegrity state of a system can shift and change, and how many different factors there are which contribute to the internal relationship patterns in a particular state of body-mind. In this particular case, the shifting of a mental and energetic perspective contributed strongly to the crystallizing of a new and healthier physical structural pattern in my body.

Movement heals. Fear and limitation do not. I've also experienced this outside of the yoga practice. When I was in my early 20s, before I had started practicing yoga, I injured my left groin while on a multi-day backpacking trip. A friend and I were attempting to cover what seemed like a never-ending amount of distance over a particularly challenging section of terrain on the West Coast of Canada. We had already taken several hours longer than we had anticipated to cover the distance required to arrive at our next destination. The only way I could will my body to keep going was to imagine that my legs were like powerful pistons, pumping up and down into the earth. Somehow, the image allowed me to ignore the muscular fatigue that had set in long before. We finally arrived near dusk at the beach where we were to camp for the night and we both threw off our heavy packs and collapsed in a heap on the ground. We lay still for a long time, enjoying the flood of endorphins rushing through our systems. When I finally got up some time later, there was a deep ache in my left groin. The pain got worse as the evening went on, and it was still there the following morning. I had no choice but to strap on my pack and walk again the following day, as our feet were the only way to get back to civilization.

The injury stayed with me for some time, and I began to grow concerned. I had plans to soon embark on my first trip outside of Canada, and I had a flight to Indonesia booked for a few weeks later. I'd never experienced such a persistent pain at that point in my young life. Eventually, I went to see a doctor. The doctor didn't order any scans or tests, and after a brief examination told me that I would be fine in 6–8 weeks. I expressed my concern about my upcoming trip to Asia, as I planned to be very physically active. I wondered out loud whether I should "limit myself and rest more." The doctor grinned broadly at me and replied, "Iain — Never limit yourself, you'll be fine." Those words had a powerful healing effect, and filled me with confidence. I went home in a good mood and happily continued to plan for my trip. Though the pain was still there, I no longer focused on it or thought about limiting myself because of it. A few weeks later, I had landed in Bali and the pain in my groin was completely gone.

Over the next months, I traveled through several of the Indonesian islands and eventually flew to India and began to travel around the subcontinent. I kept up my usual habit of vigorous physical activity, and the groin injury seemed to be a thing of the past. I never thought about it. I eventually wound up in Hampi. One day, I was lying on one of the giant boulders in the late afternoon, enjoying the sensation of the heat that still radiated out of the sun-warmed rock and into my body, even though the sun had faded into the horizon some time earlier. I was completely relaxed and at ease and peace. Suddenly, I felt a "sproing" in my groin and the pain returned, just like that. I was stunned. I hadn't been very active at all that day, and in the moment that the pain returned, I was lying down, completely relaxed, enjoying a nice heat radiation massage from the rock. I walked back to my guest house worried, and my concern grew as the pain persisted over the next few days.

I immediately defaulted to the dogma of limiting my activities again, figuring that resting my body would be the wisest thing to do. I decided to make a beach my next destination, where I could really relax. I had plans to go to the Himalayas a short time later, where I hoped to do a lot of hiking in the mountains. I also had plans to return to Canada following that, where I would work as a tree planter for several months, saving up enough money to travel again the following year. Tree planting had been my main source of income for the preceding 3 or 4 years. Tree planting in Canada is a particularly intense and grueling job, both physically and mentally. It involves living in a tent in the Northern Canadian wilderness for months at a time, spending 10–12 hours each day planting saplings in areas that had previously been logged. A good planter could plant up to 3000 trees every day, and earn a decent amount of money doing so. Of course, to do this required a healthy and strong body. An injured leg would be a big obstacle to my plan.

I took my plans to relax on the beach seriously, and for one month I did extremely little aside from lying around, and occasionally swimming. The condition of my leg changed very little during this time. I was growing more and more worried, and pictured myself returning home with very little money and an inability to work at my job of choice, which was necessary to continue with the lifestyle I wanted to live. It was not a happy vision. My anxiety around my physical condition grew.

Eventually, I decided to travel up to the Himalayas even though I didn't feel much better. The hot season was setting in, and I wanted to move to a more comfortable climate. I stopped in New Delhi on my way up and visited a doctor. The doctor gave me the standard advice of resting completely and taking painkillers. He was quite adamant about his advice and

I left his office feeling even worse. I ignored his advice and carried on up to Dharamsala and made my way up to Dharamkot village, where I would ultimately spend the better part of the subsequent two years.

Dharamkot village is perched on the side of a steep mountain, and at that time was accessible by foot path only. Moving anywhere, for any reason, meant walking up and down the steep slope. I was pleasantly surprised to find that my leg felt no worse for this dramatic increase in activity. The mountain environment was fresh and intoxicating to me and I was filled with vitality and energy and a desire to hike and explore deep into the mountains. I began to gather information about some of the nearby trekking routes, while also bitterly reminding myself that I was in no shape to tackle them.

After some time, I heard about a famous practitioner of Tibetan Medicine in Dharamsala named Yeshi Dhonden. Curious and hopeful, I went to his clinic one morning, took a number, and sat in the crowded waiting room. When my turn came, I went in to see the doctor. I described my groin injury to him via his translator, and he took my pulse and then placed his fingers on my groin. "The doctor has found a lump," reported his translator. "A lump?" I asked. "Yes, an energy lump, something is blocked," The translator replied.

He wrote a prescription for a collection of Tibetan herbs, dried and rolled into little pill shaped balls, gave me instructions on how to take them and to return for a check-up in two weeks' time. He also adamantly explained, "And—You must remain VERY ACTIVE while you are taking this medicine!" "Active?" I asked, "Like, walking?" "Yes!" he replied, "You must walk a lot. This will keep energy flowing into the wound, and the medicine will work much better." I couldn't believe this wonderful news. "Can I go trekking up the mountain?" I asked. "Oh yes," he said, "That would be very good."

Just as when the doctor in Canada had told me not to ever limit myself,

I left the clinic of Yeshi Dhonden in a wonderful mood. I felt empowered and confident. I had my bag of Tibetan pills and immediately made plans to go trekking up the mountain. I spent the next six weeks in Dharamsala, hiking, trekking, and also practicing yoga for the first time in my life. I visited Yeshi Dhonden for a check-up every two weeks and would receive a new bag of herbal pills and the news that the doctor was very happy with my progress and that I would soon be completely cured. By the time I flew back to Canada, with enough herbal pills to last me for another month, the pain had vanished. When I started the difficult work of tree planting a short time later, the pain re-emerged briefly and jumped from my left groin over to my right hip for a day, but then it disappeared and never returned, and I continued on my journey as planned.

ANSWERS TO QUESTIONS

❧ On structure, systems and reductionism

The universe is basically composed of systems nested within systems. Each system is composed of subsystems and each system is itself a subsystem part of a larger system. For example, Gaia is composed of ecozones, which are composed of ecosystems, which are composed of organisms, which are composed of organs, which are composed of cells… Each layer is its own system, and, of course, we could continue to stretch the nesting of systems within systems in both directions.

There is value in looking at, and understanding the component parts (or subsystems) of a system in isolation from the system itself. My understanding of systems sciences is that they look at both the parts and the whole simultaneously.

The way I see it, we have lenses of different focal power. One lens would analyze the system as a whole. Another lens would analyze the subsystems it is composed of. Another lens could analyze the sub-sub-systems, and so on. Which lens is most appropriate to use would depend on the question being asked, or the problem we are addressing.

That said, and in terms of "transformational pain," which is the main theme of this essay, I don't think the reductionist approach of looking at the subsystems in isolation from the whole is effective or very helpful. But there are other situations where it could be. The problem is, most people default to reductionism, or examining the properties of the component parts (or subsystems) because they expect to find a "root cause" which is more fundamentally real than the emergent properties of the whole. Here, I was attempting to point out the drawbacks in this default approach, especially in the case of transformational pain in Ashtanga practice.

A final point is that I think there is a big difference between "artificial" (i.e., man-made) systems, such as electronics, which are designed with a particular function and purpose; and systems which spontaneously occur in nature as self-organizing or autopoetic life systems. I think the latter are much more difficult to predict based on understanding their component parts or subsystems. For example, if we were to make an experiment where we took 50 random types of living organism and a set of inorganic materials and a set of environmental conditions, and threw them all together, would we be able to predict the emergent properties of the resulting ecosystem, even if we knew everything there is to know about the component parts? I doubt it. We could make educated guesses, but they would be just that—guesses, because there is an inherent element of randomness in how the relationships between all of these subsystem parts would interact and develop over time.

❦ On diet

Lifestyle factors are extremely important in supporting the transformative process of the practice.

I have found a lot of benefit in transitioning to a more anti-inflammatory diet over the past 10 years or so. It helps quite a bit in muscle recovery in general and especially when one is going through painful periods. I think eating a more alkaline diet is a key factor, as well as getting enough of all the necessary nutritional elements to support both the removal of waste products, and the rebuilding of muscle tissue.

Salt baths are great. I used to use them regularly. Sea salt and rock salt are also good in a bath. Clay baths can be good too.

Therapeutic massage is debatable. I know some practitioners feel they benefit from it, but I find it disruptive to the tension patterning in the body. The way I see it is that most types of massage will remove tension from the system, and I usually feel good immediately afterwards, but the following day my body and practice are a mess. My internal structural integrity usually feels very off and I am also extremely stiff the morning after a massage. I feel it is because the massage has also removed "healthy" tension—i.e., tension that is functional and supporting the structural patterning—along with the excess tension—i.e., tension that is not functional and needs to be released. The result is a lot of confusion in the internal bodily intelligence. I think it confuses the restructuring process. Sharath also recommends against massage. Anyone who has practiced in Mysore in the past few years has surely heard Sharath's African massage story. B.K.S. Iyengar also mentioned in one of his books that he feels massage and yoga are incompatible. I think the exact quote was something like "If you do some good yoga practice, and then have a massage, the next morning you'll wake up like a dead person."

I do find "abhyanga"—applying of oil to the body before bathing—to be quite helpful. When I am anywhere that is not a tropical climate, I do this on a daily basis. The application of oil, followed by hot water shower or bath has an anti-inflammatory and lubricating effect which is beneficial. The traditional Saturday morning castor oil bath is also very helpful, but I don't usually use this as it is too messy.

Sleep is also important, though I find that multiple periods of shorter sleep is better than one chunk of long sleep. Taking a long *savasana* (I like to have 30 minutes *savasana*) after practice, and even again later in the day is also extremely important. It is when we are at rest that the organic intelligence processes the inputs of the practice and integrates the restructuring more deeply. In general, if the body needs more sleep during these periods of deeper transition, it will ask for it, and we should allow ourselves to rest more.

❧ On commenting on an injury experienced by a practitioner that I have not specifically known or worked with

It is difficult for me to make specific comments on injury, as each situation is different. I would also find it inappropriate to comment on an injury experienced by a practitioner that I haven't specifically known or worked with personally. Without seeing a person practice, it would be highly conjectural to make assumptions, and I think somewhat unethical. I wrote this essay in general terms, and leave it up to each individual to assess how it applies, or doesn't apply to their own particular situations.

To view all pain or injury as a normal or healthy part of the restructuring process would not be correct. Poor alignment, excessive pushing or over-practicing, unfocused or disembodied practice, etc., can all lead to experiences of pain which could have been avoided and are not necessarily part of a healthy restructuring process.

I know there are outspoken practitioners who suffered grievous injuries through the practice and as a result they no longer practice Ashtanga. I have read about their cases, where the descriptions of their practices make it very clear to me that these people were not using the Ashtanga method correctly and I would say not even really practicing Ashtanga Yoga; rather they were practicing their own hybrid form of yoga. They were experimenting on themselves and it went bad, but rather than taking responsibility and ownership for their failed experimentation, they choose to blame the practice itself.

One should always endeavor to practice in an embodied state which utilizes the organic, animal intelligence of the body and the nerves as the prime authority and decision-maker. The body knows what is good and what isn't good for it. It knows what is and what isn't possible. That is why animals make very few mistakes in their movements in nature. If we learn how to move as the phenomenologically experiencing body, rather than as a set of intellectual ideas, them we will usually make the appropriate decisions, and I encourage people to try to practice this way. Sometimes, we need a good teacher to help us access that state of intelligence.

❧ On practicing with more serious types of injury

In general, with a more serious type of injury, one definitely should back off. It certainly is possible to do a short and modified Ashtanga practice, but I strongly suggest to seek a qualified teacher who understands the practice and the injury well, and to work closely with that teacher in person.

The final thing I can say, is that when one has a very strong desire to attain a particular posture, or level in the practice, that desire can obfuscate one's ability to feel the intelligence of the body and to make appropriate decisions based on that intelligence. In all cases, I recommend trying to listen to the intelligence of the body, and make actions and decisions based on that, rather than based on a visualized goal of where one wants to be.

ASHTANGA,
EMBODIMENT
& COMPLEX
SYSTEMS

BRAHMACHARYA

*Exploring relationship from an
animist and systems perspective*

— October 2017 —

THE TERM "BRAHMACHARYA" IS FOUND in both the Sanskrit and Pali languages of ancient India. It is listed amongst Patanjali's five *yamas* and the Buddha's *panchasila*, both of which address the ethical or behavioral aspects of the sphere of spiritual practice. *Brahmacharya* is commonly interpreted as pertaining to control or restraint in the exchange of sexual energy. The specific details of this prescription of control or restraint vary from tradition to tradition and are generally biased towards the prevailing standards of the culture within which the tradition is embedded.

Human conceptualization and interpretation always occur through a cultural filter. To claim otherwise would indicate a deep misunderstanding of the nature of the human mind. My interpretations of scriptural concepts tend to be personalized. I do not perceive scriptures as unquestionable ancient truths which are carved in stone, but as malleable and fluid concepts which can be reinterpreted and molded to fit into novel and emergent contexts. I have my own way of perceiving reality and my place therein, which isn't fully consistent with any of the worldviews expounded in the scriptures of the major religions, cultures and spiritual systems of the world. I do not attempt to mold my personal behavior and inner logic in a way that makes it consistent with someone else's prescribed version of truth. Instead, I prefer to actively reinterpret some of the common concepts from certain spiritual and cultural traditions in a way that consolidates my own subjective and inwardly felt understanding. In so doing, I maintain a sense of wholeness within myself and my relationship with the world.

I use the term "authenticity" to describe the aforementioned process of giving precedence to one's innate internal logic and comprehension, especially if one allows this internally generated truth to guide one's actions and behavior in one's relationships with the rest of the world. Authenticity often flies in the face of socially and culturally accepted norms, since these cultural norms represent an external consensus rather than genuine internal truth. Attempting to adopt a worldview, a behavioral code or a way of being that is inconsistent with one's own personal nature is to do a great violence unto oneself, and to create a deep internal conflict and rift which serves only to fragment oneself. I classify attempts to shape one's behavior and worldview in a way that is inconsistent with one's phenomenological experiences to be "inauthentic." Unfortunately, most people in the world engage in this unhealthy form of practice for the sake of cultural and religious conformity and belonging. I feel that an authentic seeker of truth should avoid doing this, regardless of the social hardships which may result from expressed and engaged authenticity.

Brahmacharya is one of the concepts that I have taken liberty to actively reinterpret. Normally, *brahmacharya* is restricted to a sense of boundary and restriction in the sphere of sexual exchange between human beings. I prefer to think of *brahmacharya* as broadly applying to a greater sense of responsibility and felt awareness in the entirety of the field of our relationships with "others"—whether those others are human or not. Modern (i.e., post-neolithic) religion and spirituality are hyper-focused on human beings, and in particular on human sexual energy. This is not surprising, as modern religion arose primarily as a tool to control and coordinate large groups of human beings by uniting them under a common worldview, purpose and code of moral conduct. One of the most effective ways to control a person is to control their sexual energy.

When the concept of *brahmacharya* is expanded to bring greater awareness and feeling—and hence responsibility—to the entire sphere of our interactions with others, it allows profound insight about human nature to emerge. When *brahmacharya* is reduced to forced control in the sphere of exchange of sexual energy, it becomes shallow and misleading, and can constrain one's understanding of human nature to the sphere of social control.

Human organisms are in a continuous process of exchange with our environment. We are engaged in "intercourse" with our environment 24 hours a day, for as long as we remain alive. Our environment includes everything that could be defined as "other" than us. This includes other human beings, other animals, other forms of biotic life, and all of the "non-living" aspects of the world which we are a part of—the rocks, the wind, the water, etc. In other words, one's environment is everything that one is not.

The informational exchange that takes place between a living organism and its environment is both physical and energetic. This exchange flows both ways—we are simultaneously the giver and the receiver of energy—and this reciprocal flow within the relationship between the self and its environment doesn't pause for a moment for as long as we are alive. When one abides in an embodied state, this fact is clearly felt at the experiential level. For pre-agricultural humans with an animist worldview and a deeply felt communion with the rest of the living Earth, this fact would have been a given and would not have required explanation. In modern times, the disembodied, abstract and objectified human-centric realm that we have created, and that most of us dwell in, makes it easy to lose sight of our perpetual communion with our environment.

There is a discernible distinction between oneself and one's environment. Yet, because of the perpetual continuity of the reciprocal flow of information and substance between the self and the environment, it is truly impossible to define oneself outside of the context of one's environment. On the one hand, we are autonomous autopoietic units and we are recognizably distinct from our environment. At the same time, we ARE our environment. To truly understand human nature, it is important to be able to hold this dialectical perspective of seemingly opposite points of view.

In his excellent book *The Biology of Wonder*, Andreas Weber points out that we do not "process" the elements of our environment which we consume in the way that a machine, such as an engine does. An engine burns carbon based fuels in order to extract a form of energy that moves its pistons. The waste product of this combustion is then released into the environment as carbon monoxide. It is important to understand that the actual structure of the engine does not change through this process. The engine is not in communion or intercourse with its environment — it is using the environment to drive its function as an engine. The atoms and molecules which composed the engine at the time that it was built will still be present in the engine 10, 20 or 50 years later. The structure of the engine does not change through its process of using the environment. The engine is built with a specific purpose by a creator, and placed into its environment to complete a particular task.

Modern science and religion have both taken a similar perspective of the role of the human being with respect to its environment. However, upon closer examination it becomes clear that the machine analogy does not obtain for the relationship between a living being and its environment. We do not extract energy from our environment to fuel our bodies in the way that a machine does. Nor are we placed into a pre-existing environment to serve a particular purpose. A human being interacts with its environment in a completely different and more intimate way than a machine does.

The human being actually merges with its environment during its interaction or "intercourse" with it. During cellular respiration, the cell does not "burn" carbon-based sugar to move or fuel its parts in the way that an engine does. The cell integrates the molecules of the sugar into its actual physical structure. The food that is consumed by a living being becomes part of the structure of the body, and part of the process of recreating the being. Similarly, we do not excrete waste products from a combustion reaction type of process in cellular respiration. The cell breaks down parts of its actual structure, and excretes them as carbon dioxide. Actual physical parts of the being become part of the environment around it. If we examine a human body, the atoms and molecules that compose the structure of the human body are constantly changing. Every molecule in the body is replaced over a relatively short period of time. The human continuously recreates itself from its environment, and the environment similarly recreates itself from the human. Although there is a discernible distinction between the two, they are so intimately intertwined that they are part of a unified process and truly inseparable. I think that "intercourse" is a very appropriate way to describe this intimate process of exchange and co-creation, hence my application of the term *brahmacharya* to this process of reciprocal exchange within relationship.

Another way to understand the reciprocity of the relationship between the human self and its environment is to look at the role and function of an individual cell within a human body. Each cell has a semipermeable membrane, which serves as a boundary by which it defines itself with reference to the rest of the environment of the human body. This membrane also serves as a gradient through which it is constantly exchanging information and substance with the rest of the human organism in a complex and dynamic interplay. Francisco Varela and Humberto Maturana considered the cell to be the fundamental unit of life in their theory of autopoiesis. For them, the cell is the fundamental unit of a "self." The cell is an autonomous entity which continuously recreates itself through its relationship of exchange of information and substance with its environment. Yet, the cell does not and cannot exist outside of the context of the whole of its environment. Remove a particular individual cell from a human body, and it will quickly die. The cell is an individual, autonomous "self," yet it only exists as a self when it is functioning within relationship to the whole that it is a part of. The cell is an individual self of its own, yet it is also the human body.

Human beings have a membrane or boundary by which we define ourselves with respect to our environment. We are also semipermeable and continuously recreating ourselves through the exchange of information and substance with our environment. We are autonomous and independent selves, yet we cannot also exist or have meaning as selves outside of the context of our relationship with our environment. We are perpetually in the deepest form of intercourse with our environment and we literally ARE our environment.

One of the fundamental shortcomings of traditional reductionist science is that it approaches the environment as a static, objectified "thing" which we, as observers, can somehow remove ourselves from and study as if we are not a part of it, an influence upon it, or influenced by it. This same category of mistake is also made by the major modern religions of the world. All major post-neolithic religions view human beings as having been placed into an objectified environment for some divine spiritual purpose or mission. According to these human-centric religions, the ultimate goal of the spiritual path is to successfully abstract one's true essence out of the tangle of the surrounding environment. Whether this manifests in attaining heaven (as in Western monotheistic religions), or in piercing the illusory veil and understanding that the environment is self-projected and unreal (as in Eastern oneness religions), all modern religions make the same fundamental error that reductionist science does, by interpreting the human being as an autonomous unit, which is somehow separate from, more special than, or fundamentally different with respect to our environment. We could refer to this fundamental error as the "anthropocentric part-whole fallacy."

We shape and define our environment through our physical and informational exchanges with it. Simultaneously, the environment shapes and defines who and what we are. Rather than thinking of ourselves and our environment as subject and object, real and unreal, creator and created, or otherwise separated things, it would be more appropriate and accurate to think of our environment as a whole of which we humans are a participatory part. We aren't placed INTO this world. We arise FROM it and WITH it, and are inextricably intertwined in relationship with it.

In systems thinking, the parts and the whole co-create one another in a reciprocal circular relationship which transcends the linear causality of reductionist science and religion. The parts define and generate the whole through their interrelationships with one another, while at the same time the emergence of the whole defines and generates the parts which the whole requires in order to exist and experience itself. In a system, the parts and whole are so tightly interwoven and interdependent, that the true nature of any one particular aspect of the system can only be properly understood by examining it within the context of its network of relationships. These relationships are fundamental to any valid definition of the thing itself. Without its relationships, any given thing cannot exist. So it is also with humans and our environment. Attempting to abstract ourselves, escape from, transcend, or remove ourselves from our environment—physically, conceptually, or spiritually, is to deeply misunderstand the truth of who and what we are.

This systems perspective is currently the most accurate way to view the nature of a human being and its environment—spiritually/religiously and scientifically. A human being—whether we are examining its physical biology, its psychology, its "soul," or its existential purpose—cannot be accurately understood outside of its manifold relationships with its environment. The human being and its environment co-create and co-define one another and together they make up the greater whole of the entity of the living Earth and its journey through billions of years of organic evolution. To attempt to define or understand anything about a human being outside of the context of its living and breathing network of relationships within the whole of our organic home on this planet is meaningless and represents a fundamental error in understanding reality. Our dynamic and organic relationships to and through our environment are actually the most fundamental aspect of who and what we are and they are what gives us existential meaning.

The animist worldviews of our pre-neolithic ancestors (Sapiens, as well as our extinct cousins of the Homo genus) were likely consistent with the systems perspective of human nature. I would go so far as to suggest that certain aspects of animism are the subjectively "felt" or emotional-phenomenological dimension of the conceptual theories of modern systems sciences. The two—systems sciences and animism—fit together well, and when combined they give a fairly complete understanding (rational-conceptual as well as emotional-phenomenological) of human existence.

The mistake of abstracting and conceptually separating ourselves from our environment likely began with the advent of agriculture some 12,000 years ago or so. The engineering of human-created agricultural ecosystems and the accompanying convention of ownership and property likely initiated a sense of separation between the human world and the rest of the Earth. Thus were born the stratified concepts of "human" and "environment" which prior to 12,000 years ago, probably did not exist. This conceptual rift would have grown wider and wider as modern human civilization and its engineering technologies developed. As we lost our conception of our place as a participatory part in the system of processes of the whole of nature, we began to see ourselves as something special and separate from nature, who had the right to objectify and attempt to control nature for our own purposes and uses. The objectifying worldviews of the major religions and reductionist science evolved out of this trend of modern human thought and perception, and have reinforced and propagated this trend in a multi-millennium-long experiment in cognitive bias. After a few millennia of self-reinforcing amplification of this conception of ourselves, we have arrived at the monumental rift of separation and alienation from the rest of the planet Earth that we experience today—and the resulting precipice of climatic and environmental change which may be sufficient to extinguish human life forever.

Modern religion has traditionally done an excellent job of uniting, controlling and organizing large groups of human beings through a common purpose. Reductionist science has revealed incredible knowledge about the inner workings of the parts that compose the whole of nature and life. It has harnessed this knowledge to engineer technologies that even our most recent ancestors would never have dreamed possible. Both of these achievements—to unite massive numbers of people in working towards a common purpose and to harness the forces of nature to create truly miraculous inventions—are a testament to the power and potential of our species. Yet, in spite of (and because of) these achievements, human civilization now finds itself on the brink of real catastrophe. We have proliferated and applied our technologies so wantonly and without foresight that we have permanently altered our environment to the extent that it may well become uninhabitable for our own species within the next few centuries. This reality is now publicly accepted to the extent that very few people deny the predictions about climate change and environmental degradation. Yet, humans go on with business as usual, without even considering the very radical changes in our relationship to our environment that would be necessary to avert this ongoing disaster. From my perspective, this is fundamentally a problem of *brahmacharya*. We are not engaging appropriately or responsibly in our relationships with everything that is "other"—our environment.

The only way to alter the trajectory that we are currently on is a dramatic shift in worldview. More wonders of science and engineering or greater faith in the post-neolithic religions are not going to help us from damaging or altering the system which we are a part of to the extent that we can no longer be functionally integrated into it. The prevailing modern worldviews are not going to help us, because they fundamentally misunderstand and misperceive the existential meaning and purpose of being human. As long as we sustain our perception of the stratification of the human world and "the environment," we will remain fundamentally misaligned with reality and it won't be possible to re-establish a healthy and sustainable network of relationships with all of the other parts within the dance of life that is the organism of Earth.

We need a new worldview which recognizes that humans are real, autonomous entities, yet are also interwoven into the greater whole of "nature" or "Gaia" to the extent that we ARE nature. We are not any more special, privileged or meaningful than the other elements of the whole. The other animals, the trees, the rocks, the rivers, and the wind are all animate, and are all a part of us and who we are. Our dynamic interplay with all the parts creates the web of life, and at the same time we are all created by the web of life.

Animist cultures tend to live with an awareness of the necessity of regulating their interactions with the environment in the context of their relationships within a greater whole. By perceiving their role as a part within the context of a whole, they are mindful of the nature of their intercon-

give back to the environment—are all aspects of *brahmacharya*. For me, practicing *brahmacharya* is to take responsibility for each and every interaction and exchange that we have, and to understand that this exchange is happening 24 hours a day. We create the environment that we live in, and the environment creates us. We are inseparable from our environment. It is who and what we are. It is a reflection of ourselves. To understand this, to experience this, and to truly live in a way that honors this reality is to practice *brahmacharya* properly.

Once we understand this, we can examine every interaction that we engage in with our environment, and ask ourselves whether that interaction is reciprocal, functional, and healthy for the whole, or whether that interaction is consumptive, exploitative, and ultimately damaging to the whole, and therefore alienating and ultimately harmful for ourselves. It can be difficult to face the fact that modern human agricultural, industrial, and technological society has taken the path of exploitation, damage and alienation. As participants in modern human society, it is nearly impossible to avoid treading the path of the legacy that our ancestors have laid down for the past 12,000 years. But awareness is the first step. Only by becoming more aware of our individual interactions on small scale, moment to moment levels, and guiding our personal spiritualities and worldviews back towards the Earth and our inseparable relationship with it, can we hope to generate an ethical momentum that promotes internal and external consistency and wholeness. Every interaction we have with our environment counts. Every action we engage in is felt by the living whole and contributes to the shape and quality of the whole. In turn, this also shapes us and who and what we are. Even if the effect of each individual human is negligible in the grand scale of things, I feel we have an ethical duty to act in a way that brings awareness to all of our interactions. This ethical attitude represents *brahmacharya*.

Relationship occurs through our felt embodied existence. We engage in

nections with all of the other parts, and the necessity of keeping all of these functional relationships healthy and viable. Rather than seeing the environment as something that is "other" and something to manipulate, exploit and consume to serve their own selfish interests for unchecked growth and proliferation, they see the environment as something that they participate in and are an inseparable part of. Every aspect of the environment is something to be deeply respected. Every plant, every animal, every rock, every breath of air is something sacred, to be treated with reverence and with as much respect and care as one would treat a part of one's own body or one's sexual partner. For me, this is the essence of animism, and this is the essence of *brahmacharya*.

Reinterpreting *brahmacharya* from this animist perspective is to work with respect, awareness, and reverence in the way we play the boundary between ourselves and that which is other. *Brahmacharya* applies not only in how we conduct ourselves sexually with other human beings, but in how we conduct ourselves in EVERY interaction with something that could be classified as "other." It is to recognize that we are separate and autonomous selves, yet at the same time, we ARE our interactions and relationships with the other parts of the whole. Understanding the self ultimately means understanding how the self plays in relationship to the whole.

One could interpret the highest form of *brahmacharya* as finding the essence of interconnectedness in sexual union with another human being. But we can also experience *brahmacharya* by feeling the essence of interconnectedness which exists in every aspect of our relationship with our environment. Every exchange that we have—every bite of food and every breath of air that we consume, every piece of information that we receive or take from other humans or other animals or from the wind or the trees—is an aspect of *brahmacharya*. Every impact we make on the world around us—everything we excrete back into the environment, how we walk on the ground, how we exhale, or what forms of information we intercourse with our environment through our organs of perception and action. If we are to practice *brahmacharya* by bringing more awareness to our relationships and to our exchanges of information and substance with our environment, the only way to do so is to develop our sensitivity and capacity to feel in the embodied state.

Humans have progressively objectified and separated themselves from the rest of the organic living Earth over the past 12,000 years, so it is no coincidence that we have similarly attempted to abstract ourselves away from our own organic living bodies. Modern science has explored the theory that the body is nothing more than a linear causal process which arises out of inert, lifeless matter. Modern religions view the body and its natural instincts and feelings as an obstacle or temptation which gets in the way of our path to liberation or heaven. It is common for practitioners of yoga, meditation or other spiritual traditions to subscribe to the view that the goal is to transcend or overcome the physical body. The body is seen as belonging to the realm of the "lower self" and if indulged in, it leads in the opposite direction of liberation and freedom. Just as modern humans separated themselves from "nature" and began to view it is threatening, hostile, and something to be conquered and subdued through modern technology and civilization, so also we have come to view the physical reality of our own bodies with an identical attitude.

Our attempts to subdue and control nature for our own selfish desires and purposes are backfiring. Eventually, the living Earth will rebalance itself in a way that may make it inhospitable for human life. Similarly, a person who wages war against their own physical body cannot possibly expect to attain health, freedom or peace.

The pathway back home to the Earth must begin with our own bodies. If we intend to deepen and resensitize our connection to the rest of the living Earth so that we can form more appropriate and reciprocally beneficial relationships with it, we must first do that with our own bodies. Before we can drop back into and love the Earth, we must drop back into and love our bodies. If the Earth and all of its beautiful parts are to be revered and considered sacred, as they are in animist belief systems, then our own body must also be treated and perceived with the same quality of reverence. This means embracing our physicality as a vital and essential aspect of who and what we are. To feel this reverence for our organic physicality is an aspect of embodiment.

Embodiment does not mean paying more attention to the body. It does not mean taking care of the body, or being "in" the body. We do not own the body. It is not a house or a vehicle. These concepts, though perhaps well intentioned, still approach the body as an object which is fundamentally separate from our true essence. It is analogous to those who promote human beings as stewards or caretakers of the Earth. Again, this is a well-intentioned concept, but it ultimately perpetuates the sense of separation or otherness between human beings and the rest of organic life.

True embodiment means accepting and experiencing that we ARE the body. The fundamental essence of human nature is that we are physically embodied beings. Any spirituality that attempts to take us away from this truth by denying the ultimate reality of our physicality can only lead to inner conflict and suffering. All of the magic and wonder of human existence happens through our physical existence. Body, mind and spirit are not separate things. They are just different aspects of one flowing process which is life. Similarly, human beings are not separate from the rest of our environment. We are just another manifestation of the creative impulse of nature itself. We ARE the Earth, we ARE nature, we ARE the environment. When one establishes an appropriate experience and perception of one's own body, the experience of being in perpetual intercourse and communion with the rest of the living Earth flows effortlessly and naturally.

This is the "integration" that yoga and meditation help to bring about for me. I do not believe in eastern versions of enlightenment or liberation or western concepts of heaven. Suffering is an inherent part of being alive. There is nothing to fear about suffering and there is no way to escape from or transcend it. Coming to terms with suffering, rather than striving for an unattainable state of freedom from suffering, is a more grounded, effective and integrated way to exist. Embracing all of the joys and pains and the infinite variations in feeling that the human being is capable of experiencing, is to embrace the participatory essence of life itself. To be fully embodied in ourselves is to be fully embodied in the process of life and to fully experience this entire range of feeling. It is only in this state of being that we can practice *brahmacharya*—relationship—with the necessary sensitivity.

All of the wisdom of billions of years of organic evolution is contained within this body and this Earth. The abstract concepts and ideas that have arisen from the human intellect are much more recently evolved. The deeper, older, and wiser secrets of life can only be found—felt—by tuning in to the organic resonance of the living, breathing Earth, via our own highly sensitive human bodies. It is our bodies that are capable of listening, and receiving this wisdom. Relationships must be phenomenologically felt, and only with our bodies can we feel.

I often hear yoga practitioners speak condescendingly about others who focus on asana as a physical practice. "For him, it is just a PHYSICAL practice…" is one of the most insulting things one can say in the yoga world. I feel that ALL practices which lead us to the truth of human nature are physical. Ashtanga asana practice and Vipassana meditation are two of the most potentially powerful sensitizing and embodying techniques that exist. I have used both techniques as methods of embodiment for nearly 20 years, and for me they are simply two different aspects of the same process of spiritual and organic embodiment. The sensitivity and intuitive organic understanding which develops through long-term engagement with these practices has led me to realize that ALL of the practices are physical. *Brahmacharya* is also a physical practice. Not because we are using willpower to physically restrain ourselves, but because responsible, authentic, felt relationship can only occur through the attuned and sensitized physical body.

Animals understand this instinctively. Watching an animal move through and engage with its natural environment is pure yoga. The animal is instinctively one with its environment. There is no conceptual separation, there is only embodied wisdom in action. The deepest experiences in a yoga or meditation practice occur under the same conditions, when we fully drop into and surrender to the embodied wisdom of the organic, intuitive body and breath and simply flow in that state, free from the agonizing separation that occurs with the delusions of the conceptualizing mind. Nature is enlightened. Our bodies and breath are enlightened. We need to find our way back into that state of organic wisdom and being.

ANSWERS TO QUESTIONS

✎ On the term "brahma"

Derivatives of the term "brahma" (including "brahmacharya") are used extensively in the Pali canon, as well as in contemporary Buddhist discourse. In the Buddhist cosmology there are 31 planes of existence, 20 of which are known as "Brahmanic planes" and inhabited by beings known as "brahmas." These planes are accessed through development of various stages of *jhana* (which are analogous to Pantanjali's stages of *samadhi*). In the canon, the Buddha claims to have taught the technique to attain *nibbana* to many *Brahmanic* beings.

✎ On duality and separateness being a cross to bare

It is also trendy for those who engage in practices of Eastern origin or who subscribe to Eastern worldviews to believe that "oneness" or "universal consciousness" or "unity," etc., is the ultimate nature of reality and that anything else which is in the category of "diversity," "separateness," "differentiation," etc., is an illusion and source of suffering. The commentator has decided that I am suffering due to my belief in or acceptance of a reality that has characteristics of diversity.

I do not subscribe to the oneness ideology. As Joel Kramer and Diana Alstad have eloquently expounded in their writings, "oneness" is the ultimate form of abstraction. It is so inclusive as to include everything we can possibly experience.

One can certainly experience states of consciousness where the interconnectedness, unity, and "oneness" of everything can be tangibly experienced. These are very valuable and potentially life-changing experiences to have. They can inform us at an experiential level of one particular way of viewing reality, which can have its advantages and uses.

For me, however, this viewpoint or experience of "oneness" does not trump the other ways in which we can experience reality, and is no more valid than the experience of diversity. The human mind is capable of distinguishing between an apple and an orange, amongst many other things. There is nothing illusory about this. Apples and oranges have very different qualities, at a certain level of reality.

When I want to cross the road, I recognize that I am a separate entity from the speeding bus, and that I would not particularly wish to become "one" with the speeding bus at that time. The commentator has also recognized that he/she and I are separate entities with separate ideas. We are not one, at this time, in this framework of dialogue.

There is no rational reason to believe that the experience of oneness is any more valid than the experience of separateness. They are just different ways of seeing and experiencing reality. Both are valid, and both have their place. Eastern Cosmology tends to see Consciousness as being the ultimate basis of reality from which intellect, ego, the physical body and non-living matter then successively evolve out of Western Cosmology sees non-living matter as the primordial basis out of which living matter, ego (self-reference), intellect and finally consciousness and self-awareness successively evolve. These two viewpoints move in opposite directions.

I personally feel there is no need to choose one or the other as being ultimately right or wrong. They are just different lenses to look at reality through, and both have their place and their perspective. I would suggest that it is healthy to adopt this dialectic approach to seeing reality. Can we have the flexibility to shift our worldview and perspective based on the situation and the desired goal and experience of that situation?

❧ On yoga being about transcending the physical

This logically follows from the worldview that "oneness" is the ultimate reality which we should be striving to experience.

I do not have the goal of "transcending the physical," nor do I believe that this is what yoga is about. In fact, I find this kind of striving to be most dangerous and see many people harming themselves in various ways through it.

For me, if yoga is about "union" it can only mean a harmonious integration of all aspects of our existence. This includes "the physical." I see many aspirants striving to overcome or transcend their physical bodies and its annoying cravings for food, sex, and other things. They also tend to reject and repress their experiences of anger, desire, and anything else that they believe to be "lower" or characteristic of "separateness."

I feel that this behavior involves a strong denial of the fact that one is a human being and creates a deep inner conflict and battle. People engaged in this battle attempt to embody what they feel are the qualities of those who are permanently connected to the "oneness" experience, while repressing and denying those qualities which they see as being representative of separateness—the very qualities that make them human.

Psychologists (and the Buddha) have long taught us that repression or denial of that which is a part of us only causes deep problems and pathologies in the long run. Perhaps this is why there is so much borderline (or outright) pathological behavior in the "spiritual communities." This pathological behavior is often tolerated in spiritual communities, whilst in regular society it would not be accepted and in many cases punished by law.

My own path has led me to embrace the physical as what I am. I am a living, breathing organic being. This is a beautiful experience and at times where everything is harmonized, I experience much peace, joy and vitality in that. Any experiences I have that are beyond the physical realm are then easily integrated back into my daily organic physical reality, and I do not attempt to separate them or classify any particular class of experience as "higher" or "better" than any other. I am an animal with a very refined and sensitive nervous system. This is a wonderful gift, and I attempt to make the most out of it, and have no wish to deny or transcend it.

It is also my personal belief that the current technological age tends to make humans more "disembodied" than we ever have been. I believe that this is directly connected to the rapid rate of ecological destruction and devastation of our life support system, the planet Earth. Spiritual practices and philosophies which teach us that "the physical" is illusory, lower, or to be transcended are NOT going to help in the current emergency that we find ourselves in as a species.

I don't feel it is right to float along in my own bubble and assure myself that due to my spiritual practices I will be reborn in some deva or brahma plane in the next life, so it doesn't really matter if the planet goes down the tubes due to our self-destructive tendencies as a species.

I prefer to focus on practicing and teaching embodiment. If there is anything that is sacred to me, it is the physical, and it is the connection and relationship of my physical being to the physical planet that I have co-evolved with and am in eternal relationship with. I suppose this makes me a pantheist.

As far as I am concerned, this is the spiritual "medicine" that our species needs today. We don't need to transcend — we need to drop back into our bodies and the physical reality of our home, the planet earth. I think J.R.R. Tolkien was quite a visionary, and the "elves" were his idea of what the human species could be if it lived up to its potential.

❧ On being judgmental

I find it interesting how threatened some people feel by the concepts I write about. In many ways, that is my goal — to shake up how people see things, perhaps give them food for thought or reflection. I don't expect everyone to agree with me and it is natural that my ideas are rejected or refuted by many.

I nevertheless appreciate discourse about my ideas to remain about my ideas and concepts, and not about me as a person. It is not possible to know all about who I am from reading a few pages of my writings!

I am happy to address constructive criticism or debate about my ideas. I do enjoy this kind of exchange.

For instance, I have been accused of being judgmental. It is true, I am judgmental, and I am proud of this and do not apologize for it.

The first dictionary definition which I found for the term "judgment" is as follows:

> **judg·ment**
> noun
> 1. the ability to make considered decisions or come to sensible conclusions.

It is trendy in some yoga and spiritual circles to believe that we should strive to be non-judgmental. Given the above definition, this means we should attempt to suspend our ability to make considered decisions and to come to sensible conclusions.

Indeed, I have seen many spiritual aspirants who believe that a pre-rational way of thinking is ideal or more advanced.

I do not subscribe to this philosophy. I am proud of my ability to make considered decisions and come to sensible conclusions. Those whose opinions and ideas I value most also do the same.

I suggest that it would be wise to hone our ability to be judgmental in appropriate ways. Judgments based on rational consideration are a good thing, and we should engage in this throughout every day of our lives so that we can select and choose our decisions wisely. What we can attempt to suspend are decisions based on emotional or irrational prejudice, which by the dictionary definition, is not a form of judgment.

ASHTANGA,
EMBODIMENT
& COMPLEX
SYSTEMS

NATURE SPIRITS

— January 2018 —

SPIRIT EMERGES AND EVOLVES OUT of the complex web of relationships which comprise the self-organizing intelligence of nature. No entity or organism exists as an independent island. An entity exists by means of its participation in relationship with other entities within a dynamic higher-order system. An entity's network of relationships with all that is "other" is part and parcel of the essence of the entity itself.

Nature is an intelligent evolutionary process. She is always moving, changing and evolving. She is never static or fixed. She is a person, a being, a spirit. Her innate intelligence is an emergent product of the complex patterns which spontaneously form in her web of self-organizing networks of systems within systems within systems.

Soul, spirit and self-awareness are real, perceptible and tangible phenomena which emerge out of the complexity of this self-organizing intelligence. They are properties of all complex, self-organizing systems which occur in nature, at all levels of the hierarchy of systems embedded within systems. They are not the sole property of human beings.

The inert materialism of modern reductionist science and rational analysis views the emergent magic of soul and self to be an illusion.

Supernatural religions and spiritualties view the magic of soul and self as something separate from material nature which must be infused into the organic embodied intelligence of our material existence.

Both of these erroneous perspectives developed from the modern (post-neolithic) human trend of forsaking direct phenomenological relationship with non-human nature. Both perspectives fail to recognize that being a participant in the web of relationships within the system of Gaia is inseparable from the essence of being human.

The worldviews of those humans who remain in direct, participatory and felt relationship with the whole of the living earth apprehend the essence of soul and self correctly. It is only through one's direct phenomenological experience—which necessarily means actively feeling one's relationships with all that is "other"—that one can truly perceive the nature of reality.

All entities are people. The planet Earth is a person, whom some have named Gaia. Ecosystems, Mountains and Rivers are also people, whom some have named various nature spirits. A rock or a fallen tree, covered in colorful hairy moss and lichen is also a person. No one put the moss on the log, or gave the log to the moss. The moss and the log co-created each other through synergistic relationship within a stable but shifting system. The person that they co-create has spirit and soul.

Natural evolution never rests, is never still, and is always pulsing forward, hungry in her creative impulse. She continues to manifest novel and complex forms of spirits, souls and people. For those who spend time in consciously felt, phenomenological relation with the more than human world, this magical reality reveals itself. It speaks clearly to those who are able to open their sense doors and listen, feel and connect with all that is "other."

Matter is not inert. It is full of magic, spirit and soul. Yet, this magic emerges from within matter itself. No external agent or supernatural creator is involved.

This is the new materialism, the new animism, the magic of our existence and life amongst so many other different types of lives and people. It is a perceptual path and worldview that can lead us back into integrated and sustainable existence within our home of the living person Gaia.

ASHTANGA,
EMBODIMENT
& COMPLEX
SYSTEMS

TEACHING VS. PREACHING
*Embodiment as the gateway to authentic
understanding and integration*

— December 2018 —

ONE OF MY FAVORITE FICTIONAL characters is John Oldman, from the "The Man from Earth" movie series. In the second installment of the series, John is a university professor of religious studies. Having had 14,000 years of experience to hone his discernment, he makes a particularly effective and popular teacher. Some of his students discover that he is 14,000 years old, a fact that he tries to keep hidden from the world. One of these students is particularly enthusiastic and frames John as the next messiah, asking him to share his message with the world. Having had plenty of opportunities in his lengthy life to experiment with different ways of sharing his massive accumulation and assimilation of knowledge and experience, John has learned from his past mistakes and he dispels his student's hopes that he will be willing to fulfill the role she has envisioned for him by telling her: "I'm a teacher, not a preacher."

That particular line stood out for me, as it encapsulates an important distinction between two very different ways of spreading and sharing information. This distinction is something that I have become increasingly aware of over the 20 years that I have been teaching yoga.

During the initial years of my time as a yoga teacher (and in the years before that), I had the habit of assuming that whatever "truths" I had discovered and benefited from would naturally apply to all other people in the same way they applied to me. Enthusiastic to share my insights, I was fond of doing so by telling people what they should or shouldn't do in how they lived their lives. In other words, I had a habit of preaching.

My definition of preaching is: Giving another person instructions, based on the assumption that one understands that person better than that person understands himself, and is therefore more capable of making personal life decisions for that person than that person is himself.

Preaching is a common feature of human cultural pedagogy, and includes any solicited or unsolicited lifestyle "recommendations" that one imposes on others. Examples of this include: What religious or spiritual teaching to follow, what political beliefs to hold, what types of thoughts to think, what types of feelings to have, whom one should or shouldn't have sex with or marry, what style of yoga to practice, what type of clothing to wear or what to eat for lunch on any particular day.

As a young adult, I frequently noted how widespread the habit of surrendering one's autonomy and capacity to make informed personal decisions about one's own life to an authoritarian figurehead was—whether that figurehead was a doctor, a parent, a priest, a scripture, a god, or a teacher. It perplexed and frustrated me that this habit was so widespread. I had always avoided this habit by considering the opinions and information given to me by those whom I perceived as "experts" in their particular field; but using that information as a part of my own decision-making process, rather than blindly accepting the information given to me by those experts. I noted many examples of instances when authority figures had made mistakes in their analyses, and I learned to hold my own understanding of myself and my own ability to make decisions for myself as being of the highest authority. It was extremely rare that I ever made a decision or choice that could potentially affect my wellbeing simply because someone told me to do so, without considering how I actually felt inside, in the realm of my own embodied experience, about that decision.

I also noted the plethora of intrapersonal and interpersonal effects that resulted from the surrendering of one's personal autonomy and authority to an external authority and I recognized this as one of the main ills of fragmented, broken people and fragmented, broken societies and cultures. This unfortunate ill runs through all major societies and cultures of our world today. In *The Guru Papers, Masks of Authoritarian Power*, Joel Kramer and Diana Alstad recognize this ill as being one of the main symptoms of our species' failure to mature in our process of cultural evolution. They suggest that we are trapped in a state of adolescence as a species, reliant on authority figures to inform us how to live, rather than taking responsibility for our own lives and our own decisions.

By cultivating critical thinking, discernment and embodiment throughout my life, I have largely avoided falling into the trappings of this ill on an interpersonal level. Nonetheless, by engaging in preaching myself, I was spreading the same ill on a cultural level by sharing my own personal truths and understandings with others in a way that undermined their autonomy. Once I began to realize that sharing my own insights in this way was contributing to the propagation of a deeply rooted human cultural dysfunction, I began to consciously shift the methods by which I shared my knowledge and experience. This shift was gradual, but a key point in this process came when I read the aforementioned *The Guru Papers*. The implications of this book on my life were profound and it initiated an immediate and drastic shift in my worldview which percolated into the embodied experience of my life and actions in the world. I can pinpoint this as the time that I clearly and unequivocally understood the dangers of preaching. This was also the point where I ceased to identify as a Buddhist, which was the worldview that I had identified with (and preached to others) for the preceding decade. I also abandoned the delusion that any person, group of people, scripture, or organization in the world had any kind of special access to an irrefutable and universal "truth," with respect to the nature of life, existence and morality.

In the time since then, I have been increasingly careful in both my personal life relationships and in my professional life teaching Mysore-style Ashtanga yoga and Pranayama, Yoga and Buddhist philosophy, and embodiment to avoid preaching. Instead, I attempt to teach and share my experience in a way that empowers others to make more informed decisions about themselves and their roles within their relationships with the world, without the need to defer to an authority figure in that decision-making process. In my professional role as a teacher, I am careful to confine my teachings to the technical aspects of the practices, and to avoid presenting conjectural opinions as if they were facts. I emphasize that the aspects of the practice which I teach can be used as tools to deepen one's process of embodiment and subjective observation. This process naturally enhances one's ability to make life decisions based on one's own phenomenologically felt reality, rather than on the dictates of a scripture, teacher, culture, religion, etc.

My definition of teaching is: Sharing techniques or information in a way that allows and empowers a person to use those techniques or information to make their own informed personal decisions about their life.

A key dimension of the difference between preaching and teaching is the effect that the method of information transmission has on the recipient's sense of trust and confidence in himself. If the information has been transmitted through the process of teaching, the recipient's sense of confidence in his own subjective feeling based level of experience (which I sometimes refer to as animal or intuitive intelligence) should be strengthened. If the information is transmitted through preaching, on the other hand, it can have the opposite effect.

A key element of mind control is the undermining of the confidence of the subject in the accuracy of his own subjective experience. Once the subject is trained to stop trusting his own perceptions, and therefore his own decisions, his mind is ripe for the taking. This technique has been used by leaders of all sorts for millennia. Preaching has a similar effect. If the message of a preacher is in conflict with what one experiences at the phenomenological, sensation-based level in one's intuitive animal intelligence, then one experiences an internal dissonance. In order to alleviate this dissonance, one must either reject the message of the preacher, or reject the phenomenological experience of one's own intuitive intelligence.

A person's subjective, internal experience can be mistrusted and rejected in favor of the message of a preacher, but it cannot be completely removed. If one chooses to reject one's own intuitive intelligence and subjective experience, it becomes relegated to the background, where it lurks and exerts itself unconsciously. The self therefore becomes fragmented, with the conscious, adopted message of the preacher struggling continuously against the unconscious subjective intelligence of the self. This is how Jung's "shadow self" is formed. The shadow self is sometimes mistaken to be the composed of only "negative" qualities, which one prefers not to acknowledge. In reality, the shadow self includes any aspect of the self, including positive and healthy aspects, which are not consistent with the preaching of one's family members, teachers, peers, culture, or religion. Because these aspects of the self are not supported by the preaching of one's greater social body, one banishes and suppresses them into a "dark" unconscious corner of one's psyche and being.

One of the "goals" of yoga practice is to bring about a "union," and so it must avoid any type of fragmentation or rejection of any aspects of the self. Any form of practice or preaching which promotes rejection or mistrust of some aspects of the self cannot possibly contribute to the process of union through yoga. When yoga teachers and other types of social leaders preach, rather than teach, they contribute to this process of fragmentation of the self and deepening of the shadow. This is unfortunately common in yoga and spiritual communities of today. We frequently see practitioners and teachers presenting themselves as an embodiment of a certain set of ideals which are fundamentally in opposition or conflict with what they are actually experiencing (and repressing into the shadows) inside themselves. The result of this fragmentation is inauthenticity and it leads to intrapersonal breakdown and many of the dysfunctional interpersonal dimensions that we can observe in today's spiritual and yoga communities.

The importance of embodied, felt experience cannot be overemphasized in the process of authentically integrating and assimilating knowledge and understanding. A "truth" cannot be authentic unless we are actually feeling it in the body at the sensation-based phenomenological level; and doing so without giving preferential attention to certain feelings while rejecting other feelings. Embodiment means being aware of and immersed within everything that we feel at an organic, sensation-based level. Being embodied means BEING those sensations and feelings—not as an objective, disconnected observer, but as a subjective living, breathing and feeling experiencer.

One of the major fallacies of Buddhist practice is the assumption that it is possible for consciousness or awareness to remain objective and disconnected from the experience of sensation and feeling. Buddhist practice is often portrayed with the imagery of a battle, where objective awareness struggles to remain detached from the "enemy" of the subjective experience of volitional formations (*sankharas/samskaras*) around the field of the sensations and feelings of bodily experience. I have observed that many long-term Buddhist practitioners end up living a disembodied existence, with a deeply rooted—and sometimes carefully hidden—quality of self-loathing. The dualistic worldview of Buddhism—where the self paradoxically struggles to deny the reality of the self—ultimately produces a deeply fragmented and wounded sense of self.

Modern science falls into the same trap that Buddhism does, by working on the flawed premise of the possibility of objective, detached observation of the environment around us, without accepting that we are necessarily a subjective participant within a living, breathing, feeling environment. The result of this centuries-long experiment has been to propagate a struggle against more-than-human nature—rather than accepting that we ARE a subjective participant in the whole of nature—in the same way that the Buddhist struggles against his own volitional formations around his sensation and feeling based experience—rather than accepting that he IS a subjective part of his own sensations and experiences. The fragmented self-denial of the Buddhist is not unlike the broken relationship that we have with our dying planet, which we have created through our own deluded attempts to separate ourselves from being a part of the process of nature. Preaching—which asks one to deny one's own subjective, sensation-based experience—propagates this same process of fragmentation and disconnection from the truth and authenticity of the self.

Questions are sometimes raised about horrible atrocities, such as the mass genocides which have taken place throughout the (often ugly) history of our species. People often wonder how those who committed those atrocities could have done so. Even if they were "just following orders," how could they not have known what they were doing was wrong? How could they not have rejected the orders? The answer is that they stopped themselves from feeling. Only by cutting themselves off from being embodied and conscious in their deeper somatic feelings could they follow the orders—or preaching—of those commanding them. Interviews with those who have committed these types of crimes confirm this.

We are doing the same thing in our relationship with more-than-human world today. The murder and destruction of the living, breathing biosphere of the planet earth is no different from the horrific crimes that we have inflicted upon members of our own species. The preaching of our modern cultures, such as the primacy of economic growth at all costs, necessitates cutting ourselves off from the embodied experience of what it actually feels like to destroy and demolish everything around us as part of achieving that goal. For one who allows oneself to feel everything, the cries of pain of the embodied earth can be tangibly felt inside one's own body as one moves through the landscape of the human induced destruction of this living planet, and participating in this destruction becomes an impossibility.

The preachers of "green technology" and "sustainable growth" also fall into the dualistic trap of separation. For these people, the more-than-human biosphere is still perceived as an objective, lifeless object which is to be integrated into the structure of our current social paradigms. To place "economic value" on forests, species or ecosystems or to refer to anything as a "resource," does not help us to develop a connected, living, feeling embodied relationship with the more-than-human world. It is only through removing the dualistic separation of self and others, by subjectively feeling and participating in the embodied experience of the whole living earth, that true healing and union can take place.

Indigenous human societies (most of which are extinct now) cultivated intimate, feeling-based relationships with the more-than-human world around them. Those relationships were necessarily carried out at the embodied level of experience. Plundering and destroying the environment around them was unthinkable, because it would have felt as wrong as plundering or murdering their closest human relatives. If modern humans are to salvage a sustainable and respectable existence on this planet, we must reconnect to our own embodied feelings of aliveness and by extension of that, cultivate an embodied feeling based relationship with all that is around us. Only then, can we truly and authentically understand the nature of our lives and the appropriate ways to conduct ourselves within the network of relationships that constitutes the living system of this breathing planet.

Embodiment avoids the fragmentation of dualistic traps. Our sensations and feelings that we experience in the embodied state of aliveness are the closest thing to "truth" that we can access. When we accept all that we feel in our own embodied experience, there is nothing to reject, and an authentic process of true integration takes place. Embodied experience can only happen here and now, in the present moment. This is the place where our deepest form of intelligence—the embodied, organic animal intelligence—resides and this is the place that any teaching must be assimilated and integrated into, if it is to be fully processed into a living, breathing, authentic truth. When our knowledge and our actions are integrated at this level, we are the most whole that we can be. The true experience of union and the deepest understanding of any teaching can only happen in the subjective state of embodied aliveness.

When teaching the *yama* and *niyama* of Patanjali or the *panchasila* of Buddhism, I attempt to do so in a way that encourages empowered decision-making based on one's own internal experience. Most religious and spiritual teachings contain some form of a list of "dos and don'ts," and they are often preached as a list of commandments. Telling someone "not to kill" or "not to steal" seems reasonable enough, but if we do it in a way that promotes blind acceptance, without integration of that understanding at an embodied, feeling based level, then we still fall into the traps and dangers of preaching.

Interpretations of ethical teachings vary considerably and interpretations are necessarily rooted in the cultural conditioning of the interpreter. To avoid killing or violence, for example, seems simple enough on the surface, yet when we examine it more deeply, it becomes somewhat ambiguous. The process of being alive involves the consumption of other elements of the web of life. This necessarily means that we are involved in killing and violence on a daily basis. Is it acceptable to kill animals for food? What about plants? Or fungi? Is it okay to kill trees to use as building material for a home? What about to use as toilet paper? Should we kill bacteria that thrive on our soiled dishes and would make us sick if we consumed them and allowed them to proliferate inside our bodies? Where we draw the line to discern which forms of killing and violence are morally acceptable, and which are not, is somewhat arbitrary. Should we allow the preaching of a particular culture, scriptural interpretation or preacher dictate where this line is drawn for us? Or should we allow ourselves to be informed by our own internal sensation based intelligence in terms of which actions are appropriate or inappropriate?

The late ecophilosopher Arne Naess discussed a similar type of dilemma in his book, *The Ecology of Wisdom*. He described the situation of a person struggling with the ethics of an act which is perceived to be morally wrong in the context of his cultural conditioning. This person struggles deeply against his subjective feeling based intelligence, which wants to engage in the act. He ultimately wins the struggle and stops himself from engaging in the act. He then consoles himself that he can "sleep well at night" because he "did the right thing." But, did he really do the right thing, by suppressing some aspect of his own intuitive intelligence and wisdom so that he could remain in line with the moral preaching of his culture? Naess goes on to make a distinction between "acting ethically" and "acting beautifully." He defines "acting ethically" as shaping one's behavior to be in line with the ethical standards of one's culture, regardless of whether this honor and acknowledges the intelligence of one's embodied subjective experience. He defines "acting beautifully" as allowing one's own embodied feeling based intelligence to inform one's behavior, regardless of whether that behavior falls within the parameters of the ethical expectations of one's culture (I've paraphrased his definitions to fit into the context of this essay). The question then becomes: "Did you act ethically, and therefore preserve the preaching of your culture at the cost of repressing and denying the teaching of your own embodied intelligence? Or did you act beautifully, and follow the wisdom of your own embodied intelligence, regardless of whether you received the approval of your culture for doing so?"

Preaching prioritizes the dictates of a cultural or social entity over the subjective intelligence of the individual entity. Teaching prioritizes the subjective intelligence of the individual entity over the dictates of the cultural or social entity. Ideally, the two would be in balance, where the needs of an individual, as informed by his embodied sensation-based intelligence are somewhat consistent with the needs of his culture or social body. If there is excessive dissonance between the embodied intelligence of the individual and the standards of the social organization or culture, then it is likely a sign that the individual needs to bring about some bigger life changes in his interpersonal relationships, so that he can find a situation where the truth of his own intuitive sensation-based intelligence is more balanced with the standards and expectations of his culture or social body. In turn, the culture or social body can also attempt to harmonize their expectations and standards with those that are experienced at the feeling-based, embodied level of its individual members. If a culture or social organization can succeed in doing this, then it can be said to be teaching its members rather than preaching to them.

I attempt to teach *yama* and *niyama* as tools of embodiment. For me, they are not a set of rules to be preached or blindly followed, based on someone else's interpretation of how they apply to our personal life situations. In my interpretation, *yama* and *niyama* refer to potential situations in our ongoing relationships with our environment where we may need to bring more embodied awareness to how we feel inside, at the sensation-based level, when considering how we should conduct ourselves within those social relationships. Rather than preaching a black-and-white or right-or-wrong approach, I suggest a process of deeper sensitization and allowing one's felt experience to guide one's actions in the world. In this way, we take responsibility for our actions and relationships by continuously staying in touch with how we feel inside, and we use this embodied awareness as feedback for modifying our actions and relationships. How *yama* and *niyama* apply to our personal life situations is always going to be contextual, and we should be able to make our own decisions, informed by our subjective, embodied intelligence with confidence.

Ultimately, being taught will promote a union of the layers of the self, with the new knowledge consolidated and assimilated in the subjective intelligence at the embodied, feeling level of experience. This generates empowerment and wholeness of the self and leads to healthy and functional relationships with the world. Being preached to promotes fragmentation of the self through a rejection or repression of one's embodied, feeling-based experience. This leads to disempowerment of the self and propagates the dysfunctional social structures that rule human societies today.

WELLBEING ON THE EDGE

Learning from Mysore-style Ashtanga Yoga

— March 2019 —

The following piece is a transcript of a paper presented by Andy Davis, Associate Professor of Philosophy at Belmont University in Nashville, Tennessee, at the 25th national Asian Studies Development Program conference: "Wellbeing in Asian Traditions of Thought and Practice."

The paper is partially based on an interview that Andy conducted with me in November 2018 while he was participating in my Mysore-style classes and pranayama course.

*****

Introducing the Edge

The word "wellbeing" often suggests ease or comfort, a sense of pleasantness and satisfaction. But in my talk today, I would like to examine how a pursuit of wellbeing involves the seeming opposite, discomfort and struggle, due to wellbeing requiring intense work at the limit of one's current capability. I aim to articulate how wellbeing is linked with learning and learning with growth and growth with a certain amount of discomfort and challenge. To this end, I look at the "Mysore style" of teaching and learning from the Mysore-style Ashtanga yoga tradition to see how it supports this uncomfortable work. I then adapt some lessons from the Mysore room to a discussion of challenge and risk in the university classroom.

The general idea for this paper is inspired by some comments made by my yoga teacher, Iain Grysak. In an interview I conducted with him about teaching Mysore-style Ashtanga yoga, he remarked that, in his view, the teacher's primary task is to create an "energetic container" where students are "brought to their edge."[1] In context, this was offered as a contrast to the predominant expectation that a teacher's job is to provide physical adjustments for students.[2] Grysak takes a wider view of the learning process and the learning environment, suggesting that physical adjustment is only one of many ways that students can be "brought to their edge."

What does it mean, to be brought to one's edge? The "edge" is a term used in yoga circles to refer to the limit of a practitioner's physical ability. When I press up into a backbend and go up just about as far as I can without causing myself too much pain, I am working at my edge.

That seems simple enough. However, the same shape that brings me to my edge might be very easily accomplished by another student. He will need a deeper backbend, such as *Kapotasana*, to encounter his edge. This brings us to the crux of the problem of teaching yoga: every body has a different edge. Even the same body, on different days, will work at different edges. How does a student, a relative beginner, know when he has reached his edge? What does it feel like, and what level of discomfort or pain is acceptable? How much should I push myself in trying to get my body to take the shape of an upward-facing bow?

The yoga student, with good reason, goes to a yoga teacher for help

---

1. From an interview recorded on November 9, 2018.
2. An adjustment typically involves bringing the student's body more deeply into a particular posture (pressing the back into a deeper forward bend, helping the hands bind in a seated twist, etc.)

answering this question—that is, to someone with more experience and therefore expertise in working at the limits of the body's ability. However, the yoga teacher cannot inhabit the student's body. The yoga teacher has only external access to the limitations of the student's body. To feel something from the inside, as one's own, is meaningfully different. Even if the teacher has the skill to recognize the general nature of a limitation and also suspects what might address it, the teacher cannot do the work for the student. Being adjusted into a posture (with external pressure or support) will have important differences from pressing and supporting the body from within. This inconvenient truth underlies Grysak's concerns about teaching styles that are heavy on adjustments, and explains why physical adjustments are an imperfect tool for finding and working at a student's edge. Once a student develops some amount of bodily awareness, he will be better at sensing the contours of his personal edge.

If this is so, what use is a teacher at all? Here the rest of Grysak's suggestion comes into play. The teacher provides an "energetic container" for the student. The teacher offers a space, a room, a place, with conditions that are conducive to seriousness, attention to detail, moral support, focus, patience, calmness, and collective effort. The teacher's main work is intentional, but it is not a doing, but rather, an allowing and enabling. The student experiences the work of his practice as produced neither by himself alone nor by the teacher alone. Or rather, the work is his, but has been brought out and made possible by the learning environment and the relationships that constitute it.

An "energetic container" is created by a combination of elements that are numerous and subtle. These could include everything from the colors of the walls and the presence or absence of pictures of gurus or deities to the teacher's tone of voice, gestures and attire. We will later turn to see how this can be compared with a university classroom. The notion of creating an energetic container is applicable especially with teachers that emphasize their role as listeners rather than talkers, who view their work not as depositing packets of information, but as cultivating the student's own work at an analogous sort of edge, or rather, the edge broadly conceived.

For the edge, even in a yoga asana practice, is not just the limit of the body's ability to take a certain shape. It is also the limit of the practitioner's self-conception, the shape of his ego, the idea he has of who he is and what he can do. I may believe today that I can go further in my back-bending posture, I may be utterly convinced with righteous certainty that I can straighten my legs and arms and walk my hands closer to my feet, but today I find that I cannot. I encounter a limit of discomfort and exhaustion. How do I deal with this? Do I get frustrated and force my body further? Do I immediately back off without any exploration, content to do less than I know is possible? Or will I take interest in this limit as it presents itself and investigate it, looking for space around it? The character of the yoga practice is revealed in the way we negotiate this interaction between body and self-conception. Whether it has the character of a battle, or a friendly dialogue, a yoga practice is a constant encounter between sensation and imagination, between the body and the *idea of the body*.

Sensation and Imagination

Negotiating the encounter between sensation and imagination is essential not only to achieving bendy postures, but to our most fundamental capacities as animals. When an animal senses something (with eyes, ears, skin, etc.), the sensation is brought into relation with images of sensations that linger in the imagination, i.e., sensations from the near and distant past.[1] Take, for example, when something looks heavy. Here we are combining past tactile sensations of this object or similar objects with present visual sensations. In this way, a quality that is actually absent from sensation

---

1. "Image" here is a generic term for absent sensory elements made present and could include sound images, visual images, tactile images, etc.

(heaviness) is made present to the moment of sensation not through sensation but through the work of the imagination. Imagination completes or fills out the always-partial picture of sensation in countless ways. Much of the imagination's work is unconscious and seamlessly integrated with the work of the senses.

By making present otherwise absent elements of experience, the imagination helps an animal orient itself and move from place to place, seeking out what seems best.[1] By preserving and representing sensory images, the imagination gives the animal an intuitive understanding of the continuity of itself and of the world around it. Locomotion requires holding an action together in the imagination even as the body goes through the motion only one step at a time. The animal must believe, at each step, that even though it has not yet reached its goal, the goal remains ahead of it. Our wellbeing depends on how well we navigate these daily encounters between imagination and sensation, between memory and the present, between the various parts of a single motion, between one desire and another, between who we were, who we are and who we are becoming.

The imagination is sometimes misunderstood as a source of only fictitious notions or illusions that should always be replaced. Some yoga theorists, leaning on classical Indian sources, describe yoga practice as if it could leave the normal conditions of embodied human life behind, as if it *released* us from all imagined self-conceptions (*ahaṃkāra*) and all past habits (*samskaras*).[2] If humans are a special kind of spiritual being with an accidental animal body, then perhaps this makes sense. If, however, we grant that humans are animals through and through, then memory, imagination, desires and habits cannot be discarded or left behind. They must

---

1. It is for this reason that Aristotle reasons that all animals with the capacity for locomotion must have an imagination/ memory/ desire, while plants and stationary animals (e.g., corals) may have "pure" sensation without imagination, memory and desire. See Aristotle, *On the Soul* Book III, Chapters 9–11.

2. *Bhagavad Gita* 3.27 and *Yoga Sutras* 2.15-17 are example texts that might be used to support this problematic view (but need not be interpreted in this way).

be trained or educated. This indicates to me that meditative absorption is likely not a sudden lightning flash where the material shell is discarded but rather the cumulative result of years of re-patterning the relationship between sensation and imagination to better reflect the way things are.

For the most part, sensation and imagination integrate well. As long as the experience of navigating our world seems to be going smoothly, our retained images have no reason to restructure in relation to incoming sensation. Yet if we are striving for change in our lives, we must change from the root and begin to *sense* the world differently so that we can desire differently.[1] This seems difficult to accomplish because no amount of thinking about it will change the pleasant taste of unhealthy foods or other misleading sensations and the memories around them. If, however, we bring ourselves to an edge, a limit, even a kind of crisis of perception, we will no longer rely on retained images and we begin to acquire new sensations to become part of the imagination's repertoire. This is one reason why it is easier to change habits in unfamiliar settings. At the edge, we draft a new relationship between sensations and the images that attend them and fill them out. It is not uncommon for hard-working yoga practitioners to suddenly alter diet, sleep, hygiene or other habits without exerting any effort or "willpower" merely as a consequence of increased attention to their edge.

Therefore, finding and working at the edge of one's current capabilities is not just for adrenaline junkies, but for all of us. Further, the ability to work at the edge is a revealing definition of wellbeing. To live a healthy life, a person must be ready to respond to the environment, ready to pursue or avoid what it is best to pursue or avoid. If we do not attend to fresh aspects of incoming sensation, if we do not accept what is unexpected or even contrary to expectation, then experience becomes routine, blunted,

---

1. Aristotle implies something like this in *Nicomachean Ethics* Book VII, Chapter 3 (1147a25-1147b5).

and unintelligent. If we only work with imagination and memories, then the idea of the body becomes a fantasy, abstract and divorced from lived experience. A person may imagine that he can still run or jump as he did ten years ago, even while struggling to get up from a desk chair. Or he may imagine that he is incapable of getting up from the chair without pain, when, with practice, his body is capable of much more. Because Mysore-style Ashtanga yoga is a strenuous, six-day-per-week practice, the attentive Ashtanga student constantly refreshes his own self-conception and lives as what he is: a growing, changing animal.

Without daily meditative movement at the edge, a person lives with an outdated idea of his own body. And without an analogous kind of attentive, consistent study and inquiry, a person works with an outdated idea of his own self. The Mysore style of yoga teaching cultivates work at the edge in a powerful yet sustainable way. By reflecting on the features that make this learning environment effective, we can offer parallel suggestions for other learning environments.

Mysore-Style Ashtanga

Mysore-style Ashtanga yoga is the name used to describe the tradition of yoga practice transmitted by K. Pattabhi Jois.[1] It is so named because it was developed in the city of Mysore (now Mysuru) in Karnataka, India. Ashtanga yoga has a few distinctive features worth noting up front. First, the Ashtanga practice is a set sequence of postures (or *asanas*) performed in the same order each time. Second, the postures are interconnected by moving transitions (or *vinyasas*). Third, in each posture the practitioner is to pay close attention to the movement of the breath, the placement of internal energy (or *bandha*) and the location of the gaze (or *drishti*).

---

1. The published text outlining Jois's method is his *Yoga Mala*. The method seems to be based on the method of Jois's own teacher, T. Krishnamacharya, as he taught it to Jois in the 1930s and '40s (see Singleton, Yoga Body, p. 176). Krishnamacharya went on to teach in different ways (see Desikachar, *The Heart of Yoga* pp. 28–29).

Finally, the Ashtanga practice should be practiced every day except Saturdays, full moons and new moons. Taken together, these guidelines help to ensure that Mysore-style Ashtanga yoga is a demanding yet meditative asana practice.

Mysore-style classes look quite different from other yoga classes. In the Mysore style, each student practices independently at his or her own pace and skill level, watched over by a teacher who has mastered the series of poses. One student may practice Primary series, another may practice only half of Primary series, and another may practice Intermediate series, all in a row next to one another. The different series (Primary, Intermediate, Advanced) are fixed, and poses are given sequentially as the student achieves a certain level of competence in the previous pose. An individual practice usually lasts from one to two hours.

While students practice in the Mysore style, a teacher circles through the room watching them to see if they would benefit from brief verbal reminders about the placement of parts of the body or from hands-on physical adjustments. As noted earlier, Iain Grysak suggests that physical adjustments should be minimal. He writes that a skilled teacher will "give [students] the minimum amount of input necessary for them to understand where they should be going, and then leave it up to them to work it out for themselves." Grysak concludes that "[t]his approach produces the strongest, most stable and most integrated result in the students, and it gives the students greater strength, confidence and power in the long run."[1] This pedagogy takes the independent streak inherent in the Mysore style and amplifies it. Following this model, the teacher will tend to adjust only when a certain action is very difficult to engage without help (such as dropping back from standing into a backbend).

What stands out in the Mysore style of teaching is the combination of set structure and independence or freedom. Because the sequence of poses

---

1. See chapter 1, "You Stop There." on p. 23.

is fixed, the student can show up and practice without being told what to do by the teacher. In non-Mysore yoga classes, the sequence is invented by the instructor and is not known in advance by the student, making the student dependent upon the teacher for sequencing. In this way, the Mysore method defers a portion of authority from the teacher to the sequence itself. A student works not to follow the instructions of a teacher, nor to discover the intended insight that the teacher has in mind, but to deepen the practice of the already available sequence, sometimes with a teacher's hands-on help, but often without it.

Bringing Out the Edge

The Mysore method offers several distinct advantages for the student who wants to find and work at their own edge.

Practicing the same sequences every day offers significant benefits. From the time of birth, a human body begins to be shaped by the repetitive motions demanded of it. From the way standing and walking bring structure to the developing spine of a toddler, to the way hunching over a cellphone causes the shoulders and head of an adult to slouch forward, to the way smiles or frowns develop wrinkles on our faces, repeated motions give us our shapes. And repetition, having shaped the body, is likely the best way to reshape it. Imagine how many backbends it takes to reverse the effects of twenty years (and counting) spent hunching over philosophy books.

Further, repeated motion provides a constant against which the student can measure deviations and changes. By paying attention to sensations in the practice from day to day, the student learns how to distinguish subtle differences in himself. If the practice were different every time, it would be that much more difficult to identify patterns or changes in the sensations. The repeated sequence effectively facilitates the observed experience of the body. It provides ample opportunity for the practitioner to become skilled at self-observation, a necessary prerequisite for self-teaching.

Another advantage of the Mysore method results from its concreteness, or the lack of abstract conceptualization in its instructions. In the Mysore room, verbal cues are minimal and concern gross actions. Little instruction is offered on how to achieve "perfection" in a posture, and few external standards of symmetry or geometry are applied to the poses. Such external standards impose a normative, imaginary ideal on the shape of the body. If a yoga practitioner follows the instruction of a zealous teacher, he may achieve a specific goal. But he may also lose sensitivity in his practice, overstretch the body's tissues, and cause damage. It is easy to push towards an imaginary ideal, based on a description from a teacher, ignoring the cues of one's own body. No other person can feel the sensations of the practitioner's body, and so no one can effectively specify where the right balance of tension and relaxation will be found. The more we favor someone else's description, the harder it becomes to follow our own sensations, and the more apt we are to cause ourselves harm.[1]

Ashtanga teaching does, however, instruct the breath. The vinyasa sequence is designed to pair with inhalations and exhalations. On inhalation, the practitioner moves into one posture (usually involving spinal extension) and on exhalation he moves into the next posture (usually involving spinal flexion). In the Mysore room, the practitioner is able to move the body freely with the breath, because he is able to work at his own pace. When he arrives at a held pose, which is usually held for five breaths, he has already forged a link between the motion of the body and the motion of the breath. This means that even a pose that looks motionless on the outside will continue to move, just as the vinyasa moved, but on a deeper, more subtle level.[2] Inhalation might accompany a sensation of lengthening, expanding, or releasing, while exhalation might accompany a sensation

---

1. See chapter "Teaching vs. Preaching: Embodiment as the Gateway to Authentic Understanding and Integration" on p. 209.
2. This insight is based on comments made by Iain Grysak in a Pranayama Workshop held in November 2018.

of stabilizing, containment, or deepening. The cycle of breathing shapes the posture bit by bit, finding new space within the body. Here, it is the breath that begins to work at the practitioner's edge, and the breath that seeks out new territory in the practice. Breathing is a deeply original self-motion, so much that it seems to make a bridge between our conscious actions and our unconscious biological processes. We both do and do not control our own breathing, in the same way that we do and do not control our own being alive. In the Ashtanga practice, breath becomes the pioneer, the explorer of the edge, while the gross physical body—and the practitioner—follows.

Breathing is also closely connected to the function of the nervous system. Close work with the breath results in better awareness of the nervous system and the states of excitation and relaxation that emerge from its work. The breath thus forges a link between the imagined body and the actual sensations of the body. The practitioner's idea of the body is distorted by habitual over- and under-stimulation. An overexcited nervous system is likely to under-react to sensory stimulus and a lethargic nervous system is likely to overreact. If, using the breath, a practitioner can even out the stimulation of the nervous system, he can open up a new attitude towards sensation in the present moment, one that is not pulled towards anxious or depressive responses.

It is a difficult task to learn to breathe smoothly and without forceful exertion while putting the body through strenuous athletic motions. But it is learnable. The body gains cardiovascular endurance, and the practitioner learns not to panic and gulp for air, even if a pose feels uncomfortable or seems impossible. By learning to breathe slowly and smoothly through the course of a challenging sequence, the practitioner learns to maintain a calm and focused presence of mind. This, in turn, enables a clear evaluation of the body's sensations, influenced neither by fear nor by ambition. In this way, attention to the breath helps one see through all the distractions, the messy emotions and social cues, so that one might know best when and where to stop.

Another advantage of the Mysore method is in the one-on-one teacher-student interactions. Typical yoga classes involve instructions given to all students, at the same time and in the same way, despite the fact that every student has a different body. In the Mysore room, every teacher-student interaction is one-on-one. This means they may take place as a concrete communication referring to a given body at a present moment, with immediate relevance and applicability. There is virtually no theory in it. The adjustment or instruction from the teacher serves as a reminder rather than a transmission of knowledge. When a teacher touches the body lightly or issues a simple correction, the student is given the opportunity to realize that their attention has lapsed and he has forgotten to hold the body together in the posture. Diffuse attention leads to a scattered way of holding the body. This is often a clear reminder that the idea of the body and the sensation of the body have diverged. This is also a sign that we hold ourselves in a careless way outside of the practice as well. Repeatedly addressing these attention lapses day by day gradually reduces such lapses and increases focus.

When focus is present, sensation and imagination work together at the crest of arising experience. The focused practitioner holds each moment of sensation in relation not to an abstract standard (imagination gone lifeless and dull), but to the relevant whole of a single arc of activity or motion (imagination alive and in the moment). Focus thus tends to arise most clearly at the edge, at the limit of capability, because it is here that each arising sensation bears the most significance. It is here that each decision has meaningful consequences the practitioner may observe immediately within or soon after the practice. At the edge, a practitioner can follow arising sensation towards evolving self-understanding.

Over time, a practitioner might notice attention constantly fleeing from certain areas or actions of the body. Through repeated actions and interventions, the practitioner begins to track his dark zones and blind spots, all the places in himself that he habitually avoid. In the practice, the practitioner may discover a map of habits, and in these habits, a map of choices and values. These are not the values we articulate to ourselves and to others, the stories we tell about ourselves, but the values we enact on a daily basis. I may tell myself that I am not stressed out, that I am kind and compassionate towards myself and others, or that I do not harbor deep and unspoken angers and fears; but my body tells a different story.

Discomfort and Wellbeing

Daily Mysore-style Ashtanga yoga is an intense practice and makes consistent, systemic demands on the body. As the body begins to restructure to better support itself in the practice, the practitioner experiences regular soreness, pain and occasional strains that belong to this process and can be considered good signs rather than warnings or reasons to abandon the practice. These discomforts often indicate that the student is in fact working at the edge of current limitations and cultivating a new relationship of the body to itself.

It often seems taken for granted that the point of practicing yoga is to feel good. Yoga is popularly presented as an exercise that is balancing, centering and calming. It may be more accurate to say that the point of a yoga asana practice is not to feel good, but to feel more deeply — not to feel *better*, but to *feel* better. If there is pain, anger, tension, doubt, pride, shame, strength, stability, softness, balance, anxiety, depression or uneasiness in the practitioner, asana practice is a powerful way to become sensitive to these deep stirrings of body and soul. This is necessarily a difficult path. Nobody finds it easy. Often, what the yoga practice reveals will be encountered with frustration, despair, fear, or just plain confusion. The practice is, after all, a daily encounter with one's limits, a daily attempt to make headway into what seems—what feels—impossible. If it becomes a transformative practice, this means that it involves losing one's past self. Dying to oneself, even if it prefaces rebirth, is never pleasant, never easy. Nevertheless, it is better to know oneself than to remain blind to psychophysical habits.

It is hard to find as reliable a daily measure of embodied experience as an Ashtanga yoga practice, which is both consistent and consistently diverse in its demands. Without the clarifying light of such a practice, we are likely to feel our body-souls as mediated through shifting moods and ideas or images that have no embodied reality. Human beings act in strange ways. We will claim that everything is okay, until one day we erupt, like a volcano, from a deep swell of anger. Or we will claim that we love a partner, until one day we realize that we haven't shared our true selves with them in decades. We will do things because they are socially acceptable, without acknowledging how they trouble us to the core. We will choose what is familiar over what could lead to our own happiness. Without some kind of practice that teaches the practitioner to navigate the boundaries of potential, and to do so as a self-directed, self-sensing activity, we become helpless in the face of our unknown selves. We remain unprepared for our feelings and unequipped to respond well to them.

With such a daily practice, however, one conducts a daily survey of what it is like to be living in one's body on that particular day. One has confronted negative feelings about oneself and areas of stiffness and tension. One has taken the time and effort to practice observing oneself, being sensitive to one's limits, and persevering in the face of discomfort. This increased awareness can be carried from the practice into the rest of the day. It is difficult to assess the value of yoga practice for personal change and wellbeing because so much depends on what the student does with what he discovers in himself during practice. But the more self-directed and self-applied the practice is, the more likely it is to instill the habit of self-reflection.

It is never a solipsistic practice, however. In the Mysore room, one's practice is both self-directed, and also observed by a teacher, making it not only an incubator for insights, but also a reminder to apply those insights diligently. When teachers simply talk, students miss out on discovering insights for themselves. They become disengaged, bored, or dutiful in an instrumental way. When students work without teachers at all, they often lack the motivation or capacity for discipline and consistency. The stakes may not feel high enough, the situation does not seem pressing, one feels sore and stiff, and one's trust in the practice wavers. One is apt to postpone one's work to the next day, or the next.

This brings us to the problem of pain. Pains, from minor discomforts, to aching limbs, to chronic strains, to tissue tears, present an obstacle and a puzzle to the most perceptive of students. Animals naturally withdraw from pain. This is a healthy response that generally leads to wellbeing, as it assists in survival. However, just as the avoidance of pain can be detrimental in the pursuit of self-knowledge, it can be detrimental in the pursuit of wellbeing. Someone with experience is sometimes needed to remind us that staying with a pain can be good. Pain is not always a signal of harm, even if we are apt to interpret it as such. While, on the one hand, I must let my body be my teacher, on the other hand, bodies have their own prejudices. A good teacher, who has endured the pains and discomforts himself, helps to mediate the body's work when bodily distress prevents us from recognizing things as they are.

Learning at the Edge

From this look at Mysore-style teaching and practice, a few general conclusions arise. A learning environment should help students find their own personal edge and not an abstract target designated in advance by the teacher. To support this, the learning environment should cultivate consistency, challenge, introspection and independence.

I would argue that these qualities can be applied to liberal arts courses in modern universities to help bring students to the edge of their current capabilities. A class discussion or seminar can potentially offer a flexible learning environment where students can engage fruitfully with varying levels of competence. Unlike an interactive lecture, which rewards only those students who approach the content in a way similar to the professor, a seminar discussion can make space for divergent approaches. In a good discussion, each participant can test the differing limits of their own competence as a reader, thinker and speaker at the same time.

As in the Mysore room, a consistent learning environment should allow students to prepare properly. Continual change at the whim of the teacher invites students to stop preparing for class because it is unclear what preparation is worthwhile. Inconsistency or unpredictability causes students to feel at the mercy of the teacher, and as though they have no personal grasp on the trajectory of their learning. At the same time, the teacher should be prepared to provide diverse challenges to students. If the teacher seems easy to impress or content with a rehearsal of what is obvious—or worse, a rehearsal of what the teacher wants to hear—students are not invited to try for more. To promote introspection, a seminar group should acclimate itself to silence. If the teacher seems anxious or creates the expectation that silences should be filled, there is no space to think in the classroom. The class becomes a place to rehearse ideas rather than a place to discover or test them. Finally, independence can arise in a classroom when it is clear that the teacher does not have an agenda that must be followed. When students begin to see that their decisions and contributions have consequences on the quality of the conversation each day, personal responsibility and independence are cultivated.

While this is all somewhat formulaic, it may help us work past some prevalent assumptions. Yoga pedagogy and liberal arts pedagogy are both dominated by instructional models that treat education as a transmission of information from teacher to student rather than as a catalyst for genuine self-exploration in pursuit of holistic wellbeing. When students learn, they do not learn the subject matter in abstraction, but in concrete relation to what they already know and believe. This means that the student is in a better position to know how to integrate the subject into his own particular body and soul than the teacher. The teacher may be more expert on this technique or that book, but not at the technique in relation to my body or the book in relation to my soul.

Working at the edge demands, above all, that we—as teachers and students—be willing to endure confusion. As we push to the limits of the familiar, we are bound to become disoriented. Thus education at the edge requires trust. A student must be willing to go backwards (or what seems to be backwards), believing the path will eventually lead forwards again. The teacher must also be willing to go backwards, to accompany the student as he works through his edge, and to show by example that disorientation does not warrant despair. In Ashtanga yoga pedagogy, nothing encapsulates this need for trust better than when a teacher stops a student at a pose the student himself believes he has mastered. With time, the student may come to see the value in being set back, when it helps him rediscover his edge in a place he had stopped looking for it. Likewise, seminars abound with conversational tangents that seem to lead nowhere. But then, if pursued with a collective trust and sensitivity to the unknown, such tangents can turn up insights in places we would never have thought to look.

Both approaches are rooted in the belief that real insight transcends a person's ability to encapsulate and represent things to himself in advance. Seeking wellbeing at the edge is a matter of remaining open, loosening the ego's grasp on the self and making space for an unexpected self, an emergent self. If we seek wellbeing in this way, the self is no longer a detached image or a static representation, no longer a fantasy we have of who we are. The self becomes the work of the self.[1] In this work, there is no distinction between the body and its life, no distinction between the self and its wellbeing.

Note: I would like to thank Iain Grysak for his essays and for his energetic container, "Spacious Yoga" in Ubud, Bali. I would also like to thank Elizabeth Hejtmancik for her helpful suggestions and extensive revisions to this essay.

Andy Davis
Associate Professor of Philosophy
Belmont University

---

1. The insight that to-be-something is not a passive inheritance but an active doing can be explored in Aristotle's *Physics and Metaphysics*, especially *Metaphysics Theta* (i.e., Book IX). Two recent, helpful interpretations of these arguments are Aryeh Kosman's *The Activity of Being* and Jonathan Beere's *Doing and Being*.

THE TREE OF BANDHA

*Moving in embodied relationship
with the Earth*

— June 2019 —

WHEN I INTRODUCE THE SUBJECTS of breath and *bandha* in my immersion and pranayama courses, I begin with a description of three different layers of internal feeling and experience to which we can attend and move from during practice. These three layers of our experience of posture and movement are body, breath and *bandha*. These layers are functionally intertwined and inseparable in their roles within the experience of the whole organism, so rather than thinking of them as separate "things," I prefer to frame them as different perspectives or lenses from which we can view the whole of our experience of posture and movement.

We can consider different asanas and movement patterns as dynamic "forms" which we attempt to mold ourselves into. Backward bending, forward bending, twisting, inverted postures, etc., all have different types of shape or form. When a beginner to movement practice first attempts to perform asanas, he instinctively attempts to copy the forms that he sees with the form of his own body. For someone with little experience in consciously embodied movement, this layer of external form is the main layer of awareness from which he instinctively attempts to perform asanas. The external shape or form of the asana could be considered as the most superficial layer from which we can practice.

If we compare an asana to a building, this superficial layer is analogous to the shape and form of the building—whether it is low and flat like a strip mall, high and narrow like a tower, or elongated and curved like an arched bridge, etc. We can also note details such as whether the surface of the building is made of wood, concrete, metal, etc.

The asanas of a beginner can tend to look sloppy and unrefined when compared to those of an experienced practitioner. The beginners' posture may resemble the general form of a particular asana; however he may also appear (and feel) strained and lacking in the fundamental qualities of stability and ease—or *sukha* and *sthira*—which an experienced practitioner of the same asana often exhibits. The beginner will also lack alignment, stamina and resilience. He may fatigue quickly and be unable to incorporate even minor adjustments in form without losing his balance and toppling over.

In contrast, the asanas of an experienced practitioner will hold the same general form as the asanas of the beginner, but he will exhibit (and feel) the added qualities of alignment, stability and ease. An adept practitioner will be able to sustain a longer practice or hold particular asanas for longer periods of time without excessively tiring. He will also have the resilience to change certain features and details of the posture if he is asked to, without losing the fundamental essence of the posture. The postures of the adept practitioner will look and feel "aligned, relaxed and resilient," as Rolfer Will Johnson describes in his book of the same title.

How does the progression from the unstable and strained forms of the beginner to the aligned, relaxed and resilient forms of the experienced and adept practitioner occur?

When a beginner applies the techniques of Ashtanga practice on a regular basis—especially the vinyasa system of moving body and breath in a coordinated and concentrated flow—he will eventually begin to experience the asanas from a deeper layer within himself than the external shape and form of the postures and movements. Over time, he may begin to feel as if there is something that is supporting these external forms and movements of his body from a deeper place inside himself. He may begin to reduce emphasis on applying instructions and directions which originate from the outside intellect to the form of his body, and he may start to give precedence to an intuitive and embodied intelligence which guides and moves his body from the inside.

Some experienced practitioners say that this internal force or intelligence is the breath, and that at a certain stage of maturity in Ashtanga practice, the breath becomes the primary force in shaping and moving the body through the postures and vinyasas of the practice. There is certainly some validity in this statement, and the breath is the second layer from which we can perform and experience the asanas and vinyasas. The layer of breath is deeper and subtler than the superficial layer of external shape and form. For an experienced practitioner, the sound and sensation of the continuous flow of elongated, smooth and deep breath can pull him deeper inside himself and it becomes the most prominent feature of his embodied experience of the Ashtanga practice. At this stage in practice maturity, the superficial structural layers of the form of flesh and bone become more of an adjunct to the experience of the form of the breath.

An important discovery that some practitioners make at this layer of experience is that the breath does indeed have a shape and form to it, just as the external body has a shape and form to it. One important feature of the internal form of the breath is that when correctly applied, it remains relatively constant regardless of the variety of different external forms (such as backward bends, forward bends, twists, inverted postures, standing postures, supine postures) that the body can take in the practice. That is to say, regardless of the variation in external form of the body in the practice, the internal form of the breath should remain within one basic pattern. I call this form "the tree of breath," and will return to it later.

Returning to our analogy of a building or structure, we can think of the layer of breath as the infrastructural elements, such as the main posts and beams, which support the external structure and form of a building. The infrastructure is usually not obviously visible in a finished building, but beneath the external layers, it is what supports and holds the entire building up.

We can continue to probe deeper into the forces which support and move us in the practice. Just as the internal form and movement of the breath support the external form and movement of the body, some practitioners eventually discover that there is an even deeper layer which supports the form and movement of the breath. I call this the layer of *bandha*, and it is the deepest and subtlest layer from which we can experience and perform the forms and movement patterns of asanas and vinyasas.

In this particular context, I define *bandha* as the energetic dimension of our relationship with our environment. This vague and abstract definition will become clearer if we return to our analogy of a building: The effectiveness of the infrastructure of a building in supporting the form of the structure is highly dependent on how the infrastructure is arranged in relationship to the field of gravity and to the terrain of the earth that it is built upon. The way the structure of the building will relate to the earth below it and the space around it is the most important consideration to take into account when planning the construction of the building. I don't know very much about architectural design, but as far as I understand, the features of the environment which the building is to be built within and how the building will relate to these features are the foundations of everything that comes afterwards in the planning process. A building which works with gravity in a constructive way will be strong and stable and more likely to withstand any kind of disturbance that it might encounter during its lifespan with minimal damage. An arched bridge that is built with effective distribution of natural forces from its center will be a bridge that is safe and stable to travel upon for many years.

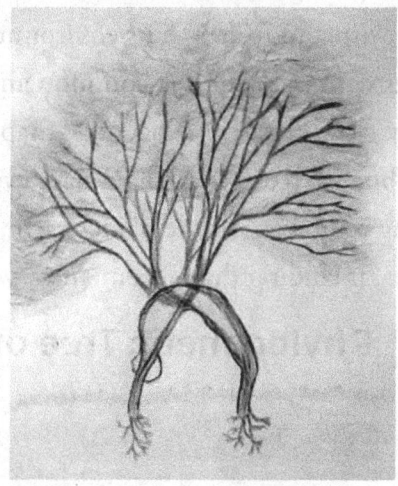

Urdhva Danurasana by Allen Enrique

Bandha is the energetic patterning which manifests in the way we move in relation to the earth below us and the space around us. This energetic movement occurs in both static asanas as well as dynamic movements of the body. When we practice in a state of embodiment and tangibly work with our relationship to the environment around us, *bandha* can be intuitively understood, and becomes the root and foundation of our entire practice experience. As embodied beings who are functionally and physiologically intertwined within—and inseparable from—the planet earth, this energetic relationship between self and environment is occurring every moment that we are alive. Formal practice is a place and space within which we can refine and cultivate the intricacies of that relationship to its maximum potential for harmonious exchange, but the actual relationship of energetic exchange between self and earth does not stop when formal practice stops. This fact can shed some light on K. Pattabhi Jois's famous statement that *mula bandha* should be applied 24 hours a day.

The energetic form of *bandha* in our postures and movements can also be understood by examining how it manifests in trees. We tend to think of trees as static entities, but a significant amount of movement takes place as a tree communicates with and relates to its environment. We share more than half of our genes with trees and the common ancestor that we share with trees is relatively close on the phylogenetic map of life, as shown in the diagram below. Though trees and humans have evolved some very different ways of relating to gravity on the planet earth, we also share some fundamental qualities, including the movement of *bandha*.

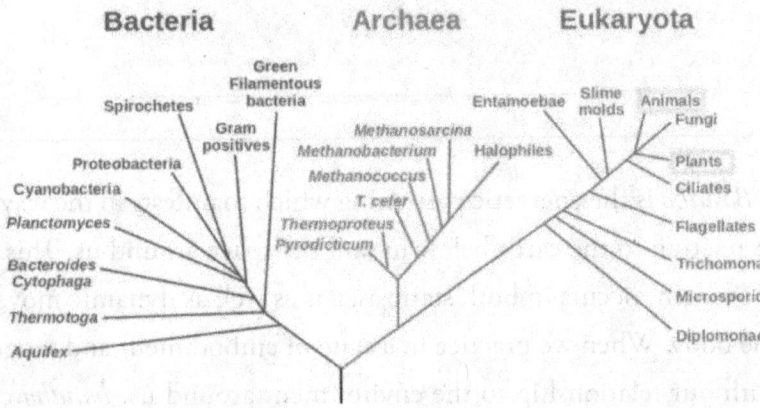

In order to see all of the movement patterns that a tree engages in, we would need to view it in time lapse, and also be able to see what is happening underneath the earth. We would also need to be able to see the chemical signals that trees exchange with one another and with animals and other forms of life. Trees form vast interconnected networks with their roots through underground fungal filament networks, which some modern ecologists have likened to the dendritic connections that are made between neurons in a mammalian brain. Trees also communicate with their peers, and with other life forms, by absorbing and releasing chemical signals through their leaves. This has led some ecologists to suggest that trees behave less like individual entities, and more like nodes in a vastly interconnected forest and planetary network. Trees are more like cells which contribute to the health and functionality of a whole forest organism, and their behavior can be more appropriately understood when viewed from this perspective. Humans, as a part of the web of life, also have this degree of connectivity with our environment. Unfortunately, centuries of the Cartesian legacy of the illusion of separateness has led us to repress and ignore this fundamental aspect of human nature. *Bandha* can only be effectively understood and felt if we allow ourselves to drop into embodied sensitivity and to feel and move as if we are connected to and communicating with our environment as participants within a network of relationships within a greater whole.

The fundamental movement of *bandha* is a co-engaging of two complementary or opposite qualities or movement patterns. In the present context, we can discuss the complementary forces of dropping downwards into the earth, and of lifting upwards and expanding outwards, away from the earth.

The rooting force of dropping downwards into the ground is the part of the movement of the tree that we cannot see with our eyes. The germination of a seed actually begins with the sprouting and downwards movement of the root. The stalk which grows upwards towards the light and air doesn't appear until after the root of the seed has already established itself. For a tree to have any degree of stability and reach its potential to expand and grow upwards and outwards, it must have space to grow downwards, penetrating ever more deeply into the earth. A tree which is kept in a pot or in a confined space where its roots have nowhere to grow, will never reach its potential to fully mature in its upwards and outwards expansion. A tree's roots are powerful. The movement of the roots happens slowly, relative to our perception, but this movement is epic in deep time. The roots of trees can eventually crack and destroy rocks, concrete foundations of buildings, roads, and other structures which are located a surprising distance from the actual trunk of the tree. If all the humans on the planet earth died today, it is the roots of the trees which would immediately begin to spread and proliferate that would reduce all of the concrete structures of our civilizations to rubble within a few decades. These deep and powerful underground movements give trees the strength, stability and longevity that they are known for, and as previously mentioned this is also where the trees become physically connected with one another through their fungal "synapses."

Humans also have the capacity to move downwards into the earth. Any action that a human wishes to perform will be executed more effectively and efficiently if the part of the body that is touching the ground first reaffirms and deepens its downwards movement into the ground prior to attempting to engage the actual lifting, pushing, pulling, or whatever the intended action is. Imagine you are standing beside a large boulder and wish to push it. You place your hands on the boulder, but before you start to push with the strength of your arms, you instinctively step back a little bit, bend your knees, and then you anchor yourself and press downwards into the earth with your feet. The earth responds to your gesture, and a reactionary force comes back up out of the earth, ripples through your entire body and you harness this force that is given to you from the earth and channel it through your arms and hands as you begin to push against the boulder. Imagine how much less effective your efforts to move the boulder would be if you didn't make these initial rooting connections to the earth through your legs and feet. This rooting action, and the subsequent channeling and harnessing of the complementary gesture from the earth is the essence of *bandha*: *Bandha* cannot be understood in this example without considering it as a function of our relationship to both the earth and the boulder.

Humans can also increase their sensitivity and connection to the rest of the web of life through the earth, just as trees do. Carl Jung is famous for having said: "It is quite possible that India is the real world, and that the white man lives in a madhouse of abstractions... Life in India has not yet withdrawn into the capsule of the head... It is still the whole body that lives. No wonder the European feels dreamlike: the complete life of India is something of which he merely dreams. When you walk with naked feet, how can you ever forget the earth?" I feel it is necessary to insert the caveat that this statement may have been true in Jung's time, or in his idealized vision of the Indian culture. In my own experience, modern India is as much of an abstracted madhouse as the West. My reason for sharing the quote is that, irrespective of culture or geographic location, engaging with the ground through bare feet, in an embodied state of perceptive awareness, is the only way to actually feel our connection to the earth and to the rest of the web of life. Without this embodied feeling, there can be no connection. Modern scientific discoveries and ecological movements which emphasize the interconnectedness of all of life on the planet earth are important, but unless we cultivate the ability to feel these connections with our living breathing body, as animist cultures have always done, then there is no possibility of authentically feeling our relationship to the rest of life, and no possibility of feeling *bandha*. I once watched a world-famous and celebrated ecologist speak at a public event. This man understands the nature of the web of life on planet earth as well as any other living human does—at an intellectual level. He has undoubtedly done very important work for the world and for encouraging humanity to understand our appropriate place in the world. Yet, when I watched him speak, as a yoga instructor I watched his body. His body was full of tension and was not connected to the ground beneath him at all. There was no *bandha* in his lived experience of the earth—at least while he was giving a public lecture.

Most modern humans are unaware of the extent of the loss of communicative skills that has occurred through our trajectory of disconnection from the earth over the last few millennia. The abstract technological universe, within which we communicate solely with other humans, has severed most of our reciprocal perceptual exchange with the more-than-human world. Though we are not able to escape our interdependence with the more-than-human earth, we operate under the illusion that we have done so, resulting in a great void and a profound lack of deeper meaning in life, not to mention the very real possibility of the collapse of all of the earth's living systems, including our own human civilizations. The few remaining extant societies of indigenous humans have spoken about the ease and regularity with which they communicate with plants, other animals, dead ancestors, etc. Modern humans tend to disregard these tales as myths from a primitive and uniformed worldview, but for those who cultivate embodied sensitivity, the richness of the network of reciprocal perceptual exchange that is possible between the human and the more-than-human becomes apparent. To perceptually inhabit these pathways of exchange is a fundamental element in experiencing the essence of human nature.

Elephants are known to communicate with each other through seismic vibrations that are picked up through their feet. I recall reading about a study which found that elephants emit low frequency vocalizations, which other elephants can receive vibrationally through sensitive receptors in their feet—up to 10 km away! If such a massive and hulking animal can be capable of such sensitivity, there is little doubt that human beings can also be this sensitive, and that our ancestral human forest dwellers also communicated with their environment through their feet.

I attempt to keep my feet open to earth as much as possible. Living in a warm climate, it is natural to keep my feet bare and free of any footwear for most of the day. The only time I put on shoes is when I walk or drive outside. A few years ago, I began to wear Vibram barefoot shoes, which allow one to retain a surprisingly large amount of tactile sensitivity with the ground. Once I became used to wearing this type of shoe, I found it very difficult to return to using regular soled shoes as the degree of tactile communication with the ground that is lost with conventional shoes becomes very apparent. Now, the only time I wear conventional shoes is when it is too cold for barefoot shoes, or if I am hiking with a backpack that weighs more than 10–15 kg. I've even considered attempting my next trekking expedition with a backpack in barefoot shoes. I've climbed all of the highest mountains of Bali in barefoot shoes, as well walked through numerous other challenging terrains. Why? Because I prefer to experience the connection of *bandha* as often as possible.

My first yoga instructor was an Iyengar teacher. He gave extremely effective training in the rooting foundation of posture, without ever using the term "bandha." A good portion of the 3–4 hour classes were spent doing standing postures on thinly carpeted flooring without the use of sticky mats. Perhaps 50 times per class my teacher would emphatically tell us to "pound your heels into the ground." And so, we learned how to connect to the ground with our feet. I spent over a year learning intensively with this teacher, and the instinctive ability to initiate all movements and forms of my body by pressing myself into the ground is something I have never lost. I've done my full Ashtanga practice without a sticky mat numerous times, as I have little need to use the sticky mat for traction. The main purpose of the mat is to provide some padding for rolling movements or movements where more sensitive parts of the body would become bruised by pressing hard against the ground. I had no idea that I was learning *bandha* in those early days of my practice. When I asked my teacher about the concept of *bandha*, he would smile and tell me, "It's happening, you just don't know it yet." *Bandha* begins with embodied movement into, and communication and exchange with, the earth beneath us.

The complementary force in the tree-shaped energetic patterning of *bandha* is upward lifting and outward spreading. This movement arises as a response to the downwards rooting force. We can think of it as the feedback that the earth gives to us when we communicate with it by dropping down into it. To understand how this force manifests, we can observe that the trunk of a tree lifts straight up out of the earth in alignment with the force of gravity for some distance, before the first branches appear and begin to spread outwards. Occasionally, we may find a tree with a split trunk, such that there are two main trunks which have split from the root trunk very close to the ground level. This can happen for a number of reasons, but trees which exhibit this feature are much less stable and doomed to a shorter lifespan in comparison to their "normal" peers who have a well-defined main trunk which grows upwards in harmony with gravity. There are two trees of the same species which stand on either side of the front door of my house here in Bali. One tree has been harvested by my landlord several times. He cuts the branches back very closely, and I believe it is for this reason that it has a split trunk. The other tree has never been harvested (to my knowledge), and its trunk is much stronger and more stable than that of its sibling. Sometimes, after a torrential rain, these trees become weighed down and bent beneath the weight of the water that has accumulated on them. The tree with the split trunk becomes much more deviated from its usual growing pattern after the heavy rainfall, and takes longer to return to its usual pattern thereafter, compared to the tree with the stronger trunk. It is clear to me which tree has stronger *bandha*. Other animals have made the same observations about these two trees. There is a lineage of white rumped munia birds which nest in the stronger tree every year that I have lived here. These birds always choose the tree which has the more developed *bandha* to build their nest in.

Trees with a stable midline—that is to say, a strong and well-aligned trunk, also have much greater capacity to spread their branches and leaves outwards in all directions. Supported by the stability of the main trunk, the branches can elongate and reach much further outwards without compromising the overall stability of the tree.

I've already spoken about the mobility of trees through the growth and connections of their roots beneath the earth. This mobility is also apparent above the ground. Over deep time, trees can grow in whichever direction and orientation will best serve them in their quest to absorb maximal sunlight through their leaves for photosynthesis. When sunlight conditions change, the growth patterns and orientations of trees change in response. Different species of trees living together in a forest also cooperate in various ways to allow each other to capture all niches available for sunlight absorption.

A minimal amount of breeze can be enough to excite all of the leaves on a tree and even cause the thickest branches of a large tree to sway back and forth lazily. In the event of a great storm with gale force winds, the branches and upper trunk of a tree exhibit a huge range of motion and will bend in harmony with the wind, without resisting the extreme forces that assail them. These movements of the branches and trunk of a tree always look very relaxed to me. The tree is so confident in the rooting aspect of its *bandha*, that it has no fear or need to hold rigidity in its branches and leaves. Rather, the tree understands that allowing relaxed and resilient movement in the peripheral parts of its structure is the path of least resistance and greatest harmony in its relationship with its environment.

Humans can also manifest the lifting and spreading aspect of *bandha* in a way that is similar to trees. Once we have established a firm and sensitive rooting movement into the earth, we can harness the force of gravity and allow the complementary lifting and spreading action to move through the rest of our body. "Harnessing" and "allowing" are terms that I have selected carefully. *Bandha* is not an active gripping or clenching of the muscles around the pelvis or lower belly. Many practitioners who have been erroneously taught to do so are not experiencing *bandha* at all. By attempting to clench abdominal and pelvic muscles without actively soliciting an embodied relationship with the ground and with gravity, these practitioners generate excessive tension which inhibits their ability to harness and allow the energy of the earth to flow freely through their bodies. The result is a state of tension and disconnection, rather than a state of *bandha*.

Just as a tree seems to relax and allow the wind to move its branches freely, relaxation and release are necessary for humans to allow the force of the earth to manifest to its full potential and move through us uninhibitedly. Once we have effectively "plugged in" to the energy source of gravity by rooting into the earth, we then must cultivate conducive receptive space for this energetic response from the earth to move through us. When we succeed in this, we can manifest movement patterns which are both rooted, stable and powerful, and yet relaxed, resilient and expansive. In this state, we are in the most harmonious and balanced possible relationship that we can have with the earth beneath us and the force of gravity around us. This represents a state of engaged *bandha*.

Effectively engaged *bandha* feels effortless, intuitive and meditative. When we cultivate embodiment and give authority to the intuitive animal intelligence within our soma, we experientially understand that the essence of posture and movement is that of reciprocal and active relationship with nature. When practicing from the layer of *bandha*, the sensations and embodied feelings associated with the "central axis" or "midline" of the body communicate reciprocally with the field of the earth and these sensations become a meditative focal point which can be carried through all of the postures and vinyasas of our practice. If we are able to feel the dropping and rooting force actively coordinating with the lifting and spreading force through the central axis of the body, and this "core alignment" is being actively solicited in every posture and vinyasa movement that we place our body and breath into, then we are successfully holding the form of *bandha* in place throughout our practice.

Allow me to emphasize again that "holding *bandha*" has very little to do with holding the anus, pelvic floor or lower abdominal muscles in an engaged state. One might ask why these particular muscle groups are so often associated with *bandha*. It is because when we do harmonize our midline with gravity and activate the tree shaped energetic pattern of balanced rooting/dropping and lifting/spreading movements, some of these "core" muscles will naturally and instinctively respond to this energetic patterning and alignment. **The muscular engagement is a product of the energetic alignment of *bandha*. The muscular engagement is not the cause of *bandha*.** This is an important distinction to understand.

I generally encourage practitioners to focus less on the science of anatomy and physiology in their yoga practice, and more on phenomenological and embodied feeling. Focusing on anatomy and physiology in isolation of engaged relationship tends to lock one into the illusion of a separate self and results in one becoming trapped in the labyrinth of abstracted mirrors which the modern human race is lost within. Moving in phenomenological and embodied relationship with the earth is something that our species has been doing for hundreds of thousands of years, and something that the ancestral lineage to our species has been doing for millions of years. I have little doubt that our hunter-gatherer ancestors moved through the forests and savannas intuitively, as if the environment was an extension of their own bodies, and were more skilled at movement than most of us are today. I am also sure that healing from injuries was an equally intuitive process which they were also skilled at. Needless to say, intellectual study of anatomy was not a part of this paradigm. Embodied sensitivity and felt relationship with one's environment provides the vast majority of the confidence, sensitivity and experiential understanding necessary to work with *bandha*, and to move safely and efficiently. The majority of injuries do not arise from a lack of knowledge in the field of anatomy and physiology. They arise from a lack of embodied sensitivity and focus in one's bodily attunement with the environment.

The tree shaped movement pattern of the layer of *bandha* also manifests in the layers of breath and external body.

As I mentioned near the beginning of this piece, the three layers of *bandha*, breath and body are not functionally separate from each other. The form of the tree should be consciously cultivated from all three layers simultaneously. I think of the relationship between *bandha*, breath and body like the concentric rings in the trunk of a tree. *Bandha* represents the innermost layer of rings, breath the middle layers of rings and the body the outermost layer of rings. Although it is possible to identify these three layers of rings as distinctly separate things, it is meaningless to think of them as being able to function separately from one another. All three layers of rings are part of the structure, form and movement patterns of the tree.

In the tree-shaped breathing we use during Ashtanga practice, the exhalation represents the downwards movement of the roots of the tree probing into the earth. In this context, the earth is our pelvis and we apply an intentional force to push the exhalation down into the bowl of the pelvis, or into the earth. In a refined breathing practice, this downwards push is not aggressive. It is subtle, yet powerful. It is possible to have power without aggression. It is also elongated. Think again of the roots of a tree, elongating in deep time down into the ground at their glacial pace, and yet with enough strength to gradually crack and move through concrete or rocks. A fully developed exhalation similarly pushes its way through all of the layers of tension and blockage in the belly and pelvis, opening them up, until it eventually connects into the floor of the pelvis itself.

The inhale begins where the exhale finishes, and represents the lifting and spreading pattern of the trunk and branches of the tree. As previously discussed, most tree trunks grow directly upwards, away from the earth for some distance, before the first branches start reaching outwards to the sides. In this context, we can think of the lifting movement of the inhale up and out of the pelvis and through the lumbar spine/abdominal region as representing this straight part of the tree trunk; and we can think of spreading of the breath through the thoracic area, including ribs and shoulder girdle as representing the spreading branches of the tree. In Ashtanga practice, when we begin inhaling upwards from the bowl of the pelvis, we do not breathe outwards into the belly. Instead, we draw the breath straight up through the lower abdominal cavity, until we reach the upper abdominal and diaphragm area. At this stage, we allow the breath to spread outwards through the entire rib cage as it continues its journey upwards. An adept breathing practitioner will eventually be able to lift and spread the inhale through the entirety of the rib cage, including the front, back and sides—all the way up to the sternum and along the width of the collarbones at the front, up to the top of the thoracic spine and between the scapula at the back, and into the armpits at the sides.

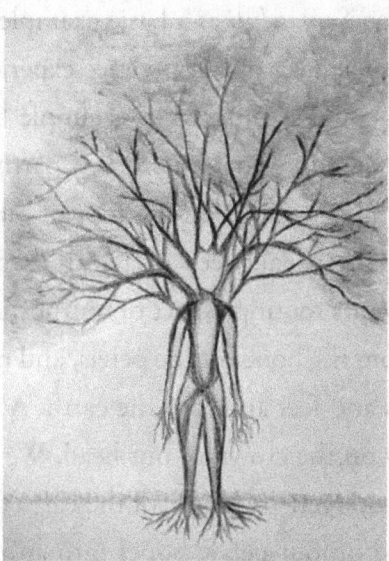

Samasthiti by Allen Enrique

When we apply the tree form to our breathing in this way, we sometimes find that the lower part of the abdomen does stay drawn gently inwards, due to a natural negative pressure that is generated in the abdominal cavity. Once more, I will emphasize that this negative abdominal pressure is not due to a conscious and rigid tensing of the abdominal muscles. Just as actively gripping these muscles will inhibit the free flow of energy in the state of *bandha* from manifesting, it will also inhibit the free flow of breath from manifesting. Sharath Jois says that we should apply "free breathing with sound" to our practice. I have also heard him define *bandha* as meaning "to lift up." Sucking in and holding the abdomen muscularly will not contribute to free breathing or to lifting up. When we are able to find relaxed and natural alignment with gravity and we can breathe freely from the roots of the floor of the pelvis to the tips of the branches at the outer reaches of the upper ribs then a natural negative pressure manifests in the abdominal cavity and "lifting up" happens naturally and with relatively minimal effort.

Finally, we can return to the layer of external structure and form of the body. We can examine *Samasthiti* as a basic example of how the form of the tree manifests at this layer of our practice experience. In my immersion and pranayama courses, I like to do a simple but effective exercise to demonstrate this: Standing in *Samasthiti*, a partner comes behind us and uses his hands to press down on the tops of our iliac bones, with a fair amount of force. This usually feels pleasantly "grounding," and allows us to feel the downwards rooting aspect of our posture. This downwards movement begins from the bones of the pelvis, and moves down through the bones of the legs and feet and into the earth. A second partner then rests his hand lightly on the crown of our head. We can then attempt to actively channel the energetic response of the earth from the downwards pressure being placed on our pelvic bones into an upwards growth and expansion through our central axis, spine and rib cage. When we succeed in this, we are able to lift straight upwards through the crown of our head. Our second partner will actually feel the top of our head growing upwards into his hand. During this exercise, most students find that they can tangibly feel the structure of their body growing taller.

If we learn how to engage with gravity and the earth through the three layers of *bandha*, breath and body in every asana and vinyasa of our practice, we actually will grow taller over time. I spent 4 years away from my native Canada when I began my yoga practice in India in the late 1990s and early 2000s. When I finally returned home, my friends and family who had not seen me during those years all commented that I had grown taller. Though I did not understand it as such at the time, this was due to long-term cultivation of the pattern and form of *bandha* in the structure of my body.

We can examine the tree-shaped movement pattern of the external body in any other posture or vinyasa movement that we choose to engage with. *Utpluthi* can serve as another example: When I give instructions for this posture at the end of a led Primary series class, the first thing I say is: "Place your hands on the ground and connect deeply with the earth." Then, I say: "**Press down** and lift up." It is the same principle as in *Samasthiti*. Lifting up cannot happen effectively unless pressing down happens first. *Utpluthi* is a strenuous posture, but it is most effectively and least strenuously performed by working primarily with our energetic relationship with the earth, rather than muscular gripping. When I am holding *Utpluthi* for a longer count and I begin to tire, the first thing I do to recharge the dynamic process is to re-establish the contact of my hands with the ground, and press down more. When I do this, my pelvis and torso immediately lighten and lift up higher with less effort. There is no conscious clenching of my belly or pelvis in this application of *bandha*. While the core muscles in that area certainly do engage, this engaging is a natural by-product of the cultivated relationship patterns between my body and breath and the earth. Lifting up to jump back to *Chaturanga Dandasana* from a seated posture follows identical principles.

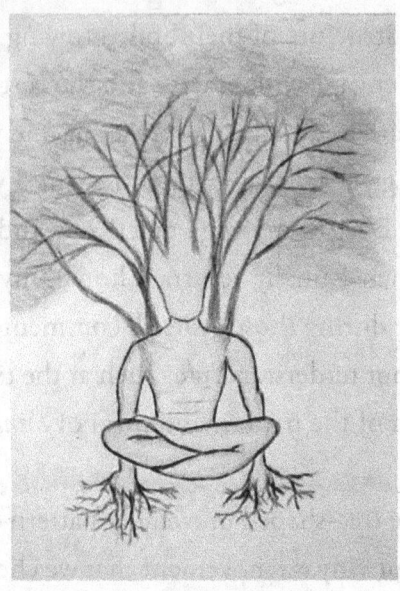

Utpluthi by Allen Enrique

To experientially understand the tree shaped movement in *bandha*, breath and body, it is necessary to work with our reciprocal relationship with our environment from an embodied, phenomenological place of tactile feeling and sensation. Every gesture and movement of body and breath generates a response from the ground and from the space around us, and we need to be receptive and sensitive enough to feel that response from the earth. When we are able to accept, feel and transmit this response through our own body and breath, this informs the next gesture and movement that we make. This reciprocal feedback loop between the self and the environment builds up in intensity and focus over the duration of our practice as body, breath, *bandha* and earth become intertwined in an inseparable web of reciprocal communication and exchange. The vinyasa system of coordinated and concentrated flowing movements of body and breath is one of the unique features of the Ashtanga practice, and is indispensable in order to experience *bandha* in this way. In a deep experience of *bandha*, the boundaries between self and environment—body and Earth—begin to dissolve, and we begin to experientially understand the fundamental truth that we are not separate from our environment. We begin to identify less with the abstracted, isolated conception and experience of self and more with the felt reality of an embodied organic organism embedded within a rich web of relationships of reciprocal exchange that is the whole of the living, breathing Earth.

ASHTANGA,
EMBODIMENT
& COMPLEX
SYSTEMS

REFLECTIONS ON TODD HARGROVE'S

"A Guide to Better Movement" in the context of Ashtanga Yoga practice

— August 2019 —

I RECENTLY READ TODD HARGROVE'S book, *A Guide to Better Movement*[1]. I don't recall who initially recommended Hargrove's book to me, but it was after I had mentioned that I was reading Katy Bowman's *Movement Matters* a few years ago. I bought *A Guide to Better Movement* around that time, and it has sat in my book box (regrettably, I can't keep my books displayed on a bookshelf in Bali as they quickly become degraded by dust and mildew) waiting to be read until I picked it up a month or so ago.

I enjoyed Hargrove's book even more than I expected to. The focus is not on the specifics of biomechanics or kinesiology (which I usually find to be boring, dogmatic and fallacious), but more about the "top-down" influence of the nervous system on our experience and performance of physical movement. I appreciated that he avoids reductionist and dog-

1 *A Guide to Better Movement: The Science and Practice of Moving With More Skill and Less Pain*, Todd Hargrove, Paperback, Better Movement (May 21, 2014), 978-0991542307. Extracts reproduced under Fair Use Copyright for illustration purposes.

matic principles of what constitutes "safe" movement and alignment, and instead focuses on a more general consideration of the multitude of factors beyond anatomy and physiology which constitute the whole of our experience of body movement and comfort/discomfort.

One drawback to his approach is that he does perpetuate a clear distinction between body and brain, whereas I prefer a more integrated and "enactive" approach to human experience which discourages the artificial and imagined separation of the component parts of the human organism. Nonetheless, the book was enjoyable and I look forward to reading his recently released second book, *Playing With Movement*. I appreciate the optimism and absence of fear mongering in the perspectives of movement therapists like Hargrove and Greg Lehman (whose recovery strategies PDF book[1] is also well worth reading).

Hargrove's book is not at all about yoga, but while reading it, I found myself interpreting many of his ideas and principles in the context of Ashtanga Yoga practice.

Each quote below is a passage from Hargrove's book, with my commentary directly underneath.

* * * * *

> *We want awareness to be mobile, to be able to generalize, to be able to receive information that is both local and non-local; we want our awareness to be versatile. We want our sensation palette to be full and rich.*
>
> *Much like a painter with brilliant colors, we are informed by the pulsations of tones that effervesce in any situation. Our capacity to know anything is not just cerebral but includes what we can feel is going on. Our sense perception becomes tentacular, spreading itself far and wide, allowing a new circumstance to take place within us.*

---

[1] https://www.greglehman.ca/recovery-strategies-pain-guidebook

When we narrow our perception, no matter how justified, we create a form of paralysis. Although we are still ambulatory, our awareness becomes truncated and unable to move. We are the living dead, unable to respond at the most basic level of our system. We become cut off from the information around us as our systems become increasingly muted.

Habitual responses, whether painful or delightful, are basically maneuvers of our defense system to maintain status quo. A habitual response can be ecstatic or difficult, it doesn't matter. What matters is that our awareness is trapped in circulating familiar responses, no matter what they are.

For example, fear can immobilize awareness, and there is now a feedback loop that ensures safety from new information or communication. Our systems are now in a highly compensatory state.

Can a paralyzed person practice Ashtanga? Can a zombie practice Ashtanga? Absolutely. I see people practicing Intermediate, Third series and beyond as paralyzed zombies. They are the practitioners who are most resistant to feedback — from the practice, from their teachers and from their own somatic experience.

Practice can be a way to dissolve paralysis, or it can be a way to deepen paralysis. It all depends on how we use the tool of practice.

* * * * *

✎ *Imagine the excellent feeling of hitting a golf ball or baseball right in the center. There is a perfect transfer of force from the club or bat into the ball. The ball moves away at maximum speed in a straight line with very little sense of effort or feeling of impact through your hands. By contrast, an off-center hit sends a horrible feeling of vibration through your hands and arms. The ball goes in an unpredictable direction, with minimal speed.*

The same dynamics are at play in your joints when they accept a compressive load. If you push a heavy object such as a door, or punch a heavy bag, proper alignment of the wrist, elbow, shoulder joint, scapula, spine and hips, all the way down to the feet will ensure a clean transfer of force from the hand to the ground. The force passes through you. There are no energy leaks in the transmission which will create friction, shearing forces and other stresses that impair efficiency and cause microdamage. The same dynamics are at play each time we take a step.

In an erect posture, proper alignment of the bones allows the force of gravity to "pass through" the body to the ground cleanly. Just as blocks that are well stacked can resist gravity from pulling them down, bones that are well aligned can hold us up with only a minimum of muscular effort to maintain the alignment. Visualizing skeletal connections is an interesting way to simplify ideas about what movements are efficient.

This is *bandha*. Note that it has nothing to do with gripping, squeezing or holding certain muscle groups, as many Ashtanga practitioners are erroneously taught to do. Aligned fluidity creates energetic efficiency.

* * * * *

🍃 *Good movement is not just about harmonious interaction or coordination between the different parts of the body. It is most fundamentally about how the system interacts with the environment, particularly in response to unexpected changes. In other words, good movement implies a quality of adaptability and responsiveness to a changing environment.*

As a teacher, I would say that the most capable students are not the strongest or most flexible ones, but those who are most receptive to, and able to assimilate new information. This may include information from their external environment (including their teacher) and their internal environment. Students who are strongest and most flexible are often the least capable in this respect.

Those who have cultivated *bandha* are able to intuitively adapt to changing internal and external conditions with fluidity and effortlessness. *Bandha* represents a seamless relationship with one's environment.

*****

We can also tune in and out of the different streams of sensory information that are continually arising from all the different parts of the body. Very few of these sensory signals will result in any actual awareness, but you can create awareness in any locality by focusing your attention there.

For example, right now you can focus on:

* *The sensation of air passing over your nostrils as you breathe*
* *The contact of your left sit bone with a chair*
* *The feeling of your shirt touching your back*

Sensory information that was previously being ignored is now processed.

This excites neural activity in the parts of the brain responsible for perceiving these areas. And so you perceive things that were previously missed.

This is why focused attention is one of the key requirements for practice that maximizes neuroplasticity and associated motor learning. The type of deep practice or flow state that produces the greatest gains in skill is characterized by tunnel vision on the activity at hand. World-class performers have an exceptional ability to spend a great deal of time in this state. People who are less skilled at focusing their attention will learn more slowly. Interestingly, some performance experts argue that what appears to be inborn natural talent at a particular activity is actually better described as a natural ability to engage in deep practice.

Physical techniques and information are of very minor importance in the process of deepening one's practice. Teachings which focus on physical techniques and an overload of information often end up being a distraction from actual practice.

Cultivating meditative phenomenological awareness of embodied breath and sensation is the key factor in deepening one's practice and one's relationship with oneself.

*****

🔖 [...] It is simpler for the nervous system to rely on a small number of general movement patterns that can be assembled together to form more complex movements.

One implication of this system is when a foundational building block is missing or compromised, the entire structure built on top will suffer. If you are missing some very basic words or letters in your language vocabulary, there are many sentences you will struggle to make. Similarly, if your movement vocabulary is missing one or more important motor primitives, many everyday movements will be compromised.

Thus, if you had the choice of improving one movement, you would choose one that had broad carryover to many other movements, as opposed to one that is highly specialized. For example, if I improve my squat, I will probably also improve my golf swing, my jump shot, and my tennis serve, because these activities are all supported by a basic squat pattern. I will also be more comfortable and functional in my activities of daily living, because I am getting into chairs and picking things off the floor all day. Better squatting could reduce mechanical stress on the hips, knees and low back.

By contrast, if I improve some specific skill, like hitting a tennis serve, I will be better at serving... but probably nothing else. So if we want to train movement, it is a good idea to train foundational movements, as opposed to highly complex and specialized movements that are specific to only one context. It is therefore no surprise that in corrective exercise, physical therapy, and functional training, it is usually fundamental movements that are emphasized.

This is why a good Mysore-style teacher will demand mastery of the foundations contained in the first part of Primary series before moving students on to more advanced postures and vinyasa.

Advanced postures are simply novel and more complex combinations of fundamental movement patterns. For those who have truly mastered all of the fundamental movement patterns, the advanced postures will come easily and with little need for instruction or support from a teacher. Those who have failed to learn fundamental movement patterns will struggle endlessly and need a teacher to put them into more difficult postures.

Rather than continue to adjust students into a number of difficult postures that they cannot perform without assistance, a good Mysore-style teacher will ask the student to go back to a more basic practice until the prerequisite movement patterns are mastered. This may feel frustrating and less immediately gratifying for the student in the short term, but will produce a much healthier, independent and empowering practice in the long run.

* * * * *

🖎 *During the first two years of life, babies develop from a quivering blob on the floor, to creatures that can roll over, sit, crawl, squat, walk, manipulate objects and drive their parents crazy. The rate of motor learning is extremely fast and very impressive. Toddlers squat with the perfection of Olympic weightlifters. Their head carriage and posture would please any physical therapist. And their movements have the grace and simplicity of a Zen monk. The amazing thing is these optimal movement patterns emerge without any instruction whatsoever.*

For hundreds of thousands of years, our Homo sapiens ancestors skillfully moved through the forests and savanna in ways that would probably make today's Olympic athletes envious. The intuitive animal intelligence of the human organism does not need rational, intellectual instruction in order to learn how to move in efficient and functional relationship with its surroundings.

It mystifies me that so many modern yoga practitioners and analysts assume there is a necessity for the modern science of anatomy and physiology to inform our postural yoga practice. To me, "99 percent practice and 1 percent theory" refers to the relative contributions of phenomenological, intuitive, animal intelligence (99 percent) vs. rational, scientific anatomical knowledge (1 percent) to our practice experience.

The suggestion that all yoga practitioners and teachers should be trained in anatomy and physiology is as absurd as suggesting that babies need to study anatomy and physiology in order to safely progress in their learning of movement skills as they develop and mature in their first years of life. Our prescientific era ancestors did just as well at mastering movement skills as babies do. What has caused us to forget this obvious fact?

Postural yoga is a beautiful opportunity to rekindle the flame of the embodied, intuitive, animal aspect of movement intelligence which we all are born into this world with, but so many modern humans tend to neglect and discard with their maturation into the adult world of civilized domestication. Reducing postural yoga to anatomical formulas and prescriptions strips it of its very heart and soul… as we have already done with so many other aspects of our lives.

* * * * *

🪶 *The part of the brain that stores memories reports this is the exact same position the body was in, last year, when it experienced extreme back pain that lasted for several weeks. Another part of the brain remembers a statement by a doctor about a "slipped disc." Another part recognizes that he may be unable to do his job, and that he will need to file for worker's compensation.*

This immediately causes emotions of intense worry and anxiety about the future, and thoughts of catastrophe.

All these inputs are instantly processed and filtered and analyzed and integrated unconsciously in the brain, which will then ask essentially two questions. How dangerous is this really, and is pain necessary for protection? The resulting pain depends on how the questions are answered.

Are you skeptical that your brain could think this fast, and without you being aware of any of it? Recall the optical illusion with the checkerboard.

In interpreting the meaning of the light bouncing off the board, your brain instantaneously took account of the alternating color pattern and the existence of the shadows. The pain alarm system involves just as much unconscious calculation and interpretation as the visual system.

Now consider another person who does the same forward bend, suffers the exact same mechanical damage and resulting nociception, but has a completely different set of proprioceptive and cognitive inputs.

This person moves with good balance, has no memory of any previous back pain, is not afraid of back injury, knows from pain education that back pain does not necessarily imply tissue damage, has excellent financial and social support and is optimistic about the future. Will this person have the same kind of pain? Probably not!

And to further illustrate the complexity and individuality of pain, let's remember that pain is not the only "output" the brain can choose to protect the body. It can choose between several other kinds of protective outputs, such as movements (flinching, limping, muscle guarding, stiffness), autonomic changes (fight or flight), or immune responses (eg. inflammation). Or some combination of all three in varying amounts.

It is relatively rare that pain experienced during a particular postural movement (in yoga practice or otherwise) is directly caused by poor alignment or soft tissue damage. There are multitudes of interconnected and interrelated factors from all layers of our being, which contribute to our conscious experience of any given phenomena, including that of pain.

I find pain and discomfort to be a fascinating opportunity to observe and transform various layers of my own reactive habit patterns (*samskaras/sankharas*) during practice. Slight and subtle shifts in the structure of my conscious awareness in the embodied state can completely transform my experience of asana practice, including the perception of pain (or more often generalized unpleasantness). This provides fuel for a fascinating journey deeper into myself on the mat every morning.

I can't recall the last time I addressed my experience of pain with a shift in alignment or superficial technique (though this can certainly sometimes be appropriate). The relationship of how the various body parts are organized with respect to one another and with respect to the earth is only one minor ingredient in the complex soup of our conscious phenomenological experience at any given moment.

It baffles me when I see many yoga teachers and practitioners focusing solely on one superficial aspect (alignment/tissue damage) of our multi-dimensional experience of yoga asanas and vinyasas. I've witnessed several teachers who claim to understand the source of a student's pain before even watching that student practice, let alone inquiring into other dimensions of the student's being. This is usually followed by application of whatever dogmatic alignment principles the teacher happens to subscribe to. Needless to say, this approach is usually ineffective.

* * * * *

> *Similar involuntary protective mechanisms may be at play in modifying or governing flexibility, endurance, and coordination patterns. These mechanisms mean that one limiting factor in reaching your physical potential is the extent to which your nervous system is in a protective mode.*
>
> *Imagine an overprotective mother riding in a car with her teenage son, and putting her foot on the brake whenever she thinks he is driving unsafely.*
>
> *The speed of the car would be limited not by how much horsepower is under the hood, but Mom's perception of danger.*
>
> *Similarly, your ability to fully express your potential strength, flexibility, endurance and coordination is limited by your brain's perception of threat associated with the chosen movements. We may not consider a sprained ankle or torn hamstring to be really scary, but our nervous systems evolved in an environment when these injuries could mean the difference between life and death. Preventing them is a major concern.*
>
> *Thus, your brain is always acting as a governor on your performance, to protect you from yourself, ensuring that you do not move too powerfully, too fast, too far, for too long, or with certain movement patterns.*
>
> *In this section we'll discuss the science behind central governors related to strength, flexibility, endurance and coordination, and how one of the best and quickest ways to increase performance is to reduce perceived threat.*

In this chapter, Todd Hargrove discusses the protective mechanisms of the CNS, which prevent us from ever reaching our full potential in strength, flexibility, endurance, etc.

I deeply appreciate and enjoy Hargrove's perspective on human movement, which recognizes the multiplicity of factors aside from simple biomechanics which contribute to the whole of our experience of physical movement. One shortcoming to his approach is usage of language which suggests that the brain/CNS and body are distinct entities. In my own explorations, I have come to the conclusion that the tendency to separate components of humanness—such as body; brain; mind; spirit, etc.—represents a fundamental flaw in human reasoning, which has been exacerbated by the scientific reductionism which has proliferated since the time of Descartes. Entities are wholes whose parts are separable in theory, but not in actual functionality. Unfortunately, modern science does not yet have language which can effectively support exploration within this framework.

Sharath Jois is fond of stating that the body is okay, and the mind is stiff. This is similar to what Hargrove is getting at here, and is certainly an underappreciated aspect of performance—in asana or anything else in life.

As I have matured over 16 years of daily Ashtanga practice, I have come to understand that physical biomechanics is of very minor importance in comparison to the perception of the conscious and subconscious mind in terms of what is and isn't possible in physical movement. The fuzzy boundary between the perceptions of the conscious and subconscious are particularly fascinating and this is where the real "openings" are taking place which allow the physical expression of difficult asanas to manifest over time.

Cultivating equanimity towards all of our embodied experience—especially towards the experience of our perception of what is and isn't possible—is a golden key to unlocking potential. When I step on the front of my mat at 2:30 a.m., feeling fatigued or achey, and think, "I can't…" My very next step is to stop reacting to that thought and to enter a non-reactive state of "let's see…" And then, 99 percent of the time, I find that I can…

"MOVEMENT HOMEOPATHY"
In Ashtanga Yoga practice

— November 2019 —

I RECENTLY LISTENED TO A PODCAST interview with movement therapist Greg Lehman. Greg's perspectives on movement, pain and pathology resonate strongly with my own, and I have shared his ideas on my Spacious Yoga Facebook page numerous times. I found some interesting concepts in the interview which are applicable to my approach to Ashtanga Yoga practice.

The concept of "movement homeopathy" was my favorite takeaway. The concept is that we can train/retrain ourselves to perform movements that are painful and/or have been injurious to us by giving ourselves small or mild doses of the movement in question. "Movement Homeopathy" effectively describes my approach to recovery from injury or excessive pain in the Ashtanga practice. It also applies to how I approach the learning of new and difficult or intimidating new postures.

Standard professional medical advice after an injury or excessive pain/inflammation is either complete rest, or complete avoidance of the particular movement pattern that is associated with pain or injury. The application of ice to the injured or inflamed area is often included as part of the recovery protocol. Those who have experienced pain or injury while practicing with me know that I recommend against these standard procedures. Both the avoidance of movement and the application of ice to a painful or injured part of the body will encourage the trauma pattern (including the emotional and perceptual aspects of the trauma) to become locked into the body/mind/nervous system. Long-term healing or resolution is inhibited.

When we follow standard advice to avoid a movement pattern (or to avoid movement altogether in the case of complete rest), we generate a belief that continuing to engage with movement will cause us to deepen the damage or pain that we are already experiencing. This belief creates an emotionally reactive pattern (*samskara*) of fear, anxiety and aversion, which further compounds and complicates the discomfort that we are already facing. Moving (or not moving) in a perpetual state of fear and anxiety about our condition is highly unlikely to lead to healing or positive resolution of discomfort. The negative and apprehensive emotions we feel will tend to increase the overall tension levels in our body/mind/nervous system, and a negative feedback cycle, which perpetuates discomfort and inhibits healing, is created. I have seen numerous cases of yoga practitioners who report consistent chronic pain that does not improve, even though they are practicing carefully and mindfully and often avoiding or eliminating the movements which were originally associated with pain. In every one of these cases, I have observed high levels of fear, anxiety, and self-distrust around particular movements or aspects of the practice.

Another common approach to pain or injury is to look for issues in the alignment of the body, and to expect that shifting to a "healthier" alignment pattern will resolve the discomfort. I have also observed many cases of practitioners with chronic pain who fixate on following certain alignment dogmas (which they have been told are healthier) in their practice, and yet continue to experience chronic pain and discomfort. Again, there is an emotional rigidity and fear which develops around the possibility that they may slip into "bad alignment" which will cause their pain and discomfort to worsen. The emotional and physical rigidity which develops around this obsession with certain alignment principles also serves to lock the pain and trauma into the body/mind/nervous system, and in some cases the pain and discomfort actually worsen.

In the above examples, something which began primarily as a "physical" discomfort, is propagated and maintained by psychological fixations and emotional reactive patterns (*samskaras*), long after the initial physical trauma (if there was any to begin with) has dissipated. Techniques which are intended to protect us from our pain end up creating a complex system of negative feedback loops which often intensifies and unnecessarily prolongs the experience of pain.

Freezing a part of the body with ice will temporarily reduce inflammation, which can be useful for emergency pain relief in the case of a severe injury. Reducing inflammation, however, does not generally contribute to long-term resolution, especially in the case of chronic symptoms. Inflammation is a natural healing response of the human organism, and we could say that inflammation is creative in nature. Inflammation is a functional response of the intuitive organic intelligence of the body, and is part of how the autopoietic, self-organizing human organism repairs and rebuilds itself. Freezing a part of the body cuts off the circulation of creative life force and awareness to the injured part. Blocking this creative flow of life force into a part of the body through freezing with ice is quite similar in principle to blocking the creative flow of life force by avoiding movements which stimulate that part of the body.

Avoiding or restricting movement or certain movement patterns; fixating on "correct" alignment; and aggressively reducing inflammation through the application of ice or allopathic anti-inflammatory agents can have limited and temporary usefulness in certain contexts, but in general

I de-emphasize their importance and in many cases I recommend against them completely. The short-term benefits of decreased pain from these therapeutic techniques are transient in nature and do not contribute to long-term resolution or aid in the creative process of self-transformation that Ashtanga practice brings about. In essence, all of these therapeutic techniques block pain to some extent, but this necessarily means that they also block the creative flow of awareness, intuitive intelligence and life force. This ultimately leads to stagnation and inhibits long-term resolution and complete healing.

The blocking techniques all work on the principle of avoidance of the phenomenally embodied experience of the movement (and pain) in question, and through this inhibition of awareness and embodied intelligence, they generate a complex of fear and aversion which runs deeply through all the layers of the body/mind/nervous system. The lack of trust in bodily movement patterns ultimately represents and deepens a lack of trust in the self, a lack of trust in the practice, and a lack of trust in the relationship of the self with the practice. The intuitive, embodied intelligence of the animal self—which is where embodied understanding and natural healing intelligence arise—is forced into slumber and the ideas of the abstract and rational mind are imposed on the movement experience of the body. The result is a highly disembodied practice and disembodied experience of the self with strongly etched grooves of physical and emotional tension.

The other point that Lehman made in the interview which is highly relevant to the present discussion, is the fallacy of the goal or expectation of being pain free. Many branches of medicine and physical therapy ask patients to rate their pain on a scale of one to ten, with ten representing the highest amount of pain, and one representing the lowest. Lehman mentioned that expecting everyone to reach "a level of two or three" is completely unrealistic. The fallacious expectation of being pain free also percolates through the postural yoga community. It is common to hear certain well-respected yoga authorities say things like, "If it hurts, you are doing it wrong." I disagree with this trend. Lehman's perspective resonates much more strongly with me.

When we allow ourselves to actively engage with movement and with our discomfort or pain, rather than applying the previously discussed blocking techniques, we allow the creative response of the human organism's innate intelligence to work most effectively. As blood, life force, and both intuitive and conscious awareness flow into the wounded or painful area, so do aspects of the intuitive intelligence which are related to the reconstructive process of healing and transformation. Inflammation and pain are an unavoidable aspect of this process.

We may wish to keep the ideal part of the process (creative healing energy and intelligence) and avoid the unpleasant part (inflammation and pain), but, we can't have one without the other. The human organism is a highly refined, self-organizing system which has attuned itself to function as it does over two billion years of evolution. These phenomenally pleasant and unpleasant components of the healing process work together, and we cannot separate them with a few simple bio hacks. Pain is one dimension of the innate intelligence of the human organism, and attempting to block or avoid pain necessarily causes us to block and subdue other important aspects of our innate animal intelligence.

Striving for a pain-free practice or a pain-free life is undesirable if we are aiming for self-transformation and self-evolution. The saying "no-pain, no-gain" is more appropriate than "if it hurts you are doing it wrong." Without pain, an important stimulant for increased awareness and for the mobilization of creative intuitive intelligence is removed. A pain-free life and a pain-free practice would be a life and practice that easily slips into complacency and stagnation. For me, pain is the creative juice that keeps self-evolution flowing. Without discomfort, there is no challenge to overcome, and hence no stimulation to change. Evolutionary biology recognizes this principle on a broader scale. One of the main driving forces of biological evolution is adaptation, and this force becomes more relevant and important when the environment is shifting and changing in a way that makes life more challenging. Adaptation occurs as a creative response to a problem (which is likely a painful problem) and this dynamic perpetuates the evolutionary process. Without pain—problems and challenges which require adaptive response—the entire creative process of the evolution of life would stagnate. If we wish to continue to grow and change, we must consciously experience the discomfort involved in problems that we face, in order for the creative flow of adaptive response within us to occur and lead us forward.

The creative flow of adaptive response to problems effectively describes the process of restructuring the human organism through the sequential learning of the asanas and vinyasas of the Ashtanga system. In the essay titled "A Systems-Thinking Perspective on the Resolution of Pain in Ashtanga Practice," I describe the restructuring process in more detail. The long-term process of changing how the different parts and systems of the human body relate to one another and to our environment is a highly creative and nuanced process. The self-regulating system of the human organism must continuously reorganize and rearrange itself in novel and creative ways, in response to the controlled pressure we place upon it through the repetitive application of asana and vinyasa sequences. There is no doubt that this creative process involves inflammation and the experience of pain. To expect to experience creative transformation of the structure of the self without some degree of pain and inflammation to flow along with the mobilization of creative energy and intelligence, is to completely misunderstand the nature of the human organism and how it participates in the endless process of change. I am highly skeptical of the depth of understanding of teachers who state, "If it hurts, you are doing it wrong."

The art and skill that comes with experience in working with a system like Ashtanga Yoga is to understand how to adjust the parameters so that we can experience creative transformation—and corresponding pain and inflammation—to a degree that is sustainable and does not overly inhibit our ability to function normally in our day-to-day lives. The main factor is how much of the series or which series we practice and how quickly or slowly we should add to that series. In my opinion, the main role of a Mysore-style teacher is to determine this for each student. How much of the series, or which series, is appropriate for each particular student to experience a sustainable level of creative transformation. Or, to provide a healing response to an injury or excessive pain.

The Mysore-style teacher is overseeing the long-term transformational dynamic which occurs between each student and the particular set of postures or series they are practicing. Many students believe that the main benefit of going to a Mysore-style class is to receive a few good adjustments in the postures. An experienced and effective Mysore-style teacher will give much subtler, deeper guidance using their own experience with the dynamics of how the system of Ashtanga reorganizes and restructures the human organism, to monitor this aspect of the student's practice. I sometimes receive emails from prospective students that say things like "I only have time to practice with you for one or two days, but I'd like to learn as much as possible in that time." I usually don't say anything, but I chuckle to myself and think: "Nothing. I can't teach you anything about this practice in one or two days, all I can do is give you a safe space and good energy to practice in. If you really want to learn about how this practice works, one month is a bare minimum for the transformational dynamics within your practice to start to really respond to my guidance." The process of relationship between the self and the asana sequences requires deep time to evolve and manifest in life-changing ways. So also does the influence of a teacher on this process and relationship.

Let us return to the specifics of "movement homeopathy" in Ashtanga practice. My advice to practitioners who are experiencing pain related to injury or to an excessive amount of structural transformation is usually to continue practice, but in many cases to back off to a more basic, shorter practice. The homeopathy is that we are "treating" the pain or injury with the same thing that has caused or aggravated it. We are reducing the intensity or quantity of the movement, to a degree that the human organism's intuitive intelligence is better able to process and integrate it. This ensures that the creative intelligence is flowing into the process of structural reorganization or healing, but at a moderate level and rate, so there is a reduced amount of pressure on the organism to shift and evolve in the restructuring process. This slowing-down and de-intensifying of the process allows the intuitive intelligence to adapt to the movement patterns in question more effectively and with less pain. Because we are still moving, and even performing movements that are painful, we are still presenting the adaptive intelligence of our animal selves with a problem to address. And so, the creative adaptive response of the organism will still be engaged. This stimulates evolution and change which will eventually generate an enduring resolution to the pain or discomfort which is present.

As the pain and discomfort dissipate, and correspondingly the level of confidence in the self and in the movements of the practice increases, the intensity of posture and movement can be gradually increased again. In other words, as the adaptive intelligence of the animal becomes stronger and more capable, we can again increase the pressure we place upon ourselves to change with more asanas, or more intensive depth in the asanas.

There is no set formula for how much or how long this "homeopathic" process needs to be continued for. In severe cases, one may need to switch from a practice of a full series or even multiple series to a very short practice of just a few *Surya Namaskar* and standing postures. In other cases, one may need to simply back off on the intensity of the last posture of their practice for a little while. In some cases the reduction to a homeopathic dose of practice may only be necessary for a few days or a week. In other cases, it may need to be applied for months or even years. It all depends on factors unique to each individual case, and a good teacher should be able to help a person determine the exact prescription. Ultimately, it is one's own embodied experience of, and familiarity and willingness to engage with the phenomenal experience of pain, inflammation and structural change, which allows one to adjust the homeopathic dosage accordingly.

The same principle can also be applied to learning new postures and movements, even when no pain or inflammation is present. Very difficult and intimidating movements, which may seem impossible from the outset, can be experienced to be much more palatable, when tasted in small, homeopathic doses. When I give a difficult new posture to a student, and that student cannot perform the posture to its full expression, I rarely give strong adjustments in the beginning. I let the student play around with the preliminary versions of the posture, and watch how the intuitive intelligence of the student adapts to those movements. Only if I see a real capability to move into the final version of the posture without excessive strain or shock, will I use some physical manipulation to put the student there. Otherwise, it is much better, and more sustainable to allow the intelligence of the student's own organism to work it out naturally and gradually. I have learned over many years of teaching that less adjusting and more observing is a more effective method for students to learn the postures in a way that is enduring and sustainable. I feel that a student has fully learned a posture, or portion of the practice, when I am confident that they can go away and do it on their own, just as effectively as they could do it in my shala or with my help.

One example of this process from my own practice is in the difficult Third series posture *Gandha Berundasana*. I began to practice this posture with my former teacher Rolf more than a decade ago. There was no possibility of coming even close to completing this posture under my own means, but Rolf would be sure to put me into the final version of the posture every day. It was always an extraordinarily terrifying experience to prepare for this posture, but over time I began to trust my ability to experience the full version of the posture—with Rolf's assistance. There was no homeopathy involved. I don't think he ever let me try to work my way into the posture alone—not even once. It was an all or nothing experience. When I was practicing with him, it would be "all" and when I would be back at home, practicing on my own after my visits to my teacher, it would be "nothing." On my own, I would simply find it too intimidating to even attempt without help, and for more than a decade I resigned myself to the fact that this was one posture which wasn't for me to experience on my own in this lifetime.

My attitude changed last year, when I realized that I might have to practice *Gandha Berundasana* with Sharath on my subsequent trip to Mysore. I dreaded revisiting the posture, and wondered what Sharath's approach with me would be regarding it. I gave myself an easy out, by telling myself that Sharath wouldn't expect me to be able to do it. Many students do get moved past this posture in Third series without having to complete it.

While I was beginning to contemplate this, a friend of mine visited my shala, and it so happened that he had recently been given that same posture by Sharath. We talked about it and my friend felt that "Sharath will expect both you and I to be able to do it." I knew he was right. A short time later, another friend of mine who can do *Gandha Berundasana* very nicely visited my shala. Both these events inspired me, so I decided to begin working on it in my home practice.

I began in earnest, and without any real expectation of success. I started with very small homeopathic doses of the posture, and would only work as far into it as felt safe; and to a point where I felt like my body's intelligence would be able to understand, process and integrate the structural changes which were taking place and would be necessary to continue to move deeper into the posture. In the beginning, I was certainly nowhere near even the first stages of completing the posture. Not surprisingly, with daily homeopathic application the organic intelligence did begin to take over, and a surprising amount of progress took place. After about six months of daily application, I succeeded in being able to catch both of my feet with my hands and to be in the most rudimentary version of the final posture. This continued for about a month, and then suddenly it was completely gone. I was back to square one, perhaps even further back than when I had first begun to tackle the posture six months earlier. What to do? Nothing, but to start the homeopathic process over again, which I did. This time it took five more months of homeopathy to attain the final stage of posture again. Only this time, I did not lose it, and I was able to continue to perform the final version of the posture every day for several months. Interestingly, I have now had to stop it again because I am currently in Mysore practicing with Sharath, and I am still a few postures away from reaching *Gandha Berundasana* in my practice with him. It will be interesting to see, if he gives me *Gandha Berundasana* on this trip (or if not, when I go back to doing it at home after the trip), whether I will be able to return to doing it straight away, or whether another homeopathic process will be necessary. I no longer have any fear or apprehension about the posture, as I can feel the deeper embodied understanding and integration from my practice of it over the past year, so I do expect that it will come back fairly quickly the next time I tackle it.

* * * * *

As I was finishing up this piece, I came across another sports-therapy-based article which resonates with what I have just written. It provides an interesting footnote and complement to Lehman's statements from the interview, and my own interpretation of those statements: *Putting ice on injuries could be doing more damage than good.*[1]

Disclaimer 1

I don't claim to represent the work or teachings of Greg Lehman. I have never met or directly learned from him. He may very well disagree with how I have interpreted his own perspectives on pain and movement. Or he may agree with me. The views expressed in this essay are my own, and are based on my own experience with the practice of Ashtanga Yoga.

Disclaimer 2

This essay is conceptual in nature, and does not represent specific advice for any individual reader. Each situation is unique, and involves many factors, and I can only give specific advice in the context of a personal relationship with a student who is present in my shala.

---

1. https://www.smh.com.au/national/putting-ice-on-injuries-could-be-doing-more-damage-than-good-20191011-p52zw0.html

REFLECTIONS ON THE NEW SHALA

And my fifth trip of practice in Mysore with Sharath Jois

— December 2019 —

I RECENTLY COMPLETED MY FIFTH trip of practice with Sharath Jois in Mysore, India. It's been a few trips since I wrote an anecdotal account of my experiences in Mysore. After my preceding two trips, I didn't have much that was new to say about Mysore or practice with Sharathji, but this trip felt different. I had the opportunity to be in the first batch of students who practiced the full schedule in the new shala that Sharathji has recently opened. Something about this trip felt special for me, not just in terms of being part of the inauguration of the new shala, but also in the context of personal development. It was my best trip so far and I feel it is appropriate to share some of that positivity, especially in light of all the negative sentiment that has been propagated by a disgruntled minority of the Ashtanga community on social media over the past year or two.

The new shala is located approximately 10 km outside of Gokulam.

Sharathji began conducting led classes there in the previous practice session—which I did not attend—but this was the first session when the full schedule of classes was held at the new shala. When it was announced that all of the classes would be held there, I was not looking forward to the daily commute for practice. On previous trips, I enjoyed the fact that all of the facilities we need as students, including accommodation, decent restaurants and shops have all been developed in Gokulam. One could stay close to the shala in Gokulam, without the need to travel further than walking distance for most of one's daily needs. It was always pleasant to stroll to the shala on foot in the early hours of the morning and I wasn't very keen about a 10 km scooter drive for practice.

The drive took 10–15 minutes in the early morning hours, which are mostly traffic free. I drive faster than most people, as I am accustomed to a similar scooter commute from my home to the shala where I have taught in Ubud, Bali for the past five years. The roads on the main route from Gokulam to the new shala are all in decent condition and it only took a few days for me to get used to the drive. It wouldn't be possible to have a shala of the size of the new one in the Gokulam area, and it quickly became apparent that the drive-in was an acceptable trade-off for the benefits we experienced at the new shala.

The most notable thing about the new shala is its size. It is very large and can easily accommodate all 300 students for a led class. It seems to have previously been some sort of warehouse. A nice floor has been installed, which is similar to the floor that was installed at the old shala in Gokulam a few years ago. The property surrounding the shala is also sizable and the folks from Depth N Green restaurant have set up a refreshment and snack stall in an adjacent side building. The coconut guy has also set up there during practice hours.

The interior of the shala is well organized. There is a central stage on the east side, where Sharathji sits, and there are 76 mats spaces, individually marked out by construction tape, in front of the stage. The mat spaces are of ample size and in total, the 76 mat spaces take up approximately one third of the total floor space of the shala. Tall students, like myself, are requested to practice in the back two rows. I ended up claiming the back right corner spot, which I enjoyed quite a bit. It gave me even more room with no one on my right side or behind me.

There is a large space between the main entrance on the north side and the marked mat spaces. On the south side of the mat spaces, there are a few removable dividers, which section off a good-sized space for finishing postures. The changing rooms lie on the Southern most end of the shala.

Everything was impressively organized, especially considering this was the first run of a very sizable move of everything into a new space. The system for Mysore classes ran smoothly. Each new shift would wait outside the main doors, and eventually be brought in all at once to sit in the back right corner, where they would wait to be called to the vacant spaces one by one, as each practicing student finished and moved to the finishing area. As usual, I was on the first shift, which officially began at 5:30 a.m.—one hour later than it did in the old shala. Arrival was very casual. The doors would open at 4:45 a.m. and I usually arrived on my bike right about that time. We would all walk in and set up without any rush or fuss and begin practicing. Sharathji would come out of his office at 5:30 for the opening mantra.

Led classes were also smooth and it was enjoyable to practice with everyone together. All 300 students easily fit in the shala space, without any feeling of being crowded. Hence, there were no long line-ups or jostling for spaces like there was in the old shala. Led Primary series began at 6:30 a.m. I don't know what time the door was opened for led class, but I would usually arrive between 5:45 and 6 a.m., and about one third of the students would already be in the room and setting up. Conference would be held after led Primary class, with a 30-minute break in between.

On Mondays, led Intermediate was at 8:15 a.m., after led Primary series finished.

One of the main benefits that I enjoyed in the new shala was the feeling of more air and specifically more oxygen in the room. While I enjoyed the intimate intensity of the old shala, I always found the air to be depleted of oxygen, and I would tire easily at the end of my long practice. I always felt that the oxygen levels in the old shala were somewhat akin to practicing at 3000+ meters in elevation (which I have plenty of experience with), except one didn't ever get a chance to acclimatize to the lower oxygen content because the rest of the day outside of the shala was spent at normal oxygen levels. At the new shala, this was not an issue at all. The space is so large and the ceilings so high, that even when all 300 students were practicing at once in the led classes, the space felt airy and the oxygen levels felt normal. I immediately noticed the difference in my stamina, and I did not experience oxygen-related fatigue, even though my practice grew to the longest and most intense level it has ever been in Mysore.

Finishing was also very relaxed. There was always space for everyone to finish, and no sense of having to rush through finishing postures to make way for the next batch of people that needed to finish. We were welcome to take a long relaxation at the end, which I am accustomed to doing.

During October and November, the temperature in the shala was near perfect on the first shift of Mysore-style classes and for led Primary series class. Some people complained that it was too cold, and it certainly was colder than it was in the old shala in Gokulam. This wasn't an issue for me, as I am used to practicing in the chilly early morning hours at home in Bali. I don't rely on external heat to open my body up, and I usually feel better practicing in a slightly chilly environment than I do in excessive heat. Even in these slightly cooler conditions on the first shift, I was always sweating heavily by the end of my practice. I can imagine how it might get uncomfortably cold in the colder months of December and January, however. For led Intermediate at 8:15 a.m. and also for a conference at approximately the same time on Saturdays, it felt uncomfortably hot in the warmer month of October. Once the morning sun hit the roof of the shala, things heated up very quickly. Apparently, a better ventilation system is one of the next projects to be implemented, so we should see this improve by next season. The climate in Mysore cools down in November, so the heat was never an issue towards the end of my trip, even during led Intermediate and conference.

During the first week or two of practice, I felt there was an intimacy and certain energy that was missing in the new shala. The place felt too big and "cold" energetically, but this perception shifted by the time we had all been practicing together in the space for two weeks. It takes time for energy to accumulate in any new space, and this was no exception. By the second half of the first month, I felt perfectly at home and comfortable in the new shala, and this feeling was reflected in my practice experience. No doubt the energy will continue to build in the room as different batches of students develop their practices there.

Sharathji himself was very sharp and seemed to be in a positive and vibrant mood for the duration of the two months. In the old shala, I believe we had 50–60 students practicing at a time for Mysore classes, so the numbers were only slightly increased here at 76 students. In the old shala we had 2–3 assistants at any given time for Mysore classes, and here we had 5–6 assistants. There was never any waiting for postures like *Supta Vajrasana* or for catching, as someone was always close by and ready to help. Sharathji was attentive and the increase in student numbers did not seem to affect his ability to monitor everyone's practice. I certainly received ample attention from him. Other students that I spoke to felt the same in this respect.

For Sharathji himself, I feel this move made the teaching process more sustainable. I always marveled at the amount of work he did at the old shala, teaching from 4 a.m. to 11 a.m. for Mysore practice and teaching three led classes in succession on the led class days. Though he did it extremely competently, and I cannot think of any other living human being who could have done so, it also seemed like it would not be sustainable for him in the long run. He still has to work extremely hard in the new shala, but his work hours are slightly reduced, with a later start time in the mornings, and only one led class on Saturdays and two on Mondays. I hope he feels like it is something that he can continue to do, so that we can continue to benefit from his teaching for years to come. He certainly seemed to feel good about the move, and we all benefited from that positivity.

Overall, the energy and mood in the shala were high. I am a hermit by nature, and don't socialize very much in Mysore, so I can't claim to have access to a very wide sampling of perspectives from other students, but all of the people that I did talk to, shared similar opinions. We all enjoyed practice in the new shala and felt as if we had an extremely positive experience there. The move seems to have been beneficial for both Sharathji and for the students.

The past one to two years have seen a certain amount of negativity directed towards Sharathji on social media. I have no interest in publicly commenting on the specific issues that have been brought up, except to say that I fully understand and support the changes that Sharathji has made. His actions all make complete sense to me. As a trained psychologist and Buddhist, I have found it extremely interesting to witness the vehement negativity in the accusations that some people have publicly leveled against Sharathji. A teacher of any authentic system of self-transformation has a difficult job, in that he becomes an easy object for the projection of the internal *samskara* (habitual patterns or grooves that we generate in the ways that we unconsciously react or respond to the world around us) patterns which naturally arise for the students in the practice.

Any authentic practice will bring our *samskaras* onto the surface of our conscious experience. When this occurs, a practitioner has three choices: 1) Run away from or avoid experiencing the *samskara*; 2) Add fuel to the fire of the *samskara* by reacting more strongly to it and increasing the depth of its groove in our subconscious patterning; 3) Attempt to consciously observe the manifestation of the *samskara* without reaction and with as much objectivity/equanimity as possible.

Some members of our community have engaged in dramatic public displays of self-immolation, burning in the flames of their own unresolved *samskaras* for everyone to witness. Certain opportunists from outside the Ashtanga system have capitalized on this mess and encouraged the performers to deepen the drama of their performances. I have felt both entertained and embarrassed for these social media circus acts over the last year or two. Other people have left the organization in quieter and more respectful ways. The most unpalatable aspect of the entire spectacle for me has been the number of people who have jumped onto the bandwagon of blatant social media virtue signaling, as a means to promote their own self-interest.

The positivity of our experience in the new shala with Sharathji over the past two months has solidified my perception that what has occurred has been a very healthy process of weeding out those who are no longer benefiting from, nor wish to continue to engage in the practice of Ashtanga Yoga in the way that Sharathji teaches it. I wish all of the people who have weeded themselves out the very best, and I hope that they can find a healthy and fruitful way to engage with themselves and with their lives which makes it irrelevant for them to criticize those of us who still very much enjoy and benefit from our practice and especially from our relationship with our teacher, Sharath Jois.

The above is all I wish to publicly say about recent controversies. I request those who hold a different opinion from my own to refrain from attempting to engage with me on this subject. This is not because I wish to exist in an echo chamber. I am well aware of all of the issues and accusations, and my own opinions are well developed and considered in light of all of the information that has been shared. I am comfortable and happy in my own relationship with the Ashtanga practice, and my relationship with my teacher, Sharath Jois, and with my students. I simply don't wish to devote any of my time and energy to debating with those who hold a different opinion from my own, and who are unable to move forward from the quagmire of their own *samskaras*. There are issues and problems facing the human race and the entirety of life on the planet earth which are of far greater magnitude and importance than the internal politics of the Ashtanga system of yoga practice.

To sum up this section of my reflections on the past two months: The evolution of practice with Sharath Jois in Mysore feels very positive to me, and seemingly to most of the students who were there in October and November. We all enjoyed and benefited from practice in the new shala very much and it was a privilege to practice with a group of 300 people who were all grateful for the opportunity to be present at the inauguration of the new shala and to benefit from Sharathji's teaching.

Part of the positivity I experienced on this trip came from the development in my personal practice. I've written about some of the struggles that I experienced in my personal practice on my first two trips of practice with Sharathji, as well as the insights and benefits that I gleaned from working through those struggles. The subsequent three trips have been much smoother on a practice level, and the sense of ease in my asana practice at the shala culminated in this fifth trip. I feel that Sharathji and I have learned a lot about each other, in spite of the fact that we rarely exchange words, and we understand how to work with each other effectively and with mutual respect. The evolution of this relationship is a major factor in my increased sense of ease and progression in my asana practice under

Sharathji's guidance.

I began this trip on *Koundinyasana*, which is about halfway through the arm balance section of Third series. My only major stumbling point in my previous trip was *Eka Pada Bakasana A*, which is the most difficult arm balance and one of the weakest links in my Third series practice. Sharathji demanded that I develop the ability to lift the foot of the bent leg up higher and that I straighten the arms in the posture. These expectations required me to study and rework the entire posture from the ground up, which I did in part by watching YouTube videos of the few advanced practitioners who are able to execute this posture adeptly (thanks to those who have shared their practice of this posture in this way). I was stuck on *Eka Pada Bakasana A* for a few weeks on the previous trip. Once I had worked out how to do the posture in line with Sharathji's standards, he moved me forward with a few more postures at the end of the trip.

I continued to develop my *Eka Pada Bakasana A* in my home practice over the past year and was happy to experience continued progress in it. On the first day of Third series practice on this most recent trip, I think I heard Sharathji make an approving comment from somewhere nearby while I was executing the posture.

A large part of my asana development with Sharathji over five trips can be summed up by the following general description: I consider the full manifestation of Difficult Asana X to be beyond my physical capabilities due to structural limitations in my body. When I reach Difficult Asana X in my practice with Sharathji, he points out that he wants me to be able to do it anyway. He then leaves me to work it out myself. I grumble and moan about it for a few days, and then put my head down and attempt to figure it out. With persistence and effort, I eventually manage to improve my ability to manifest the full version of the posture, and then feel happy about having attained something which I had previously considered impossible. Due to the conscious engaging with, and eventual transformation of my most challenging structural limitations, the positive effects of having attained Difficult Posture X reverberate to deeper layers of my being for a significant period of time afterwards. My overall understanding of the dynamics of how the practice works on the human organism deepens as a result. There aren't any other teachers out there who would force me to encounter these blind spots within myself through the necessity of encountering Difficult Posture X, and I wouldn't have the willpower or motivation to do it on my own without it being made a requirement by a teacher. This is one of the main reasons that I return to practice with Sharathji each year.

My focus for this trip was the intimidating Third series posture *Gandha Berundasana*. After returning home at the end of the previous trip, I realized that if Sharathji continued to give me new postures at the standard pace he has developed with me, I would probably reach *Gandha Berundasana* at the end of this trip. *Gandha* is a physically challenging posture, but it is the psychological intimidation which makes it the most difficult posture in the series for me.

I first learned *Gandha Berundasana* more than a decade ago with my former teacher, Rolf. At that time, I did not have the ability to attain the final stage of the posture on my own, so my teacher would put me into the posture every day, by holding my legs for me while I brought my arms around to catch them. I practiced *Gandha Berundasana* with Rolf in this way for several trips over a period of a few years, but I never cultivated the ability to practice it on my own, at home. Without assistance, I would find it too intimidating, and eventually left it out of my practice altogether. At the end of my previous trip with Sharathji, in August 2018, I hadn't attempted to practice *Gandha Berundasana* since my last trip with Rolf, which was in 2013. I realized that I would have to re-encounter the posture soon enough in my practice with Sharathji and I wondered what his expectations would be for it. Few people develop the ability to do the full version of it, and some do get moved past the posture without having attained the ability to catch the feet without assistance.

Sharathji has always set very high standards for me, and I realized that *Gandha Berundasana* would be no exception. *Gandha Berundasana* thus became my Difficult Posture X for 2018/2019. I began to work on it at home in earnest, not really expecting to attain the final version of the posture on my own, but hoping to at least gain some experiential familiarity with it before I had to attempt it in Mysore. I surprised myself by cultivating the ability to bring my left arm forward and to catch my left foot with my hand within a few weeks of commencing my daily attempts. Bringing the second arm forward was a completely different story. Once the second arm comes forward, the psychological vulnerability comes into play, as the entire body is then in an extremely compromised position, with all of the weight of the body being born on the upper chest and chin. If the posture is done incorrectly, the breath can be completely cut off and blacking out is a possibility. This happened to me once when I was practicing it with Rolf, and I have heard of other practitioners who had a similar experience. Not wanting to repeat this sort of experience added to the intimidation factor for me.

It took me at least another month to gain the courage and skill to bring the second arm forward. The breakthrough came when I watched a few YouTube videos of advanced practitioners who can do the posture well (thanks again to those who shared…) Sharathji's own technique of bringing the second arm forward very quickly appealed to me the most when I watched his Third series practice video, so I decided to apply this method in my practice the following morning. When the moment came to try, I whipped my second arm around, and was happy to find that it worked—for a moment. In the next moment, I lost my balance and fell sideways out of the posture, which is quite dangerous considering the compromised position and weight distribution of the body and neck.

Fortunately, I didn't injure my neck in the fall, but I did land heavily and uncontrolled on one foot and bruised a toe, which resulted in the necessity of modifying my practice for a few days afterwards.

Once a particular physical movement is completed for the first time, it sticks in the cellular memory of the body, and one is much more likely to be able to complete the movement again on subsequent attempts. From the next morning onward, I was able to bring the second arm forward every day, with greater control and no sense of risk of falling.

The final step, of catching the right foot with my right hand took the longest for me to attain. After bringing the right arm forward, the right foot still hovered what seemed like a vast distance from my hand. Due to the intensity of the stimulation of the nerves in the compromised position, I didn't feel I could stay there very long and there wasn't much progress in either lifting the hand up or bringing the foot down. I remained stuck at this stage for at least a month or two. Eventually, my comfort in that particular stage of the process increased and I made some progress by playing around with how I shifted my weight on my chest. I learned that I was allowing my weight to fall back too far. This helped with the sense of comfort and balance, but to bring my right foot down, I had to allow my weight to tilt more forward. I also learned that by pulling my left foot closer to the ground with my hand and then more forward and away from my head, the weight of my entire body could shift more forward, and subsequently, more arch would become possible in the right hip and leg. I also began to cultivate the ability to move my right arm and shoulder more freely by focusing on deepening the mobility of the shoulders in twists like *Bharadvajasana*, *Supta Urdhva Pada Vajrasana* and *Viranchyasana B*. Increasing the mobility of the shoulder and chest in these postures felt very similar to what was required to move the shoulder and arm more freely in *Gandha Berundasana*.

Finally, about 3 or 4 months after I began to work on *Gandha Berun-*

dasana, my right hand caught the right foot, and I had completed the posture. For the next week, I was able to complete the posture each time I attempted it. I then had a scheduled trip to Canada, which is a long and exhausting journey from Bali, to visit my family for a month. I was surprised to find that my ability to complete the full posture hadn't been lost in the 30 hours of air travel and arrival in sub-zero early spring weather. I retained the ability to complete the posture fully for the following three weeks in Canada, but then I suddenly lost the ability in my final week in my home country. The series of return flights to Bali was tougher physiologically than the flights to Canada were, and I arrived feeling stiff and exhausted. When my physical condition did not open back up very much after a few days of settling in, it became clear that I was entering into a "pull back and integration phase," which often follows a period of deeper opening. After more than 15 years of daily Ashtanga practice, one becomes accustomed to the dynamics of the cycles of structural shifting and integration.

When one enters into a phase of tightening up, as the structural intelligence of the body integrates the deeper changes that have begun to manifest, it is good to respect the process by letting go of any attachment one may have felt to the achievements and feelings of the open state, and to work intelligently with the new reality of the body as it manifests each day. In this case, I continued to practice only Intermediate series for much longer than I usually would after a period of travel. Intermediate felt like enough of a struggle and Third series felt completely unpalatable. A few weeks later, I began to work back into what had been my regular practice of the preceding six months, which was all of Intermediate and Third series up to *Gandha Berundasana*. Once I started working on *Gandha* again, I was back to ground zero, and I had to repeat the entire process of learning the posture step by step as I had done six months earlier. It took another three months of patient daily application to arrive back at the stage where

I was catching both of my feet and completing the posture. By this point, it was June or July, and I had two or three months of being able to execute the posture fully again before my trip to Mysore in October.

The three months of practice at home before my Mysore trip were quite strong. A deeper phase of structural change and integration was taking place and I had been maintaining a long daily practice of nearly two full series on three of my practice days per week for over one year. The opening and strengthening felt good, but there were also the inevitable transient aches that come with deeper integration, such pains in the ribs (especially on the right side) and shoulders. The right side of my body had changed significantly from the process of teaching myself how to catch the feet in *Gandha*. I was a little bit concerned that I might experience another "pull back" or burnout once I reached Mysore, but fortunately this did not happen at all. In fact, my practice in Mysore became much easier than it had been at home, and all the little aches disappeared completely within my first two weeks of practice in Mysore. Starting practice at 4:45 a.m. in Mysore means I get to sleep in a few hours longer than I do at home, and being able to go home after practice and relax, instead of going to teach for several hours probably contributed to the increased ease that I felt my practice in Mysore. I felt strong, open and vibrant right from day one in the new shala.

After the customary first few days of Primary and then Intermediate series practice, I started my full practice in the second week. Sharathji began giving me new postures right away, and also helped me with catching at the end of backbending a little more frequently than he had in previous trips. For most of the trip, he did catching with me at least 3 days per week, leaving the assistants to do it only occasionally. Deepening my catching became the focus of the trip and my interactions with him. The postures of Third series that he added to my practice each week seemed to be superfluous, and he rarely even watched me perform them before giving me the next ones, but catching my legs seemed to be something he was adamant about deepening with me.

Catching has never been easy for me. My previous teacher did not do it very often with me because his wife was strongly opposed to the procedure altogether. So, when I began practice with Sharathji in 2014, I had only rudimentary experience with catching. Catching is a big focus in Mysore, as those who have practiced with Sharathji know. Over the five trips, I developed in catching significantly. I went from catching my ankles and lower calves on the first trip, to regularly being able to catch just below my knees, and being able to stand and straighten my legs on my own by the time I was at the end of my third trip. A few times on my third and fourth trip, Sharathji adjusted my fingers right up onto my kneecaps, which was terrifying. The first time I was successful in holding my kneecaps was towards the end of my third trip when we did catching at the end of led Intermediate. Sharathji was accustomed to me bailing out of the posture pretty quickly when he moved my hands higher up, so this time when he put my hands on my kneecaps he loudly commanded, "Now STAY! Everyone is watching." It worked, and I managed to balance holding my kneecaps for a good 5–10 breaths on that day. Each new stage of development in catching has always felt very healthy for me structurally, and no one is better at adjusting this posture than Sharathji.

Holding the kneecaps was a rarity in my third and fourth trips, and usually he left me at the standard holding place of just below the knees. This trip was different. By the middle of the second week, he was already bringing my hands onto my kneecaps. The first time he did it, I didn't feel ready, and I bailed out. We smiled at each other when I came up and he asked, "Why? It came so nicely today." As he pressed me in *Paschimottanasana*, he jovially inquired, "Why you fear so much?" The next day he tried again and this time I disregarded my habitual fear reaction and I managed to stay and hold my kneecaps. Sharathji is correct about the fear. Once I let go of the fear reaction and try my best to work with the adjustment, I experience the reality that there is nothing physiological which prevents me from being capable of it. It is the aversion to the intense feeling in the nervous system that drives me to avoid it. This is the wisdom of a teacher like Sharathji, who can see exactly what one is capable of, and expects one to encounter whatever *samskaras* are preventing one from achieving one's full potential.

From the second week onward, catching the knees became the standard each time that Sharathji did it with me. As with each of the previous stages of catching, the more often I did it, the easier it was to become comfortable and to stay there. Sharathji is also adamant about squeezing my elbows inwards while holding my legs. It always feels great on my spine and shoulders and being adjusted skillfully into catching is truly the best way to end the practice. For most of this trip, I was finishing after a long sequence of apanic postures, and the deep catching was a wonderful counter posture to end with.

It soon became clear that the focus on catching was preparing me for the deep backbending in *Viparita Salabhasana* and *Gandha Berundasana*, which were soon to come. This is another aspect of Sharathji's teaching that I admire. He isn't interested in simply adjusting postures. He teaches according to a long-term plan that he makes for each student, given the amount of time the student is spending with him on any particular trip. He is also aware of whether he will see a student again on a subsequent trip or not. He knew that he was going to take me up to *Gandha* on this trip, and his focus for the weeks before that happened was not so much on the other Third series postures that he was giving me, but on cultivating the necessary depth in my backbending for me to be able to perform *Gandha* well.

There were very few backbends in my practice for most of the trip. After the backbending sequence at the beginning of Intermediate series, the subsequent two thirds of Intermediate series, and then the first two thirds of Third series are all apanic postures, featuring mainly leg behind the head variations and arm balances. In order to help myself in the process of going deeper into catching at the end of this long apanic sequence of postures, I focused strongly on pulling my sacrum and tailbone deep into my body with each and every upward facing dog posture that I did in my practice. It was a nice meditative thread to sustain, and the degree of mobility I could cultivate in the sacrum and tailbone would be a good yardstick to measure how I would feel in backbending at the end of my practice. As long as I could feel a natural ease in the mobility of my sacrum and tailbone in my upward facing dogs, I knew it would be no problem to straighten my legs and move deeper into catching at the end of the practice.

Sharathji added the two *Viparita Dandasana* variations, which are the first backbends of Third series, near the beginning of my second month of practice. It was a relief to have this extra preparation for catching after stopping on the *Viranchyasana* postures for the preceding week or two. As soon as *Viparita Dandasana* was added to my practice, Sharathji upped the ante for catching. After bringing my hands to the customary position at the bottom of the knees, and then waiting for me to straighten my legs, instead of bringing my hands onto my kneecaps—as I had grown accustomed to in the preceding weeks—he brought my hands entirely above my knees, so that all of my fingers were on my thighs. After the first hand was moved into position, my mind reacted with a familiar "You've got to be kidding! No way!" sort of revolt, but having grown accustomed to pushing my limits over the preceding weeks of practice with Sharathji, I was able to remain fairly calm and was shocked to find that it was physically possible. After the second hand was brought into position, I was able to remain there for a few breaths, though my balance was shaky, and Sharathji had to keep his hands on my hips to steady me. When I came out of the posture, I had a unique and interesting experience. I felt like something "snapped" energetically somewhere deep inside me. There was no physical pain or discomfort, but my entire body felt like it was made of rubber. The structural tension that I was accustomed to feeling in my relationship with gravity had been completely shifted and I felt loose and untethered. Although it wasn't a painful feeling, it was mildly disturbing to have the foundation and base of my relationship with gravity suddenly vanish, as if a rug had been pulled out from under my feet. I walked over to the finishing area with wobbly rubber limbs. By the time I was done with finishing postures I felt relatively normal, and the wobbly feeling was replaced with the familiar pleasant feeling of deeper structural opening.

I felt relatively "normal" in the next morning's practice, but I was not surprised to find that I couldn't lift out of *Karandavasana*. In my previous trip, I had also found that deepening my catching had inhibited my ability to lift out of *Karandavasana*. This is natural, because catching and *Karandavasana* are polar opposites in their physiological and energetic patterning. On this trip, it was only that particular morning where I could not do it. By the following morning, the changes had been sufficiently integrated and I could once again lift up out of *Karandavasana*. From then onward, catching with my hands completely above the kneecaps became the standard when Sharathji did catching with me. I no longer experienced the wobbly rubber man effect after the first time.

Interestingly, he kept me on *Viparita Dandasana* for two weeks, which was the longest stretch of this trip that I did not receive new postures. In the second last week of the trip, he added *Viparita Salabhasana* and *Gandha Berundasana*. On the day he gave me those postures, I had already finished *Viparita Dandasana* and all of the finishing backbendings. I had done three backbends on the ground, three drop backs, three "tic toks" and I was in the middle of executing *Vrischkasana*, when I heard him say, "Tsk tsk… what did you do?" I knew he was talking to me, even though I couldn't move my head to see him from the compromised position that

I was in. I came down and looked at him and he asked me again what I did. "*Viparita Dandasana*," I replied.

"Show me *B*," he said. Having already done all of Intermediate series, three quarters of Third series, and the entire backbending sequence, I was shaky and exhausted. But it was easy enough to pop back into *Viparita Dandasana B*. Afterwards, I looked up and Sharathji was nowhere to be seen. I knelt on my mat for a few seconds, unsure of what to do, and then I saw him walking back towards me. "Show me," he repeated. So, I did *Viparita Dandasana B* for the third time of the morning. When I finished, he said "*Viparita Salabhasana*."

Though my focus for the past year had been *Gandha Berundasana*, and I consider it much more psychologically intimidating than the posture that precedes it, *Viparita Salabhasana* is more difficult for me in terms of flexibility. Though I had managed to teach myself how to catch the legs in *Gandha Berundasana*, I hadn't developed the mobility to touch my feet onto my head in *Viparita Salabhasana*. *Viparita Salabhasana* requires a different kind of movement than *Gandha*, and this movement has always been very difficult for me. The posture is less psychologically intimidating due to having the support of the arms behind the body, but I feel like it does require more flexibility in the spine and hips. *Gandha* is a more complex combination of flexibility, balance, coordination and courage.

All of the extra backbendings that I had done that morning was exhausting, but it was a blessing because, along with the sustained preparation of all the deep catching over the preceding six weeks, it created the conditions where I couldn't have possibly been more prepared to attempt one of my most difficult postures than I was in that moment. Whether Sharathji had made me do the extra repetitions of *Viparita Dandasana* and the whole backbending sequence first on purpose, or whether it was just a fluke is unknown, but he certainly did have a plan to prepare me for this by relentlessly pushing my limits in catching over the preceding six weeks.

Not surprisingly, it was the easiest and deepest *Viparita Salabhasana* that I have ever done. As I began to work my way into the posture for the first time in two months, I found entirely new qualities and degrees of movement. I was shocked to find my feet plant themselves on my head, with my toes in my eyes. Sharathji had been watching me intently, and demanded, "heels together!" I lifted my feet a bit, pressed my heels together and drew my knees in, and was then able to reposition my feet on my head again. After I jumped back to *Chaturanga*, I looked at him, and he silently made the motion of moving his arms around as a signal for me to attempt *Gandha Berundasana*. I made my way into the posture and caught the first foot fairly easily. "Catch the other foot quickly!" he demanded. I was accustomed to taking a few breaths while I gathered my courage before bringing the second arm around. He repeated his demand: "Catch it quickly!" I brought the second arm around and managed to grab my foot immediately. As soon as I had caught my second foot, I saw him turn around and silently walk away. I then did the closing backbending sequence for a second time, to complete what was probably the strongest morning of practice that I had ever had with Sharathji.

A key feature of Sharathji's style of teaching the Ashtanga system, is to ensure that the foundations are properly and deeply developed, so that the subsequent postures are much more likely to be easily attained. When I had first learned *Gandha* with my former teacher, I did not have enough foundational development to be able to accomplish the posture, and even when he helped me do it, the intensity of the experience was overwhelming. This is why I had dropped it altogether in the interim years before practicing it with Sharathji. The depth of Sharathji's understanding of how the system will work on each individual person, is that he is able to prepare you for what is to come, and he feels no hurry, allowing the preparations to take root over time. The five years that he focused intently on catching and backbending in general with me, the preceding one year that I had personally placed so much emphasis on cultivating *Gandha* in my own home practice, the six weeks of this trip where he was having me catch my legs much deeper than I ever had before, and finally, all the extra backbending preparation (whether it was accidental or not) on the day I did it, led to the moments of finally practicing *Viparita Salabhasana* and *Gandha Berundasana* in the shala to be an almost effortless anticlimax. There were times where I had imagined what practicing these postures in the shala with Sharathji would be like, and I never anticipated it would be anything less than extremely intense. In the end, because of the cumulative preparatory work that had been done, there was no struggle or special emphasis, aside from the fact that Sharathji watched me do them intently that first time.

The only downside to my first day of practicing *Viparita Salabhasana* and *Gandha Berundasana* in the shala was that I injured my toe jumping back from *Viparita Salabhasana*. A confluence of factors contributed to the injury: The fact that I was fatigued from all the extra backbending on that day; the fact that I had not practiced the posture for two months; the fact that I was much deeper into the posture than I had ever been before and due to the unfamiliarity of the increased bend in my body, I had less of the strength and control I was accustomed to experiencing in the jumping back to *Chaturanga*. The transition from *Viparita Salabhasana* to *Chaturanga Dandasana* is always a bit tricky and usually involves a harder landing than in most transitions. On this occasion, I landed extra hard in *Chaturanga*. It didn't seem like an injury at first, I simply had a feeling of: "Oh! That was a bit hard on my toes," but no pain seemed to linger as I carried on with *Gandha Berundasana*, backbending and finishing. When I got up from relaxation, however, my toe had begun to swell and feel painful and I figured it would be sore for a day or two. Throughout the day the swelling increased dramatically, spread to half of the foot, and the toe itself cycled through most of the colors of the rainbow. I went to a homeopathic doctor around noon and got some arnica cream and pills, and figured I'd have to modify my practice for a few days, as I had when I had fallen out of *Gandha* and hurt my toe in my learning process at home. It turned out to be more serious than I anticipated, and for the remainder of that week, I was not able to place any weight on my left foot at all while jumping forward or back and had to modify the postures which required me to bear all of my weight on one foot. I still managed to maintain the intensity of my full practice jumping with one leg and it didn't dampen my mood at all. I even managed to continue my daily 5 km walks around Kukkarahali Lake, albeit at a greatly reduced pace and with a pronounced limp for the subsequent week. After a few days, the swelling began to subside somewhat, the color began to normalize and I began to be able to bear more weight on the foot and needed to modify less. It's been slow healing, though. At the time of writing, it has been more than one month since the injury and the base of the toe is still quite swollen, though my movements are 95 percent back to normal. I still avoid landing on it in the most difficult transitions.

I didn't expect to be moved past *Gandha Berundasana* on this trip. From what I understood, Sharathji usually likes to keep people on that posture, with a marathon practice of all of Intermediate and three quarters of Third series for at least one whole cycle between trips. I was surprised when he told me to half-split Intermediate the following day. From then onward I would only do either the first or second half of Intermediate, on alternating days, before doing all of Third series. Even with the added strain of my toe injury, the shortened practice felt rejuvenating and invigorating. I was even more surprised the day after that when he told me to add *Hanumanasana* the following week, which was the final week of the two-month trip. He added a few more postures in that final week, and I ended the trip on *Digasana*, which is only four postures away from the end of Third series.

The trip ended quite fittingly with the deepest and most stable catching I had done so far. As had become the standard in those final weeks, he placed my hands on my thighs, above my kneecaps, and I was able to stand quite steadily, draw my elbows inwards, and remain stable for a good 10 breath. "Last day," he smiled, as I came up. "Thank you!" I replied.

The trip felt like a maturation of all of the work I have done with Sharathji over the preceding trips. It was my favorite trip, and the smoothest one I have had. One final reflection to share about this experience is that at age 44, I feel that I am still making deep progress in my practice on all levels, including strength, flexibility and stability. I hear a number of longer-term practitioners talk about how they are "feeling their age" and that something is lost when they reach their late thirties and forties. I have not experienced this at all. I also "feel my age," but this is not a negative or detrimental feeling when it comes to my *asana* practice. I do feel that a certain… vigor… has declined over the past decade or so, but other important factors, like concentration, stability, and overall maturity have increased over the same time period, and the net effect of the increase in these positive qualities far outweighs the decline in vigor. Overall, my practice feels orders of magnitude stronger and more open than it ever has. Vigor carries immaturity and recklessness with it, and this leads to many pitfalls. I don't miss that, most of the time. The "sthira bhaga" (steady strength) that has come with aging is something I value more than immature vigor, and this is why I continue to make deep progress in my *asana* practice.

I feel that lifestyle factors have a major influence on the sense of wellbeing or lack thereof in the fourth and fifth decades of life and beyond. I can understand how teachers in their forties and fifties who live a lifestyle of constant travel, consume a less than ideal diet and add excessive strain to their bodies through engaging in frequent *asana* displays (outside of their usual practice routine) for Instagram and YouTube would feel the negative effects of aging on their *asana* practice much more readily than I do. Anyone who leads a busy, high stress lifestyle is more susceptible to a sense of decline as age increases.

Stability in my life, which includes traveling as infrequently as possible, has become increasingly important for me over the past decade. The subtleties of structural transformation and integration require a stable background in order to manifest in a way that is healthy and assimilable. I love the feeling of landing back at home in Bali after traveling and realizing that I won't have to move for the next six to nine months. This is when I feel I can really settle into myself and sink deeply into the intricacies of my practice. It is one of the main reasons that I almost always decline invitations to teach workshops in other places. There are other reasons that I don't enjoy short-term teaching gigs in new places, but the disruption to my own lifestyle and my own practice is first and foremost.

It boils down to a question of emphasis. I prioritize my personal practice and I still enjoy engaging in a longer and intensive daily practice. I work my teaching habits around that emphasis. I still practice one and a half to two full series on three or four of my six practice days per week. I completed Fourth series with Rolf Naujokat in 2013, but since I started practicing with Sharathji in 2014, I've chosen to mainly focus on what I am practicing with him in my personal practice at home. Usually, in between trips to Mysore, I practice what I think Sharathji will give me in the shala on my subsequent trip. That means that over the past year, at home, I maintained a daily practice of all of Intermediate, and Third series up to *Gandha Berundasana* on at least 3 days of the week. For the other 3 practice days, I practiced one series—one day each for Primary, Intermediate and Third. There is no possibility that I could have sustained this kind of practice if I was traveling around and teaching in different places, or if I was engaging in additional display sessions for Instagram and YouTube. Maintaining a high level of depth and intensity in personal practice before teaching for several hours each morning requires being grounded in one place, and cultivating a disciplined, regular lifestyle and diet. I enjoy this form of asceticism.

From where Sharathji left me at the end of this trip, I will probably start to work back into Fourth series in my home practice over the next year. I look forward to this, it should be interesting to revisit Fourth series, after all of the changes that have manifested from my practice with Sharathji in the years since I last practiced Fourth regularly.

I feel that diet is also extremely important in maintaining a high physical and energetic level into my forties. Diet is a vast subject, which is far beyond the scope of this already lengthy piece.

In brief, I eat a vegan diet, based on nutrient dense whole foods with approximately 50/50 ratio of raw and cooked food. I avoid all processed foods, most common allergens, most forms of sugar (including "natural" sugar) and most kinds of fermented food. I rarely consume heavy pulses or nuts. I consume moderate, but not excessive, amounts of starchy grains and vegetables. I consume a moderate, but not excessive, amount of fruits. The most important and prominent components of my diet are fresh fibrous vegetables, lighter legumes, "pseudograins" and seeds. My diet tends to be alkaline overall. Brendan Brazier's *Thrive Diet* is the published dietary system which is closest to my own. Brendan has written several books about his Thrive Diet, and I feel it is conducive to deep yoga practice.

I feel that it is also important for Ashtanga practitioners, and especially teachers, to monitor the effects of the quantity of food that they eat. Most people are aware that overeating is detrimental to progress in the practice, but undereating, or following an overly restrictive diet, will also lead to weakness and inhibit muscle recovery. Undereating over a long period of time will certainly contribute to a sense of decline as one ages.

Appropriate quantity and timing of food are highly individual and dependent on one's personal constitution. I have a very rapid metabolic rate and need to eat a high quantity of the right kinds of food in order to sustain my high level of physical and mental activity. I never skip dinner, and I would rather eat dinner too late than not at all. My last meal of the day is typically around 6–6:30 p.m., and I begin my practice around 2 a.m. I finish my practice at 4 a.m., and take a long relaxation until 4:30 a.m. I then have two hours before I start teaching at 6:30 a.m. Those two hours are dedicated to preparing a calorie-dense and nourishing breakfast — typically buckwheat porridge (or raw dehydrated buckwheat granola when I can get it), with lots of nutrient dense toppings and a fruit and herb smoothie, followed by a nuclear-strength coffee. I then shower and drive to class.

Many Ashtanga teachers don't leave any time gap between the end of their personal practice and the beginning of teaching. Their first meal of the day doesn't occur until after teaching, when they have already engaged in 4 to 6 hours of heavy physical and mental work. I believe that this lifestyle will weaken and deplete a person if sustained over a long period of time. I have witnessed older Ashtanga teachers become weaker and unhealthy due to this lack of self-care. Many give up regular Mysore-style teaching because of it. Paying more attention to diet — especially in the important junction between practice and teaching — is a way to prevent this.

I use a lot of herbal and whole food supplements, and this experimentation becomes increasingly important as my age increases. I focus on three categories of herbal supplements — anti-inflammatory, adaptogen and tonic strengtheners. My favorite anti-inflammatory foods include cissus triangularis, varieties of the ginger family and turmeric. In the adaptogen category, ginseng, maca and shilajit are my favorites. For tonic strengtheners, muira puama, Thai black ginger and tribulus terrestris are the most effective for me. When I am consuming any of these strengthening herbs on a regular basis, there is a tangible increase in strength and stamina that runs through my entire practice. Many powerful herbs and foods overlap between the three above-mentioned categories. I also include a high quality vegan protein powder on a daily basis, blended into a smoothie with homemade coconut cream, bananas, coconut water, and a few of the above-mentioned herbs. Vega Sport Performance Protein (formulated by Brendan Brazier) is the best one available on the market. One needs to be careful with protein supplements, as many contain inferior sources of protein and contain filler ingredients which can upset the digestive system and increase inflammation in the body. Whey protein in particular should be completely avoided. On this most recent trip to Mysore, I also began to experiment with adding pure L-glutamine powder in several doses throughout the day. This seemed to have a positive effect overall. I am currently experimenting with L-arginine, and 2:1:1 BCAA powders as well. These amino acids are also found in any good quality protein powder supplement, as well as in a healthy regular vegan diet. I have found that adding additional supplementation is quite useful for supporting a 2-to-3-hour advanced daily Ashtanga practice. There is much, much more I could say about diet and supplementation, but I will save all of that for its own dedicated discussion in another time.

It should also be noted that the aging process is undoubtedly different for men and for women. I think much of what I have written above applies generally to both sexes, but the intricacies of the different hormonal changes would certainly lead to different experiences and probably to different foods and herbs that would be most helpful. As always, one's own phenomenal experience is the best teacher.

A final factor that I attribute to helping maintain my strong *asana* practice is my daily pranayama practice. I've been practicing pranayama for nearly as long as I have been practicing *asana*. My current pranayama routine was taught to me over a 5 year period by Rolf Naujokat approximately 10 years ago, and according to him, it is the pranayama sequence that K. Pattabhi Jois taught to his advanced students in the 1990s. The entire sequence takes about 45 minutes to complete, and I usually do it in the late morning or early afternoon. It has a powerful rejuvenative influence and it brings immense depth and subtlety to the cultivation of breath and internal form in the *asana* practice itself. It is said that pranayama practice becomes stronger with age, and I can attest to that. For me, it works hand in hand with the *asana* practice, and the two are part and parcel of a single process of self-cultivation.

In summary, my fifth trip of practice with Sharath Jois was my best trip so far. I enjoyed practice in the new shala immensely, and my own *asana* practice has never felt better. I am deeply grateful for the influence and guidance of Sharathji on the evolution of my practice, and my respect for him as a teacher and as a person grows with each trip. I look forward to the months ahead of continued self-exploration in my practice, in the dark, damp early morning hours at home in Bali, and I look forward to my next trip with Sharathji in Mysore.

ANSWERS TO QUESTIONS

❧ On diet; more specifically on fungus, mold, or cultured/fermented foods, yeasts, etc., and soy products

I've never been very tolerant of fungus, mold, or cultured/fermented foods, yeasts, etc. I used to have quite a bit of trouble with Candida overgrowth and many fermented foods tend to stimulate those symptoms for me. I rarely eat mushrooms and avoid overripe fruit for the same reason. I do use powdered extracts of reishi, cordyceps and lion's mane, and they don't give me any issues in this form. Once in a while I cook some fresh mushrooms in pasta, but if the mushrooms are even slightly old, I will feel bad the next day. I know a lot of people find benefit in fermented foods, but for the most part, they are not good for me. Even the smell of kombucha makes me want to vomit. There is a very good Ayurvedic doctor in Panaji, Goa, that I used to visit regularly when I was practicing with Rolf and having chronic digestive issues. He always told me to avoid fermented foods, which confirmed what I already intuitively felt. I can tolerate, and do enjoy some of these kinds of foods in small doses, on occasion, but definitely not regularly.

Regarding soy, it is a common allergen, and I don't consume very much of it. I do enjoy fresh tofu in moderation—once or twice a week. Tofu quality varies. Fortunately, here in Bali we do have access to nice, fresh tofu. Tofu is definitely a strengthening food and it contains a lot of arginine, one of the amino acids that I mentioned I also supplement with. Tempeh is out of the question for me. I can't even stand the smell of it cooking. I don't prepare miso myself, but on occasion when I have it, I do enjoy it. I also like fresh edamame once in a while. I don't ever use soy milk, as there are better alternatives for that sort of thing. So, I do consume moderate amounts of soy products. Many new vegetarians and vegans tend to rely on soy products as the backbone of their diet, which I think is less than ideal.

❧ On developing your own lifestyle

My current lifestyle had been gradually developed over the past 20 years. Step by step, I have arrived at where I am today. The changes were small and incremental, and time was taken to adapt to each stage. I didn't start out with a "master plan" or ideal lifestyle that I wanted to emulate, I simply made changes as I felt they were necessary, to support the ongoing process of evolution in practice and teaching. I think making an abrupt shift from a "normal" lifestyle to something like the lifestyle that I live today would be too much of a shock to the entire system to be sustainable for anyone. So, I don't recommend that anyone try to "copy" what I do, but if it provides "food for thought," and inspires natural lifestyle exploration, that is great.

My need for sleep is certainly less than it was 15 or 20 years ago, and less than the average person. I typically am in bed for 4–5 hours on days I am teaching. I also take a 30-minute-long rest at the end of my practice, which ends up being something that I would classify as "Yoga Nidra," and I usually have a 30–60-minute "Yoga Nidra B" in the late morning, after all my teaching work is finished. This rest is also taken in the traditional "*Savasana*" position, which I find provides a much deeper rest. I am in a deeply embodied and focused state when I take these two "naps," which also brings more restfulness than normal sleep. This sleep schedule gives me plenty of rest to do what I want to do with my life. I can even miss the second *Yoga Nidra* from time to time if necessary. Once a week, I like to get a longer sleep of 7–9 hours, on the night before the day I don't teach. I find that being mildly "sleep deprived" puts one into a bit of an edgier state, which can be worked to one's advantage, if one is able to work with the sensations and feelings non-reactively. I find it brings a sharpness which can be more useful than the dullness and lethargy that comes from oversleeping.

It isn't possible to pinpoint one aspect of practice which brings about the need for less sleep. It is a synergistic effect of all the elements of practice and diet together. One key theme would be equanimity or non-reactivity. I have devoted a lot of time and energy to cultivating this quality through my Buddhist practices, and "Sampajanna" is the thread that links all of my practices together. Reactivity is the biggest energy drain of all, and training oneself to let go of reactive patterns is the biggest aid to increased energy, in my experience. So, asana, pranayama, meditation, diet, all linked together by the thread of Sampajanna is the main element leading to decreased need for sleep.

Regarding whether getting up shortly after midnight and practicing at 2 a.m. is "unnatural"... I would say it depends on how one defines "natural." For me, natural means wild, and the human species has been a domesticated species for tens of thousands of years. Domestication is the opposite of wild, and hence to me, the opposite of "natural." The degree of domestication has increased as civilization has developed, and so I don't think there is anything about the human species that can be considered "natural" in the sense of being wild and instinctual. We are highly conditioned by the culture and society we are born into. That is not necessarily a bad thing, as cultural influence is a part of human nature. But I think this fact makes it very difficult to say what a natural sleeping pattern (or diet, etc.) is, or should be, for a human being.

We are certainly diurnal, not nocturnal, so I think that getting one's main sleep in the dark period of the 24-hour cycle is natural. I do this, as I go to bed shortly after sunset (in most parts of the globe…). The only difference is that I don't sleep the entire night. I have read some interesting theories which suggest that it is more "natural" for humans to sleep in shifts, rather than one big chunk of 7–9 hours. These theories suggest that this is what our ancestors did, up to the time just before the Industrial Revolution. This makes sense to me, as it is the sleeping cycle I have adapted to. It is a challenge because it goes against what most other humans around me are doing, but does feel natural in a way that it is sustainable and feels healthy when I disregard the influence of other humans around me.

One thing that is clear is that human beings are highly adaptable. We can adapt to many different kinds of lifestyle conditions, and if one is sensitive and exploratory, one can learn how to thrive within a varied range of lifestyles and environments. Would I get up that early if I didn't have to teach at 6:30 a.m.? No, I wouldn't. I would say the "ideal" time to begin practice would be 4 or 5 a.m.

✎ On practicing the same sequence every day over a long period of time

When we practice the same sequence of postures and vinyasas every day, over a long period of time, the deeper layers of the structure of the body will shift and change in order to accommodate these movements into the permanent structural framework of the body and nervous system. At times we can feel we are really "opening up" or becoming stronger, more stable, etc. This could be thought of as the first phase of structural change as we assimilate new movements into the structural repertoire of the body. As we continue to practice, those changes take root at a deeper level, and at times the body can elicit a healing response, which can include inflammation, tightness, tiredness, etc., as the deeper elements of ourselves rearrange and reorganize in their relationship to one another. When this happens, we often lose the abilities to perform certain asanas or movements that we had when we felt more open. This is what I mean by the integration phase. The sense of "progress" in the practice is never linear, and any phase when we feel we are making a lot of progress, will almost always be followed by a period when we feel we are regressing. This can feel frustrating, but with long-term practice, one comes to understand that this is part of the process, and if we patiently work through these integration phases, we come out the other side feeling open again, but this time in a way that is more permanent and stable.

THE ROLE OF THINKING IN ASHTANGA YOGA PRACTICE

A conversation with Andy Davis

— January 2020 —

A FEW MONTHS AGO, I engaged in an email discussion with Andy Davis, Associate Professor of Philosophy at Belmont University in Nashville, Tennessee and an Ashtanga practitioner. We explored the subject of thinking during asana practice. Many practitioners hold the erroneous assumption that the goal of yoga and meditation practice is to stop thinking. Andy and I discussed this assumption and some of my alternative viewpoints based on reactivity:

Andy: I'm wondering about the stray thoughts I have during practice. By "stray thoughts," I mean thoughts not directly related to the asana at hand. Yoga teachers often define or describe asana practice in relation to *citta vrtti nirodha [cessation of the fluctuations of consciousness]*, which is the stated goal of Patanjali Yoga. On one understanding of *citta vrtti nirodha*, all my stray thoughts are signs of deficient absorption in what I am doing. But in my experience, sometimes stray thoughts seem to get in the way of practice and sometimes they don't. I'd like to ask you some questions about this.

How would you describe the general relationship between thinking and asana practice? Is practice a form of thinking? Is it opposed to thinking?

Iain: I suppose the answer to this would depend on a precise definition of "thinking." For example, can we consider actions and responses in movements of the physical body as a form of "thought"?

The abstract, disembodied process of mental conceptualizing, which we commonly refer to as "thought," must have gradually developed over time in our Homo sapiens ancestors and our other ancestral species. What were the experiential precursors to the abstracted and disembodied thought processes which characterize much of our lived experience today? Can we still feel these sorts of ancestral precursors to thought at an organic, embodied level, where the boundaries between physiology and psychology become blurred? Can we refer to these phenomena as "thinking"? Can we/should we think in this way during our asana practice?

If you prefer to stick to a definition of thinking as something that is inherently disembodied and abstracted from our phenomenal level of experience, then I suggest that asana practice is a method through which we use a formulaic set of conditions to objectively observe whatever habitual patterns (*samskaras*) tend to manifest within those conditions. If abstract thinking is one of those patterns which arises, then we accept and observe that. So, I wouldn't say asana practice is biased either towards or against this form of thinking.

Andy: One type of abstract thought is what is sometimes called the "inner monologue" or ego-based narration of past and future events. Will Johnson suggests that when we are fully present in our lived, ongoing sensations, the "inner monologue" shuts off completely (*Aligned Relaxed Resilient* pp. 19–20). Should we work to diminish this form of thinking?

Iain: In general, I would say that physical practices which promote embodied concentration within a limited field of awareness will—over a long period of continuous practice—tend to reduce the degree of *unnecessary* *or superfluous* thinking. Having the inner monologue "shut off completely" is a relatively rare phenomenon, which represents a very deep form of concentration that leads into the first stages of *samadhi*. This is unlikely to be experienced by most practitioners—even those who have engaged deeply with their practice for many years. To suggest that this should be the case would be discouraging to the vast majority of people, who are likely experiencing the opposite of this form of "cessation."

Superfluous or unnecessary thought tends to be based on reactivity. The phenomena of having certain thought loops and themes which we revisit again and again—and that we can't let go of—tends to be caused by a deeper reactive pattern (*samskara*) which is playing out on the surface of our conscious awareness. A long-term practitioner should train himself to concentrate on—and ideally become absorbed within—the experience of sensation and feeling in body and breath for the duration of his daily practice. If this absorption within embodied experience is coupled with the intention of objective (non-reactive) awareness, the reactive *samskara* patterns will become weaker, as will the persistence of superfluous or excessive thought.

Is the goal to eliminate thought completely? No. Thought is useful, and essential to function in the human world today. I feel that practice can help us to avoid falling into the trap of reacting to our thoughts, and building those reactions up into grooves and loops which we become trapped in. But I don't feel that practice should be viewed as an attempt to eliminate thought.

Andy: I find your emphasis on reactivity helpful. Instead of performing a classification of thoughts, sorting them into categories of good and bad, helpful or harmful, we might attend to the manner in which we take up the thoughts. An otherwise "good" thought can become obsessive. Even something that begins as embodied awareness can become a reactive loop. Sometimes the concern for alignment in a pose can become a loop that sucks attention away from the lived conditions of the body into an abstract, ideal body. I've certainly aggravated my body by pushing a pose to the place it was yesterday, rather than the place it wants to go to today, using an abstract marker like whether my chin touches here or there on my leg. By contrast, a thought about something very unyogic can arise and dissipate without any problematic reactivity. Does the awareness or observation of a reactive loop as such naturally diminish or dissolve it over time or have you found additional steps necessary?

Iain: The cultivation of equanimity is central to the teaching of the Buddha, and also plays a role in Patanjali's Yoga Sutras. "Upekkha/Upeksha" is the term in Pali/Sanskrit which refers to this quality of non-reactiveness. It does require some degree of effort and awareness to cultivate. In fact, cultivating increased sensitivity without a corresponding emphasis on cultivating equanimity can be detrimental, as reactiveness will naturally tend to increase with sensitivity. Some Ashtanga practitioners become highly sensitized as a result of their embodied concentration in the energetically stimulating practice. This sensitization can lead to emotional and energetic imbalance if they have not cultivated an ability to experience their increased sensitivity in a relatively non-reactive way.

Attempting not to react to a thought is slippery. In the Vipassana meditation technique, it is understood that the locus of sensation/feeling on the body is where reaction actually takes place. We may feel like we are reacting to a thought, or an emotion, or an external object, but what we often fail to realize is that with every experience that we have, there is a corresponding sensation and feeling in the body. *Samskara* is formed through reaction to this sensation/feeling on the body. So, a central part of the Vipassana technique is the conscious attempt to decrease reactivity towards sensation on the body. I apply this technique to all of my practices, including asana and pranayama, and I feel it is extremely important to develop.

For powerful and deeply rooted *samskaras*, it can take months or years of cultivating non-reactivity before we start to feel their power and influence over our lives begin to diminish. With long-term and regular cultivation of increased embodied sensitivity and non-reactivity towards that sensitivity, we should experience that the influence of our *samskaras* gradually diminishes over time.

Andy: Are there kinds of thoughts (or ways of having them) that you have found to be beneficial to asana practice?

Iain: Any thought pattern which arises during asana practice creates the potential for a reactive tendency or *samskara* pattern to manifest. The point of asana practice is to encounter these reactive patterns and become more consciously aware of them, so that we can learn to work with them more effectively. One could argue that *any* thought pattern which arises is beneficial, because it gives us the opportunity to encounter and potentially transform a habit, which is certainly more beneficial than ignoring or repressing it.

The question becomes: What do we *do* once that thought pattern arises in our practice? Do we allow it to distract us from the experience of being absorbed in embodied sensation? Or, can we allow the thought to play itself out in the background with minimal disturbance to our process of embodied absorption in the process of asana? The second option is the field where authentic transformation can take place.

Andy: Are there thoughts (or ways of having them) that you have found to be obstacles to asana practice?

Iain: Being extensively trained in Buddhist practices, I see all practice as a method of observing "reality as it is." Any thoughts which naturally arise during our practice are helpful, as they represent some tendency that we have. In other words, by observing those thoughts which naturally arise, we are observing a natural part of who and what we are—whether we like that part of who and what we are, or not.

What can be contradictory—and even dangerous—to mix with the above-described process are thoughts which are intentionally conjured up, because we feel it may be good for us to try to think in a certain way. If we are "trying to think" certain things, or even "trying not to think at all," then we are not observing ourselves naturally, and we often end up repressing or avoiding what is actually there. We hide the reality as it is with a "suggestion." I consider this to be inauthentic practice. Unfortunately, this process is widely taught and promoted in the name of "spirituality."

Andy: A thought which is natural to me might be forced for you and vice versa. This suggests that teaching yoga is very difficult because the likely result of a specific teaching is that the student will "try" to have a different practice than he naturally has, i.e., he will try to have a practice that looks like the teaching. The problem with "spirituality" you identify also seems to be a problem with teaching more generally. By attending to the teacher's insight rather than our own, we get to avoid ourselves and believe that we have found our true selves at the same time!

Iain: Absolutely. Accepting any form of dogma without having experienced the truth of it ourselves—at the embodied, sensation/feeling based level—is fallacious. I feel the main role of a teacher should be to train people how to experience and feel things for themselves.

Andy: Do you take specific precautions to reduce certain kinds of stimulus or certain kinds of thoughts during asana practice?

Iain: I think it is helpful to practice in a space that is as neutral as possible. A neutral environment will promote concentration and the lack of strong stimulus will promote natural arising of *samskara* patterns which are normally hidden in the deeper layers of our subconscious.

Andy: Can you say a bit more about what you mean by "neutral" here?

Iain: By neutral, I mean attempting to remove stimuli which promote reactivity. For most people, that would mean things such as one's phone, or any external object which will tend to draw one's attention away from being present with embodied breath and sensation. In places like Southeast Asia, it is common to find yoga shalas in stunning beachfront locations. I find this distracting. A shala should be simple, and mostly enclosed by walls. It should be a protective "container" which keeps one's awareness and energy within the room, and ideally within one's own body and breath. Even excessive instruction from or interaction with a teacher can take one's attention away from being present with embodied sensation and breath. A good teacher should also strive to be "neutral" in their presence.

Andy: Have you found that there are separable "stages" of awareness (e.g., like the four *jnanas* of Buddhism or Patanjali's *Dharana-Dhyana-Samadhi*) that one climbs like a ladder as the asana practice deepens?

Iain: Not really. I don't feel that there is a particular end goal to yoga practice and therefore, I don't feel there is any form of linear path to reach a goal. All eight of Patanjali's limbs can and should be experienced together. I don't really consider them to be separate things. They all support and loop back into one another and should not be thought of as sequential or linear. The ability to observe oneself and one's own *samskara* patterns with less reactivity will gradually develop over time, but this manifests within all forms of consciousness and awareness, from the mundane to the sublime.

Andy: Do you have advice for students who find themselves easily distracted by stray thoughts of such a powerful nature that they derail practice or cause them to lose their place in the rhythm of the practice?

Iain: This is the power and beauty of the vinyasa count. If we hold ourselves accountable to "staying with the count," we will be much less likely to be pulled completely out of our embodied experience of practice by distracting thoughts. When one forces oneself to stay with the count, one must necessarily pay more attention to the breath. This will lead to a deeper phenomenal experience of the sound and sensation of breath and body. As a teacher, this is the main thing I look for when assessing the maturity of a practitioner. Is a student able to remain absorbed in the vinyasa count—and therefore absorbed within themselves for the duration of their practice? Or, are they constantly slipping out of that flow (flow of body and breath and flow of concentration) and losing their focus? I see beginners doing half Primary or less who are very focused and absorbed in the vinyasa count and within themselves. I see long-term practitioners doing Intermediate or advanced series who seem to give no importance at all to the vinyasa count and are constantly distracting themselves with superfluous movements, props, and unnecessary fidgeting. They seem to be doing everything that they can to avoid their phenomenal experience of the practice. It is clear to me which practitioners are experiencing the deeper benefits of working with the unique tool of embodied absorption within the flow of the vinyasa count. This has little to do with which postures or series they are practicing.

A group Mysore class is usually conducive to this process. A good Mysore-style teacher will promote an atmosphere which is conducive to concentration and accountability towards the vinyasas count. The main benefit of a once or twice a week led class is also to teach students how to be accountable to the vinyasa count.

If one is unable to practice in a Mysore class, then creating a neutral space at home—where external distractions which might tempt one to drift away from the essence of practice are kept out of sight and out of reach—is helpful.

Andy: This makes me wonder about led classes. They would certainly encourage accountability to the vinyasa count, but they can also pull the practitioner away from the timing of their own breath. I have experienced them as mixed blessings, helping me focus in some regards while disrupting my focus in others. What role do you think led classes play in the process of developing a non-reactive, embodied awareness?

Iain: Led classes can be tricky in the way you described. We are often forced to move in a way that is not in harmony with our natural rate of breathing or counting. But this can also be a good thing. We can become attached to the habits we develop in Mysore-style practice, and unwilling to move in a different way. The led class shakes up these attachments (reactions) by forcing us to let go of our own particular pace and habitual way of moving through the sequence. If we allow ourselves to be open to the insights that this brings, it can then have a profound effect on how we practice Mysore style. Practicing led Primary series and led Intermediate series with Sharath Jois profoundly influences the way that I move through the vinyasa count in my own independent practice. When I am practicing on my own, I don't necessarily move at the same pace that Sharathji uses in the led classes, but I find that I do hold myself much more accountable to the integrity of the vinyasa count due to the influence of his led classes. As a teacher, I have observed that students who do not regularly experience led classes often have something missing from their practice, which is connected to the integrity of the vinyasa count.

Andy: For counterpoint: do you think some students are, in fact, not thinking enough during practice?

Iain: There are practitioners who are able to stay within the framework of the vinyasa count effectively, but who are not absorbed in concentration on their internal experience, because they are coasting on autopilot. A teacher can sense this when nothing about the student's practice ever changes—even after a long period of time. There is no inquiry, no receptivity to information that is coming from the embodied experience of practice. Practice should promote evolution of the self, and this can only happen when we are paying attention to the information we receive in the form of embodied sensation. Subtle and gross changes within the structure of one's practice should occur over time if one is paying attention to feedback and "thinking" about it. This form of thinking is similar to what I described in my answer to your first question. It is as much a property of the responses of the body to its environment, as it is an abstract, disembodied process.

Andy: Do you think there is tension between embodiment and some forms of thinking or is all thinking part of the body and therefore part of being embodied?

Iain: Over tens of thousands of years, we have manufactured a human world of conceptual abstraction, which has nothing at all to do with the physical reality of rocks, wind, water, trees, animal bodies, etc. Most modern humans spend most of their hours of conscious awareness immersed within this abstract, conceptual human-made world. We treat it as if it has an objective reality of its own, independent of humans. As human society becomes more complex, our absorption within the abstract, conceptual human world seems to increase, to the point where it feels more real than the physical world of rocks, trees, wind, water, and animal bodies. This is largely why our planet earth is in such a critically unhealthy condition today.

The interesting thing is that if all the humans died tomorrow, the abstract, conceptual human world would vanish along with us. It has no objective existence of its own, and it means nothing to the rocks, wind, trees, water, and animal bodies. The reality of the abstract, conceptual human world of thinking and thought is entirely dependent on the world of animal bodies. But, the reality of animal bodies, rocks, wind, water, etc., is not dependent at all on the abstract conceptual world of human thought. It is unfortunate that the legacy of Descartes's fallacy of dualism is so strong and enduring. Mind and matter are inseparable and any distinction between them is illusory. I feel that the "union" of yoga is to remove the illusion of separation between body and mind. We can experience all thought in an embodied state, and we are much less likely to become lost or deluded by our thoughts when they are grounded in conscious, phenomenal, embodied experience. Paying more attention to the rocks, water, wind, trees and animal bodies can help with this.

Andy: If we reject dualism, what does it mean to say that a certain sort of thinking is "disembodied" or "abstract" activity? You seem to identify some human activities as natural and others as unnatural or as out of sync. Can you say more about this and how you aren't suggesting some form of nature/culture dualism that follows from a body/mind dualism?

Iain: I don't think nature and culture are separable, just as I don't think body and mind are separable. Culture is an inherent part of human nature. We are social creatures and culture simply represents our way of social interaction, just as it does for other social animals such as primates, wolves, ants, etc. I think the "out of sync" problem refers to an overemphasis on social interaction within our own species, and specifically through our abstract ideas. We have narrowed the sphere of our social interactions to such an extent that we have almost completely fallen out of awareness of our relationship with all that is more-than-human. We forget that our environment has shaped who and what we are over millions of years of biological evolution. Our environment is part and parcel of being human (this is also why I think the idea of colonizing other planets is a form of madness). The agricultural, industrial and technological revolutions have progressively diminished our awareness of this fact, to the extent that we are now destroying our environment and our heritage. We are thus losing touch with and destroying an integral aspect of who and what we are as a species. A person who cuts off his own legs would be considered insane, yet this is essentially identical in nature to what we are doing by destroying all of the other species and aspects of the more-than-human world which we are structurally coupled to. This is the fundamental reason for the "void" and lack of meaning that pervades so much of modern human culture and society, and the necessity of inventing religion as a means to anesthetize the discomfort of that void. We have abandoned something that has accompanied us for millions of years. I don't think it is a matter of nature/culture dualism, I think it is more of a lack of inclusiveness of the sphere of our ancestral social interactions with the more-than-human world within our "culture."

Andy: Would you describe *bandha* as necessarily bringing with it a certain kind of focus, attention or equilibrium of thought or is it possible to have "aligned fluidity" in the body without having it throughout the fields of attention and thought?

Iain: Embodiment and intuitive phenomenal awareness are necessary conditions for a true experience of *bandha*. It can be difficult to teach this concept to students who are fixated on intellectual, biomechanical analysis of what constitutes *bandha*. *Bandha* is a deeply felt continuity between self and environment, where the borders between where one ends and the other begins becomes blurred. This certainly requires a degree of concentration and focus. The illusion of discontinuity between body and mind must be yoked for the illusion of discontinuity between self and environment to be yoked. So, I would say that a true experience of *bandha* takes the union of body and mind one step further by creating a fluid union between body, mind, and environment (see the essay titled "The Tree of Bandha" for an in-depth discussion of this).

Andy: I'd like to thank you for taking the time to explore these questions. As I have continued my practice, I have found your responses helped guide me away from self-criticism that perpetuated reactive thought patterns. It has been a valuable discussion for me.

Iain: Thank you. Your questions are a valuable opportunity for me to examine and clarify my own beliefs and biases. I look forward to the next discussion.

THE ENERGETIC DYNAMICS
Of Ashtanga Advanced A
(Third series)

— September 2022 —

IN SEPTEMBER 2020, I DECIDED to turn on the video camera, along with a few more lights than usual, and film my Third series Ashtanga practice. The video[1] takes place in the dark early morning hours of 2:25–4:15 am, at home in Bali, before going to teach my Mysore class in Ubud.

The video is not meant to be a perfect demonstration, but rather an accurate documentation of what an average practice looks like for me, as it is and as it has been each and every day since I began to practice the Ashtanga system of Asana in 2003. I chose not to select my "greatest hits" (scripted performances of my best asanas) nor did I edit out any mistakes or weaknesses. There was no staging, editing, retakes, music, enhancements, or anything else. This is real and raw practice.

The video is the entire Third series from *Surya Namaskar A* to *Utpluthi*. I made three cuts in it—editing out a toilet break, a break where I had to chase the dogs out of the room when they decided to play around my

---

1. See videos on Iain's YouTube channel at https://www.youtube.com/@iaingrysak4001

mat (the brighter lights usually aren't on and it seemed to make them more active than they usually are at this time of the morning), and lastly I cut out the section of Fourth series postures, so the video jumps from the last posture of Third series to final backbending. Aside from those three cuts, there are no further edits.

I also cut the video up into six separate sections, and over a period of several months in late 2020 and early 2021, I posted the segments to my Facebook page, along with an extensive commentary for each section. I have collected all of those commentaries and wrote them below, alongside each of the video segments, so the entire series has a home as a collected whole. Each commentary focuses on some of the fundamental principles of the energetic dynamics of the Ashtanga system. The principles that I discuss in each section are inspired by that particular section of Third series. However they are also principles which apply to the Ashtanga system as a whole, and therefore should be of interest and relevance to practitioners of all levels.

Part 1: Surya Namaskar A & B and Standing Sequence
- 5 x Surya Namaskara A
- 3 x Surya Namaskara B
- Padangusthasana – Padahastasana
- Trikonasana A & B
- Parshvakonasana A & B
- Prasarita Padottanasana A–D
- Parshvottanasana

In the Ashtanga system of asana practice, we always begin with 5 repetitions of *Surya Namaskara A*, 3 repetitions of *Surya Namaskara B* and the Standing Sequence, regardless of which series we are going to practice on that day. These first 25–30 minutes of practice are the same for all practitioners, regardless of whether one has yet to complete Primary series, or whether one has been practicing Third or Fourth series for decades.

I've begun my daily practice with this 25-minute sequence each morning for the past 19 years. The repetitive nature of the Ashtanga system and the simplicity of this introductory section of the practice is a feature which some aspiring practitioners consider to be boring. The necessity of working through this initial aspect of self-encountering (the tendency to become distracted and bored while craving for gratification through novelty) dissuades them from delving deeper into the system. At my shala in Ubud, Bali, I frequently receive inquiries from practitioners with varied backgrounds who are interested in giving a trial to the Ashtanga practice. For someone who does not already have an established, daily Mysore-style practice, the minimum requirement to join my class is one week of daily practice. One week of practice is actually not enough to begin to experience the essence of the Ashtanga practice's influence on the human organism. A more appropriate initial trial length would be one month. Due to the transient nature of travelers passing through Ubud, I make a concession for one week. This requirement of time commitment is still enough to dissuade many potential students. It weeds out those who are not interested in cultivating focus and commitment.

Those who do commit to join for at least one week encounter the next requirement—which is the ability to memorize the vinyasa sequences of *Surya Namaskara A & B* and the Standing Sequence, before they are moved on to begin learning Primary series. In today's era of fragmented attention and instant gratification, memorizing this 25–30 minute sequence proves to be a challenge for many new students, and they often do not accomplish it within one week. Those who consider themselves to already be accomplished and advanced asana practitioners from other systems of practice—and who perhaps expect to be practicing hand stands, arm balances and advanced backbending—sometimes find that being asked to repeat the Standing Sequence three or four times (or until mistakes in memorizing the sequence are resolved) and then to lie down and take rest is not very gratifying for the ego. They often do not return for a second week of practice.

For those who persevere, and apply themselves to this style of learning, a rich universe of authentic practice and self-cultivation opens up for exploration. *Surya Namaskara* and the Standing Sequence become the cornerstone of a lifelong practice. It is the ground and the roots upon which we build the structure of the core series of asanas. It is the foundation that we can always return to in order to stabilize and recalibrate when the transformative process of the core series of asanas become overly intense or overwhelming. This is ground zero of Ashtanga practice.

Surya Namaskara A & B introduce the fundamental process of coordinating the movements of body and breath in the vinyasa system of practice. For a true beginner, this alone can be enough to grapple with for at least a few days. The key postures *Chaturanga Dandasana, Urdhva Mukha Svanasana* (Upward Facing Dog) and *Adho Mukha Svanasana* (Downward Facing Dog) are introduced here. The sequence linking these three postures together is often repeated 50 times or more in a full series practice, so it is imperative that we cultivate some degree of experiential understanding and ease in these three postures.

During the practice of *Surya Namaskara*, we can focus on the three core postures without the added complication of the other postures of Primary, Intermediate or Advanced series. In particular, it is important to cultivate some degree of comfort in *Chaturanga Dandasana*. For those who begin the Ashtanga practice with a lack of strength, or with certain injuries or disabilities, we can certainly modify *Chaturanga* in the beginning stages. In the majority of cases, I prefer that a student applies himself to develop the ability to practice *Chaturanga* properly (without the knees or belly on the ground) before I begin to teach them the seated asanas of Primary series. I've had students join my shala who have been taught full Primary series, and yet they cannot perform *Chaturanga–Upward Dog–Downward Dog* without touching their knees or belly on the ground. Cultivating a 90 minute full Primary series practice of movement and flexibility without a corresponding cultivation of strength is an extremely imbalanced way to go about progressing through this practice, and I deem it to be incorrect. Also consider that asking someone to begin to cultivate a proper *Chaturanga* at this stage—when they are already practicing it in a modified way 50 or more times per session—would be overwhelming and destabilizing. It is much more appropriate to cultivate it properly from the beginning. The same philosophy applies to jumping. It is fine for beginners who lack confidence, strength and control to step forward and back—rather than jumping—in the beginning stages. However, by the time one is working on the first seated postures of Primary series, I do expect at least a rudimentary form of jumping to be attempted.

The importance of the Standing Sequence is often overlooked. This sequence of postures is stabilizing, balancing and therapeutic in nature. Although the postures are basic, there are infinite layers of depth to be found within them for one who practices with a commitment to embodied awareness and an attitude of exploration. After 19 years of practicing this sequence each morning, I still regularly experience new insights within these postures. The way that I experience them within myself continues to evolve and change over time. The Standing Sequence is often the most enjoyable part of my practice. I appreciate the relaxed stimulation of my body and breath opening up and aligning in a gentle way, before the more intensive postures of the core series exert their effect upon me. The way that I feel during the Standing Sequence is also an important indicator of the constantly changing state of my body, breath and nerves on each particular morning.

A fundamental skill which is essential to cultivate in the Standing Sequence is the ability to harness the force of the earth and to channel it throughout the entirety of our body and breath. This is the core alignment which is common to each and every asana that we practice. It is also known as "Mula Bandha." *Mula Bandha* is experienced when the part of our body which is in contact with the ground is able to press down into the earth with firmness and stability, while we simultaneously release tension in order to allow the resistance that comes from our engagement with the earth to spread and reverberate throughout our entire body. In essence, *Mula Bandha* is the experience of a continuous and unbroken energetic connection between ourselves and our surrounding environment. A tree drops its roots into the ground, while growing and spreading upward and outward into the space surrounding it. Similarly, our body and breath extend themselves downward into the earth, while simultaneously expanding outwards into the atmosphere around us. For me, asana practice is a cultivation of the fluidity of my relationship with my environment to the extent that the boundaries between myself and my environment are blurred. *Bandha* is a process of working with the ground and space as if they are extensions of one's own body and breath. Refining the way that we respond to the ground beneath us and the space around us—at an intuitive and phenomenal level of experience—is the key to cultivating efficiency and fluidity in our movement patterns. I have written in greater detail about this process in the essay titled "The Tree of Bandha."

Standing on the ground, and cultivating the ability to harness the earth's energy through the soles of our feet is the appropriate place to begin to cultivate the process and state of *Mula Bandha*. Those who fail to learn how to harness the earth's energy through their feet in the Standing Sequence, will most likely not be able to do so with other parts of their body in the more complex postures of the core series of asanas. I've seen practitioners who manage to get through Primary series and some of Intermediate series based on flexibility alone, without cultivating strength and stability through a solid connection to the earth. At some point in Intermediate series, these practitioners become stuck and they aren't able to move forward until they learn how to cultivate the foundational element of deepening their connection to the ground beneath them, so that effective and efficient movement can blossom from this base.

The grounding and stabilizing aspect of the Standing Sequence is also therapeutic in nature. When the structurally transformative process which is induced by the more intensive postures of Primary, Intermediate or Advanced series becomes overwhelming, and the body and nerves become destabilized and excessive pain is experienced, my advice is always to continue to practice at least the Standing Sequence—returning to ground zero—until things begin to stabilize and the system is able to manifest a certain degree of dynamic balance again. Once this balance is re-established, we can then move back into the core series of asanas.

Part 2: Lateral extensions and Leg Behind the Head Variations (Visvamitrasana to Durvasana)

- Visvamitrasana
- Vasisthasana
- Kasyapasana
- Chakorasana
- Bhairavasana
- Skandasana
- Durvasana

Third series can be divided into four distinct sections on the basis of energetic dynamics. Each of these four sections can be further divided into subsections, but the boundaries that delineate the four main sections are the most noteworthy for me and they mark distinctive turning points during my embodied experience of Third series.

The first two sections of the series are deeply *apanic* in nature, while the concluding two sections are *pranic* in nature. *Prana* and *apana* represent opposing, but complementary forms of energetic movement within the human organism. *Apana* governs exhalation and the movement of energy in the downward direction, while *prana* governs inhalation, and the movement of energy in the upward direction. An intention of practice should be to cultivate a dynamic and balanced relationship between these two movements. If we are successful in nurturing harmonious communication between these two energetic patterns, we experience a state of *bandha*.

In the previous section on the Standing Sequence, I characterized the phenomena of *bandha* as an engaged relationship with our environment. In this context, *apana* is responsible for the ability to press downward with whichever part of our body is in contact with the earth. Those who are unable to engage firmly with the ground need to cultivate more *apanic* energy within themselves and their relationship with their environment. *Apana* is also responsible for the various elimination processes. Defecation, menstruation, and the release of stress and tension through a deep exhale or a heartfelt sigh are all examples of *apanic* energy movement. The *apanic* energy pattern is cultivated through postures which stretch the back part of the body (i.e., forward bending) or move the body toward the ground. Vinyasas which are *apanic* in nature are always executed with an exhalation. In terms of working with the breath, learning how to press the breath down into the root of the belly and the pelvis at the end of the exhalation will improve our proficiency in working with *apana*. Mastery of the *apanic* pole of the breath has been attained when we are able to feel clear contact between the end of the exhale and the pelvic floor.

Prana governs the complimentary response to the downward *apana* movement. It allows us to lift and spread upward. *Apana* allows us to tap into the energy of the earth (gravity) and *prana* distributes our response to the earth's energy throughout our body. Those who are unable to feel a natural ease in lifting the ribcage up and away from the pelvis, and who frequently feel heavy, as if they are sinking down into the earth, need to cultivate more *pranic* energetic movement within themselves and their relationship with their environment. It should also be noted that *prana* requires resistance from the ground to manifest effectively. *Asana* should always be practiced on a firm surface for this reason. A rubber mat and thin cotton rug is usually firm enough, but anyone who has attempted to practice Ashtanga on a plush carpet, or loose sand has experienced the impossibility of overcoming the sinking feeling of excessive *apana*. I also recommend that seated meditation be practiced on a firm surface, for the same reason. A folded wool blanket is the maximum softness which will allow for effective resistance to stimulate *pranic* lift in the body. Standard meditation cushions are too soft and will lead to compression in the spine due to excessive *apana*. Those who experience a backache after sitting in meditation for long periods of time should experiment with a firmer meditation cushion. A similar philosophy also applies to sleeping mattresses. A night spent lying on a mattress which is too soft will result in a feeling of compression in practice the next morning.

The qualities of expansion and vitality are governed by *prana*. Asanas which stretch the front part of the body or lift us upward and away from the ground cultivate the movement of *prana*. In the Ashtanga system of practice, we execute these types of vinyasas with an inhalation. When working with the breath, we can maximize the expansion of *prana* by cultivating the ability to inhale into the entire thoracic cavity, including the top of the chest, between the scapula, and the sides of the chest below the armpits. When we can expand the inhalation freely and without restriction into these areas, we have mastered the *pranic* pole of breathing.

As one matures in the Ashtanga system of practice, a realization tends to occur: The entire practice is designed to enhance and refine the way that we engage with the complementary movements of *prana* and *apana* within ourselves and with our environment. *Bandha* is both a process and result of fluid, stable and dynamic relationship between these two forms of energy, and is a defining feature of mature practice.

There are various methods through which the dynamic balance between *prana* and *apana* is cultivated within the Ashtanga system of practice. We can first examine the energetic structure of the ordering of the vinyasa sequences. All of the vinyasa sequences—from *Surya Namaskara A* to the postures of Third and Fourth series—follow a similar pattern of oscillation between *pranic* and *apanic* movements. For example, in *Surya Namaskara A* the vinyasas *Ekam*, *Trini*, *Pancha*, *Sapta*, and *Nava* are all *pranic* in nature and executed with an inhalation. The vinyasas *Dve*, *Catvari*, *Sat* and *Astau* are all *apanic* in nature and executed with an exhalation. In other words, we alternately stimulate *prana* and *apana*, from one vinyasa to the next, for the entire duration of our practice. The net effect of this continuous oscillation is an interwoven communication between *prana* and *apana*, which builds a state of *bandha* over the duration of practice.

We can also examine the balance of *prana* and *apana* within each posture. Most postures can be characterized as either predominantly *pranic* or predominantly *apanic* in nature. To maintain dynamic balance between *prana* and *apana*—and to experience *bandha*—we must consciously cultivate the pattern that is opposite to the predominate natural pattern of each posture. For example, in a naturally *apanic* posture such a forward bend, we will predominantly experience the *apanic* pattern of the back of the body stretching and the movement of the body towards the ground. Yet, to maintain a balanced state within the posture—and thus to experience *bandha*—we should also consciously cultivate some *pranic* movement by maintaining spread and opening in the chest and lengthening the crown of the head towards the toes. We should also inhale deeply into the entire back of the rib cage. If we don't add these *pranic* elements to a forward bend, and instead allow ourselves to flop over with the entire spine completely flexed and relaxed, the posture feels lifeless. By adding active and engaged *pranic* movements to a forward bend, we experience the flow of life force and the state of *bandha* due to a more balanced internal pattern. It is worth noting here that I don't advocate the "yin" system of asana practice as a complement to the Ashtanga system. Ashtanga is not a "yang" practice, which needs to be balanced by a separate "yin" practice. The *yang* and *yin*—or *prana* and *apana*—can and should be experienced together within each posture, each breath, and across the energetic experience of the practice as a whole.

We can also consider a counter-example of the same principle: In a naturally *pranic* posture or movement, such as backbend, we must consciously apply engaged *apanic* patterns in order to bring about the desired state of balance and *bandha* that we are attempting to nurture. Backbends tend to feel exhilarating and energizing as they lift us away from the earth. If we overindulge in this phenomenon, our internal experience can resemble a manic high, which is neither sustainable nor balanced. At some point later on, we will crash and experience a "backbending hangover." I've witnessed practitioners drive themselves deeply into imbalance and pathology by repeating this process over a long period of time. In order to experience the positive benefits of backbending in a balanced and sustainable way, we must add *apanic* elements to these postures. Pressing the body downward into the earth and consciously cultivating stability in both body and breath is the most effective way to do this. In *Urdhva Danurasana*, for example, we must actively press the feet down into the ground. The next time you practice backbending and dropping back and standing up, see if you can do so without moving your feet from their initial position on your mat. This will give you a sense of how grounded (or not) your backbends are. Those who are not able to maintain a solid *apanic* connection to the ground are not yet energetically prepared to integrate the *pranic* stimulation of deeper backbending.

Another important aspect of the dynamic balance between *prana* and *apana* to consider is the long-term psychological and physiological tendencies that we carry. We've discussed how most postures have a natural *pranic* or *apanic* bias to them. People also have an innate structural bias towards either *pranic* or *apanic* energy as their natural baseline state. Those who have an anteriorly tilted pelvis tend to have a *pranic* energetic bias, while those who have a posteriorly tilted pelvis tend to have an *apanic* energetic bias. The preceding statement is a gross generalization, and each individual experience is subtle, complex and nuanced, but our natural biases are an important factor to consider. Understanding our personal *pranic–apanic* biases will help us to understand why some postures, movements and breathing patterns feel more natural and comfortable, while we struggle with others. This bias will also shift and change over time, as the practice shapes and alters our innate structure. When the Ashtanga system is applied correctly—that is, when we are required to complete each posture or movement before learning the next one in the series—we are forced to encounter, cultivate and integrate the movement patterns which are less natural and comfortable for us. This is what makes the Ashtanga system unique in its structurally transformative and balancing effects. Progress through the system must be gradual, if it is to be sustainable. Deep structural changes which shift our fundamental biases require time, patience, and often involve a certain degree of discomfort as we integrate them. A skillful teacher will ensure that his students work through this process in a way that is sustainable and not overwhelming.

Finally, we can zoom out to observe the relationship between *prana* and *apana* across the broader scale of the structure of entire series. Primary series is *apanic* in nature. Only two of the postures (*Purvottanasana* and *Setubandhasana*) are *pranic*. *Apana* represents the roots from which the tree of *prana* rises and spreads. This is why we begin our journey through the Ashtanga system by fully developing the rooting *apanic* pattern in Primary series. Once the roots of *apana* are firmly established within us, we can use this stable foundation as a base upon which we nurture the growth *pranic* energy.

Urdhva Danurasana represents a counter posture to the entire Primary series, and cultivation of *pranic* energy though backbending at the end of the series is necessary to elicit an overall balance. Developing some integrated experience of *pranic* energy through proficiency in backbending (including the ability to stand up from and drop back into *Urdhva Danurasana*) at this stage is necessary before we learn Intermediate series.

The first section of Intermediate series features a powerful sequence of eight backbending postures in a row. The net effect of practicing these postures together, with the connecting vinyasas and breathing, creates an experience of *pranic* stimulation which most practitioners are unprepared for. It is not uncommon for practitioners who begin a daily practice of this sequence to experience disturbed sleeping patterns, vivid dreams, resurfacing of old and possibly traumatic memories and emotional instability. These phenomena illustrate the extent to which the transformative influence of the Ashtanga system reaches the deepest layers of our embodied selves. It is worth repeating that a stable and integrated practice of the *apanic* Primary series, along with the initial *pranic* experience of standing up and dropping back from *Urdhva Danurasana* are essential prerequisites to attempting to integrate the more intensive *pranic* experience of the first section of Intermediate series.

The next section of Intermediate series features leg behind the head postures and arm balances. This section provides a stronger *apanic* stimulation than Primary series provides, and also counters the *pranic* stimulation of the first section of Intermediate series. It is at this stage that we can remove Primary series from our daily practice, and focus on Intermediate as a stand-alone practice, since both the *pranic* and *apanic* sections have now been cultivated within Intermediate series.

Third series reverses the order of energetic patterning that we experience in Intermediate series. In Third series, we begin with *apanic* stimulation and finish with *pranic* stimulation. Changing the order in which we stimulate the two patterns elicits a very different phenomenal experience of the practice.

The first section of Third series begins with *Visvamitrasana* and *Vasisthasana*. I consider these two postures to be advanced variations of the standing postures *Trikonasana* and *Parshvakonasana*, respectively. We could refer to these postures as *Trikonasana C* and *Parshvakonasana C*. In terms of the *pranic–apanic* energy spectrum, these postures are relatively neutral in nature. Beginning the series with these two postures functions as an extension of the Standing Sequence, which is helpful when we are practicing Third series as a stand-alone practice (without preceding it with Intermediate series). This subsection is an effective way to ease into the series before the deeper postures which follow.

The remainder of the first section of Third series features a deeply apanic sequence of five variations of *Eka Pada Sirsasana* (leg behind the head). It is essential that one has mastered *Eka Pada* and *Dwi Pada Sirsasana* in Intermediate series, before one is moved on to begin Third series. Unfortunately, this is often not the case. *Dwi Pada Sirsasana* is one of the most poorly performed postures in the Ashtanga system. I have observed very few students who are taught this important posture properly—that is, cultivating the ability to spread the feet apart with the toes pointed away from each other and to keep the head held upright. I struggled with this posture myself, and it was only when I went to Mysore to practice with Sharath Jois for the first time in 2014, that I was required to learn the correct technique. I detailed my experience with *Dwi Pada* in the essay titled "You Stop There."

Those who fail to cultivate the prerequisite depth and comfort in the intermediate variations of leg behind the head are far more likely to encounter structural issues if they are taught the five variations in Third series prematurely. Practicing these five variations in a row with the connecting vinyasas induces a tremendous amount of structural shifting—especially for those who have a natural *pranic* bias in their body structure. If the groundwork has not been sufficient to prepare oneself for this experience, there is a high likelihood of experiencing pain in the hips, pelvis and lower back as the core part of the body restructures to accommodate the daily inputs of these extreme *apanic* postures. It is also essential to have developed enough strength and opening in the upper body and shoulder girdle to safely hold the leg behind the head without strain on the neck. This sequence should not be approached casually or lightly. For those who are prepared, and who learn these postures in the gradual manner that is taught in Mysore, our understanding and mastery of the *apanic* energetic pattern is deepened and these postures provide a grounded entry into the power of Third series.

Part 3: Arm Balances (Urdhva Kukkutasana to Astavakrasana)
- Urdhva Kukkutasana A
- Urdhva Kukkutasana B
- Urdhva Kukkutasana C
- Galavasana
- Eka Pada Bakasana A
- Eka Pada Bakasana B
- Koundinyasana A
- Koundinyasana B
- Astavakrasana A
- Astavakrasana B

The second section of *apanic* postures is considered to be the most demanding part of Third series by many practitioners. This section features ten consecutive arm-balancing postures. If we count both sides the bilateral postures, the total is seventeen consecutive arm balances. Those who have a natural *apanic* bias in their physical structure will tend to have an easier time with this section than those who have a *pranic* bias. For *pranic* types, this section will undoubtedly pose the greatest challenge in Third series. The potential for profound structural transformation is accordingly high for a *pranic* practitioner who dedicates the time and musters the necessary perseverance to master this section.

A sufficient level of strength cultivation is the most obvious prerequisite to completing this section of the practice. Mastery of Intermediate postures such as *Bakasana, Karandavasana, Mayurasana* and *Nakrasana* (along with their connecting vinyasas) and deep stability and comfort in *Chaturanga Dandasana* will be necessary before tackling the arm balance section of Third series. There is simply no possibility of compromising for a lack of strength by working around, avoiding or modifying these ten postures, which represent a significant chunk of Third series. At this stage, one must fully embrace the strengthening aspect of the Ashtanga practice.

Strength is not the only necessary factor for mastery of these postures. A sense of ease in accessing the *apanic* rounding pattern of the back and pelvis is also extremely important. The rounding pattern is essential to experience the full expression of the first six of these arm balances—which are done with straight arms and the back rounded in the characteristic *apanic* shape. The *apanic* rounding is less relevant to the final four arm balances, which are done with the arms bent and the spine in a twisting pattern. The rounded shape of the back is cultivated through mastery of Intermediate postures such as *Bakasana, Dwi Pada Sirsasana* and *Karandavasana* and Primary postures such as *Baddha Konasana B*.

Eka Pada Bakasana A is the most difficult of these ten arm balances. The *apanic* rounding of the back is absolutely necessary, in order to attain the full expression of the posture with both of the arms relatively straight, the kneecap of the bent leg placed on the arm and the foot of the bent leg pulled up. Most practitioners end up doing the "easier" version of this posture, where the shin of the bent leg rests on the arm (rather than the kneecap) and the foot of the bent leg hangs down, which ultimately makes it impossible to straighten the arm that the bent leg is resting upon. This was one of Third series postures which posed the greatest difficulty for me to learn (the other being *Gandha Berundasana*, which comes in the next section). For over a decade, I did the "easy" version of this posture. It was only when I was given *Eka Pada Bakasana A* in my practice with Sharath Jois on my fourth trip to Mysore in 2018, that I was required to learn the full version in order to satisfy his standards. I am happy to have been pushed to this level of integrity in my practice, as the full version always felt out of reach for me prior to that trip. Two and a half years later, my ability to execute this posture has improved significantly, though it is certainly still a work in progress (as are all of the postures in the practice).

The third aspect of self-cultivation which is indispensable for success in the arm balance section of Third series is that of stamina and concentration. The qualities of stamina and concentration go hand in hand. They support one another and work together synergistically. It is impossible to fully cultivate one of these qualities without the other. Mastery of these qualities within the Ashtanga practice is represented by the ability to flow through all of the vinyasas and postures of a particular section or series without the need to stop and break the flow of body and breath in order to rest, or to distract oneself with anything outside of the structured flow of the vinyasa count. In other words, stamina and concentration are responsible for the ability to follow the flow of the vinyasa count precisely, without breaking or deviating from the count for the duration of one's practice.

The ability to "follow the count" is one of the most important, but least recognized components of mastery of the Ashtanga system of practice. Teachers who focus on this feature of the practice in the training of their students tend to produce the strongest and most stable practitioners. This is one of the defining features of the teaching style of Sharath Jois (and those of his authorized teachers who follow his teaching faithfully). I've noticed that the ability to follow the vinyasa count tends to be lacking in students who prefer to learn from "workshop teachers"—many of whom seem to discard the importance of the vinyasa counting system from their teaching styles. At my shala in Bali, I've encountered students who have been trained by "workshop teachers" to the level of Intermediate or even Third series. Some of these students haven't even learned what the appropriate vinyasa counts are, let alone cultivated an ability to flow through them without interruption. These same students tend to have distracted, unfocused practices, lack of stamina, and often complain of chronic pains and injuries.

In the previous section, I discussed the structure of the vinyasa count with respect to the way that it alternately stimulates *prana* and *apana*, via oscillation between *apanic* vinyasas, executed with an exhalation, and *pranic* vinyasas, executed with an inhalation. When a practitioner cultivates the ability to focus continuously on this oscillating internal pattern of breath and bodily movement in a meditation on internal form, the phenomenon of *bandha* builds up within him. *Bandha* is not something that can be turned on or off from moment to moment with a simple muscular contraction. I am sometimes asked by students if they should be "holding *bandha*." *Bandha* is not something that can be "held." Rather, it is something that is built up through sustained flow and internal concentration on the continuous movement of body and breath. For steam to build up in a pressure cooker, heat must be applied continuously, and the lid must be kept tightly sealed on the pot. If the application of heat is stopped—even for a few moments—the internal buildup of pressure in the pot will cease and the pressure will begin to decrease. If we take the lid off the pot, the internal pressure escapes completely. Similarly, if we stop the continuous oscillation between *pranic* and *apanic* stimulation via the flow of breath and movement through the vinyasas, then we remove the heat which drives the buildup of internal pressure which generates *bandha*. If our concentration wanders away from our embodied, phenomenal experience, then we have taken the lid off the pot and we lose everything. Nothing inside gets "cooked" and we don't experience the internal transformation that we could potentially have experienced.

Sharathji once made a comment during a conference that stuck with me and is relevant to the present discussion. He said that the biggest cause of injury in practice is a lack of concentration. I had never thought about this fact in these particular terms before, but the statement resonated with my understanding of the practice and injury completely. As I previously mentioned, it is often those students who have not been trained to follow the vinyasa count precisely, and who have distracted and unfocused practices, who seem to be nursing chronic pains and injuries. These students tend to address these injuries by deviating from the structure of the practice even further—obsessively squirming around, adding in extra stretches in between postures and vinyasas and skipping certain postures and vinyasas altogether. They generate a vicious circle where the very thing that contributed to their injuries (improper application of the Ashtanga system) becomes the tool they attempt to use to address their injury, which only drives them deeper into discomfort. When I encounter such a student in my shala, I usually address the issue by bringing them back to the foundational sequences—Standing Sequence and Primary series—and I train them to move slowly and carefully through these sequences with emphasis on focus and attention towards the count of the vinyasa. In most cases—for those who are willing to follow my instructions for a sustained period of time—the injuries and pains work themselves out, and the student then progresses further into the system feeling stronger and more stable. When one is deeply focused on the vinyasa count and engrossed within one's internal experience of movement of body and breath, a profoundly embodied state of being arises which is characterized by the primacy of intuitive, animal intelligence. This is a state where injury or mistakes that will lead to excessive pain are much less likely to occur.

When we remain internally focused on the sensations involved with the flow of body and breath, and we commit to staying with the continuous flow of vinyasa from one posture to the next, we encounter challenging experiences within ourselves. The state of *bandha* is not a natural experience which would occur in ordinary circumstances outside of the practice. When we build *bandha* through continuous flow of body and breath, we experience unique sensations in deep somatic layers, which are unlike sensations that we would naturally encounter in our mundane lives. These sensations can be connected to subconscious *samskara* patterns (habitual patterns of reaction which we generate throughout our lives, and which we tend to default to). These deeper sensations can sometimes feel overwhelming and unpleasant (though they can also sometimes feel blissful and intoxicating), and the default tendency will be to react to these sensations by attempting to avoid them. This is particularly common when we approach or arrive at the most difficult postures or vinyasas in our practice. Aversion and the tendency towards avoidance lead us to either stop and take a rest, or perhaps to distract ourselves by adding in extra stretches, squirming around, looking at other people practicing near us, picking our toenails, or any of the myriad of escape techniques that practitioners employ.

When the process of building *bandha* through continuous flow of body and breath is sustained for longer stretches of time, our internal experience and the *samskaras* that we encounter can become even more challenging. This is why it is necessary to build the intensity our practice up gradually, taking the time to adapt to each section of practice by training ourselves to be non-reactive towards the internal sensations that arise through the unique experience of flowing through the vinyasa count. If we hold ourselves accountable to the vinyasa count for each section of practice, and train ourselves to master the ability to flow through the count without interruption, then we can adapt to our inner experience and work through these layers of *samskara* patterns in a sustainable way. If we don't habituate gradually, and we launch into the more intensive postures and vinyasa sequences of Intermediate and Third series prematurely, the *samskara* patterns which arise can be overwhelming and destabilizing, causing serious emotional and energetic imbalance. This can lead to a full-blown breakdown which often results in the abandonment of the Ashtanga practice altogether. If one does take the time and effort to work through these layers of *samskara* in a gradual and sustainable way, one becomes stronger and more resilient emotionally and energetically. Emotional and energetic resilience and equanimity are key signs of correct long-term application of practice.

When I consider whether to move a student forward and add more postures to their practice, the ability for that student to flow through the vinyasa count of their current practice without interruption and without exhibiting signs of being energetically or emotionally overwhelmed is an extremely important factor. It is of equal importance as the mastery of the postures themselves. A student may be able to bind or complete all of the postures in his practice perfectly, but if he cannot flow smoothly through the vinyasas without becoming distracted or excessively fatigued, then I won't move him forward and teach him new asanas until his focus and stamina improve. This is also a factor that I closely monitor when judging the state of my own practice.

The arm balance section of Third series is a make or break point in terms of stamina and concentration. Most students will need to stop and take breaks during this section, especially when they are in the process of learning it. In my opinion, this section of Third series is not mastered until one can flow through it without interruption, following the vinyasa counts.

Following the vinyasa counts does not mean that one cannot take extra breaths here or there when necessary. Taking extra breaths within the flow of the vinyasa is quite different from dropping out of the flow altogether to rest, or to distract oneself. Taking extra breaths within the flow of the vinyasa count lessens the intensity of internal experience, but allows one to maintain the process of building *bandha*. If you watch the video closely, you might notice that I do take some extra breaths in my execution of the arm balance section of Third series. For example, when I jump into headstand, and then position my leg on my arm, in a few of the postures I then take an extra inhale and exhale, before I then inhale into the final state of the posture itself. Ideally, even these extra breaths should eventually be eliminated completely. In Primary series, it is possible to flow through the entire series without these sorts of extra breaths. In Intermediate, and especially Advanced series, most mortals will need a few extra breaths here and there.

Part 4: Transitions and Peak Backbending (Purna Matsyendrasana to Supta Trivikramasana)

- Purna Matsyendrasana
- Viranchyasana A
- Viranchyasana B
- Viparita Dandasana A
- Viparita Dandasana B
- Viparita Salabhasana
- Gandha Berundasana
- Hanumanasana
- Supta Trivikramasana

The third section of Third series features the transition from the *apanic* energetic cultivation of the first half of the series into the *pranic* cultivation of the second half of the series. This section also features what I consider to be the energetic culmination of the series in the difficult backbending postures *Viparita Salabhasana* and *Gandha Berundasana*.

The transition from apanic to pranic movement patterns occurs over three seated postures: *Purna Matsyendrasana*, *Viranchyasana A* and *Viranchyasana B*. These postures maintain a slight apanic bias in their nature, but help to prepare one for the subsequent backbending postures by also featuring strong *pranic* elements. *Purna Matsyendrasana* and *Viranchyasana B* are both twisting postures, which require *apanic* movements in the lower body, combined with *pranic* expansion of the upper body. *Viranchyasana A* is a variation on the leg behind the head theme, which is deeply *apanic*, but also features *pranic* cultivation with the addition of binding the arms in *Gomukhasana* style.

I find these three transitional postures to be the calmest part of Third series. They are a welcome respite after the intensity of the arm balances which precede this section, and before the peak backbending which follows these postures. These three postures are complex, as they combine elements from several different categories of posture. Provided one has completed the necessary groundwork to establish the various types of required mobility, the energetic demands are less here than in other parts of Third series, giving this section a feeling of calm between the *apanic* and *pranic* storms which precede and follow it, respectively.

Transitioning back and forth between *pranic* and *apanic* movement patterns is an important feature of the Ashtanga practice. As I have previously discussed, *bandha* manifests through a fluid and dynamic balance between the *pranic* and *apanic* energetic poles. If we are successful in cultivating the phenomena of *bandha*, one hallmark should be ease and resilience in our ability to move back and forth between opposing patterns of movement and energy. In other words, a sign of maturity and competence in the Ashtanga practice is the ability to move effortlessly and fluidly between *pranic* and *apanic* trends.

A state of *bandha* is analogous to walking upon a high and narrow mountain ridge between two valleys. From the vantage point of the ridge, we can clearly see the terrain of both valleys and if we should choose to move into either valley, we can easily do so from the central point of the top of the ridge. Conversely, if we are stuck in either one of the valleys, it is impossible to see the terrain in the other valley. If we want to move into the other valley, it requires great effort as we must first climb up the ridge, and then down into the opposite valley.

I once had a unique experience while walking along a steep and high ridge while trekking in the Indian Himalaya. I was trekking alone, without a guide or companions. It was mid-morning, and I had set off from my starting point about 90 minutes prior to reaching the ridge. I hadn't seen anyone, or any signs of human settlement since setting off, and I wasn't fully confident that I was on the correct route to my destination. The ridge and the surrounding mountainscape were stunning and I felt intoxicated by the power of the mountain wilderness. At the same time, I felt a gnawing apprehension due to the extremity of the environment and the potential of getting lost.

There were broken sections of thin rock wall upon the ridge, and the walking path meandered back and forth from one side of the rock wall to the other. When the walking path passed along the side of the wall which exposed me to the Northwest and blocked my exposure to the Southeast, I was struck by a ferocious and icy cold wind blowing from the main Himalaya range. There was no sun on this side and the path was full of patches of snow and ice, as was the steep and foreboding valley that lay on this side of the ridge and the jagged mountain peaks that stretched out beyond the valley. The icy wind stung my face and threatened to throw me off balance as I carefully navigated the icy patches of ground. I felt my fear and apprehension of getting lost increase dramatically when I was on this side of the rock wall. Then suddenly the rock wall would end and a new section of rock wall would emerge, with the foot path running on the opposite side of the wall, exposing me to the Southeast and blocking my exposure to the Northwest. As soon as I passed onto this side of the rock wall, the entire universe shifted. The howling wind was abruptly cut off by the wall and replaced with a calm stillness, punctuated only by the heartening chirp of birdsong. The sun shone warmly on this side. There was no snow or ice and the valley running down this side of the ridge towards the gentle foothills was green and sparkled majestically in the morning sunlight. I loosened my clothing and felt my mood shift just as abruptly as the wind had ceased. Here, I felt confident that I was on the right path and I basked in the gentle warmth of the morning sun and birdsong playing on my senses. Then, the rock wall would end again and the next section would take me back to the opposite side with its wind, cold and fear. My memory of walking this particular ridge exemplifies the experience of *bandha*. When we are moving from the perspective and vantage point of *bandha*, we can taste the essence of both extremes which lie on either side of the middle line, and we can effortlessly move back and forth between them. It is this vantage point and perspective which we should strive to cultivate in our Ashtanga practice, always keeping one foot on the ridge of *bandha*, while we move between the opposing valleys of *prana* and *apana*.

As we progress through the sections and series of the Ashtanga system, the macro level transitions between *pranic* and *apanic* tendencies become more intense and more challenging to navigate. The more deeply we venture into either extreme of *prana* or *apana*, the more difficult it becomes to move back into the opposite pattern. Using the example of the mountain ridge, we can say that the further we descend into one valley, the more difficult it becomes to climb back up to the ridge and then down into the other valley. One of the first places we may encounter this challenge in the Ashtanga system is after *Supta Kurmasana* in Primary series. *Supta Kurmasana* is one of the deepest expressions of *apanic* energy in Primary series. Many people will find that after exiting from *Supta Kurmasana*, the subsequent upward-facing dog (a *pranic* position) will feel a little bit stiffer than usual.

The next place we may encounter this challenge is in practicing the backbending sequence (*Urdhva Danurasana* and dropping back and standing up) at the end of Primary series. After spending the entirety of Primary series cultivating an *apanic* pattern in the body and nerves, it can feel difficult to suddenly attempt to move deeply into the opposing *pranic* pattern with *Urdhva Danurasana*. Dropping back and standing up—and perhaps even catching the legs with the hands—brings us even deeper into *pranic* expression. Some newcomers to the system complain about the abruptness of this transition and about the requisite of cultivating the ability to drop back and stand up from *Urdhva Danurasana* before starting Intermediate series. It's common for people to suggest that practicing the milder backbends at the beginning of Intermediate series is a more appropriate way to ease the transition into the deeper backbending of *Urdhva Danurasana* and dropping back and standing up. I address this issue by pointing out that Ashtanga system is designed to aid us in cultivating the skill to move between the extremes of *prana* and *apana* with ease and fluidity. As we cultivate the elemental skills of the practice, we should require fewer transitional steps to move between extremes. The transitions between deeply *apanic* and deeply *pranic* sections of postures increase in intensity as we move into Intermediate and Advanced series, so it is essential that we cultivate some skill in transitioning between extremes while we are still in Primary series.

After completing backbending, we flip back into *apanic* energy with *Paschimottanasana*. Just as upward-facing dog can feel a bit stiff after *Supta Kurmasana*, most practitioners have probably had the experience of needing a few breaths to get fully into *Paschimottanasana* after drop backs or catching the legs in backbending. The ease and fluidity with which we can move between these extremes are indicative of our state of internal balance and *bandha*. If we can easily move into a full *Paschimottanasana* without resistance after deep backbending, this indicates that our body and nervous system are relatively stable and energetically balanced. If, however, we feel stiff and it requires a few breaths to fully move into *Paschimottanasana* after backbending—and especially if this phenomenon happens for several days in a row—this indicates that our body and nerves are not in an ideal state of balance. This could be due to some deeper structural shifting that is taking place. In this case, it is appropriate to exercise increased caution and awareness in our practice until things feel more balanced and a sense of ease returns to our *pranic–apanic* transitions.

In Intermediate series, we encounter the macro level transition from the peak *pranic* posture *Kapotasana* to the peak *apanic* postures *Eka* and *Dwi Pada Sirsasana*. This can be a tricky section of the series to navigate and it is essential that the learning and integration process not be rushed. Students should cultivate ease and full integration of each posture before learning the next one in the series. An experienced teacher will usually keep a student on *Kapotasana* for some time, even after the student has cultivated the ability to catch the heels with the hands. Keeping a student on *Kapotasana* for a few weeks (at least) after attaining the ability to complete the posture will ensure that the peak *pranic* experience is deeply imprinted in the body and nerves. This integration of the extreme *pranic* pattern will make the subsequent transition to peak *apanic* movements less destabilizing. If a student is moved past *Kapotasana* prematurely, the result is often that the ability to catch the heels in *Kapotasana* is lost when the *apanic* cultivation of putting the legs behind the head begins to be developed. If one is simultaneously struggling with both *Kapotasana* and *Eka Pada Sirsasana*, the potential for the body and nerves to become completely overwhelmed—and for a painful breakdown to occur—is much higher.

Cultivation of new structural and energetic patterns in the self-organizing network of the human organism is a process that cannot be rushed. The power and depth of the reorganizing process which is induced by the Ashtanga system must be respected. Rushing through the system prematurely and without proper integration of each step is a sign of immaturity and lack of respect (often on the part of a teacher who encourages their students to move through a series too quickly), and inevitably leads to negative results such as excessive pain and emotional and energetic imbalance. The vast majority of injuries and negative experiences in the Ashtanga system are caused by moving through the series too quickly and without respect for the depth of the process. I believe this is the main reason Sharathji chose to slow down the pace at which students are taught new postures over the years after he took over from his grandfather.

In the third section of Third series, the buildup to the peak of pranic backbending in *Gandha Berundasana* occurs quickly over four backbending postures. *Gandha Berundasana* was the most difficult asana in Third series for me to learn, and is still the most psychologically intimidating part of the series for me. On the majority of my Third series practice days, I catch myself thinking "I can't do that today," at the beginning of my practice. Experience has taught me that this doubt is always unfounded. Rather than obsessing about sections of the practice which are yet to arrive, I let go of those thoughts as soon as they occur, and drop into embodied presence within each movement and each breath. I patiently complete each posture and vinyasa of the practice with this embodied awareness. Then, when I do arrive at *Gandha Berundasana*, I find there is no longer any doubt and I am always able to move into it with minimal struggle. I wrote at length about my process of learning this posture, and my experience of practicing it with Sharath Jois in the main shala on my last trip to Mysore.

A final reflection on the cultivation of the ability to transition between *pranic* and *apanic* states in our practice is to understand how this trains us to be able to shift energetic states in our daily lives off of the mat. We all have physiological biases in our bodies towards *pranic* or *apanic* patterning. Similarly, we all have habitual states of our nervous system which we default to in our interactions with the world. All states of the nervous system have advantages and disadvantages. Some states are appropriate in certain situations and inappropriate in others. If we remain limited to a small repertoire of states in our nervous system, and we always default to these select few states, we limit our ability to engage with life in the fullest and most effective way possible. If we cultivate the ability to move between all of the different possible states of our nervous system with ease and fluidity, then are able to engage with life more effectively. Cultivating the ability to transition easily between *pranic* and *apanic* postures and movements in the Ashtanga practice—and to feel equally comfortable in all of the different varieties of postures—will aid us directly in cultivating more resilience and fluidity in the way our nervous system responds to different situations in life. We use our practice to reconfigure our nervous system to function more effectively and efficiently.

Part 5: Standing Balances and Final Backbending (Digasana to Eka Pada Rajakapotasana)

- Digasana
- Trivikramasana
- Natarajasana
- Rajakapotasana
- Eka Pada Rajakapotasana

The final section of Third series consists of five postures, all of which are pranic in nature, and three of which are deep backbends. This section begins with a return to *Samasthiti*, followed by three postures which involve balancing on one leg. After the deep backbending (*Gandha Berundasana*, etc.) of the previous section, the standing balances function to restore some stability and grounding to the body and nerves. Although the three standing balances are *pranic* in nature, they also require deep focus on the standing leg and the connection of the foot to the ground. These features aid in cultivating the *apanic* qualities of strength and stability, which are essential to counterbalance the strong *pranic* stimulation of the second half of Third series.

After completing the standing balances, we return to the ground for the final two postures, *Rajakapotasana* and *Eka Pada Rajakapotasana*, both of which are deep and stimulating backbends.

Although none of the five postures in this section could reasonably be classified as "easy," they are less difficult than the peak backbending of *Viparita Salabhasana* and *Gandha Berundasana* in the previous section. The aforementioned postures are the peak "hump" in Third series, and after completing them there is a tangible feeling of winding down as one approaches the end of the series. Although the five final postures of Third series do require meticulous presence and depth, once one has attained the ability to complete *Gandha Berundasana*, there are no major challenges remaining.

All of the series in the Ashtanga system share the feature of having the most challenging postures in the middle section of the series. The final section of each series is a winding down of sorts, with relatively easier and somewhat restorative or grounding postures.

In Primary series the peak challenges of the series occur in the section from *Marichasana D* to *Garbha Pindasana*. Once *Garbha Pindasana* has been completed, the final section of postures are much easier, and several of them are performed in the *Supta* (reclined) position, lying on the back. These *Supta* Variations are restorative in nature and function to replenish one's energy reserves after the peak effort required in the middle of the series.

In Intermediate series, there are three postures which comprise the peak challenges, all of which occur in the middle part of the series. Those postures are *Kapotasana*, *Dwi Pada Sirsasana* and *Karandavasana*. Once *Karandavasana* has been completed, the final section of Intermediate series won't pose any significant challenges. The final few postures involve twisting and lateral movements, which are restorative and help to release any tensions in the back which may have arisen from the deeper peak postures. The seven *Sirsasana* variations which close the series are restorative in nature.

The phenomenon of winding down with easier postures towards the end of a series helps to stabilize the internal energetic dynamics, so that one can approach the final backbending and finishing postures in a state of relative calm and repose.

There are a total of seven deep backbending postures in Third series, all of which occur in the second half of the series. In my discussions of Third series thus far, I have focused extensively on the dynamic balance between the opposing patterns of *prana* and *apana*, and how the two patterns collaborate to create *bandha* via their antagonistic energetic movements. I'd like to conclude my discussion of Third series by acknowledging that there are also antagonistic patterns within both *pranic* and *apanic* categories of postures.

It is natural to assume that if a person is competent at performing certain backbending postures, this competency will extend to all backbends. This is untrue, and it was the seven backbending postures in Third series which gave me an experiential understanding of this fact. Although all seven of Third series backbends are *pranic* in nature, and all seven postures involve deep extension of the spine, there are also antagonistic movement patterns within this subset of postures. For example, when I first began to practice Third series, well over a decade ago, I noticed that on days where *Viparita Salabhasana* felt quite deep, *Rajakapotasana* would feel more difficult than usual, and vice versa. This is extremely counterintuitive. If we examine the two aforementioned postures, we can see that the shape of the body itself is nearly identical in both postures, with the only major difference being the orientation of the body with respect to the ground. My experience of the antagonism between these two postures makes little sense, if one approaches the analysis from a reductive, mechanical perspective.

I no longer experience the antagonistic dynamic between the aforementioned two postures. However I do experience antagonism within the seven backbends in Third series in other ways. When I filmed the practice that I have presented in the videos—in September 2020—I was able to press my heels onto the ground in *Gandha Berundasana*. This had been the case for several months prior to the filming of the video. However, at this time I had difficulty in keeping my heels together and touching the entire foot on my head in *Viparita Salabhasana*, as well as in *Vrichikasana* (both the variation in the final backbending sequence and the variation in Fourth series). I could touch my toes on my head, but I struggled to keep my heels together, and could not fully press my heels to my head. *Gandha Berundasana* is structurally very similar to *Viparita Salabhasana/Vrichikasana*. However I found the former to be easier than the latter. Then, a short time after filming, the bias between this antagonistic set of postures switched. Over a period of several weeks, it felt like my ability to keep my heels together and press my feet more fully into my head was improving dramatically, but at the same time, my ability to press my heels on the ground in *Gandha Berundasana* became more difficult. By November, I found it very easy to keep my heels together and was able to fully press my heels on my head for a sustained period of time in both *Viparita Salabhasana* and the two *Vrichikasana* variations. This represented a depth of movement I had never previously experienced. At the same time, I completely lost the ability to touch the heels to the ground in *Gandha Berundasana*. I could still catch my feet with my hands, and I could press my toes on the ground, but I could no longer bring the heels all the way down. At the time of writing—in February 2021—this antagonism and bias between these two very similar types of *pranic* posture remain in the state I have just described.

Maturity in the Ashtanga practice should lead one to the experiential understanding that antagonism and trade-offs between moving parts are a fundamental property of self-organized living systems. An even more important realization is the fact that we have very little control over how these trade-offs and antagonisms manifest themselves. I have observed that relatively few practitioners and teachers possess this important insight. More commonly, I see reductive biomechanics being erroneously applied to the Ashtanga practice, and to the human organism in general.

The pioneering systems biologists Humberto Maturana and Francisco Varela beautifully described an important property of complex living systems with the following statement:

"You can never direct a living system. You can only disturb it."

A complicated system, such as a machine, is fundamentally different from a complex system, such as a cell, a human being, or an ecosystem. All living systems are complex systems. They self-organize, behave nonlinearly, and are fundamentally less predictable than complicated systems. We can direct the behavior of a complicated machine such as an airplane or a factory. One who devotes the necessary time to study and fully understand the mechanics of how these complicated systems function is able to manipulate certain parts of the system, in order to attain a predictable and desired result. It is for this reason that airplanes generally succeed in transporting millions of people through the sky without disaster each day of the year. Complicated systems are predictable and they can be directed by one who has the skill and knowledge to do so.

The fundamental fallacy of modern biomechanics and medical science is the assumption that complex, living systems will also behave predictably if we attempt to direct them. In the postural yoga and Ashtanga world, we often see this philosophy applied. If one experiences tightness, or discomfort in the shoulders, for example, a teacher who applies biomechanics philosophy may recommend adding in some "shoulder openers" before key postures or outside of the usual practice routine. These well-intentioned recommendations rarely give the desired result, because they fail to take into account the non-linearity and lack of predictability inherent in complex living systems.

If one develops tightness or pain in the shoulders during the course of their Ashtanga process, this may very well be a natural result of the deep and complex structural reorganization involving the network of relationships between all of the parts and systems of the human organism. The shoulders may develop tightness or discomfort due to other parts of the body opening up or strengthening in order to accommodate particular postures or movement patterns which have been added or deepened in the practice. Adding in extra shoulder stretches may temporarily relieve pain or stiffness in the shoulders, but the deeper and unpredictable costs of doing this may be to completely sabotage the intelligence of the underlying structural reorganization which is under process. The result will be that the pain or stiffness in the shoulders will simply re-emerge in a different form elsewhere in the system a few days later. One may end up feeling a pain in the back, or the hips, or the knees, and other postures or movements will then suffer. The ignorant practitioner or teacher will again apply symptomatic linear treatments to the afflicted part, in a never-ending cycle of futile attempts to exert control over the direction of the evolution of a complex living system. I consider this an immature and erroneous way to approach the Ashtanga system and its influence on the human organism.

An approach that represents matured wisdom and understanding of the dynamics of the evolution of complex systems, is to recognize that our practice—and especially adding new postures / elements to our practice—is simply a method of "disturbing" the complex balance of our internal structural dynamics. After consciously choosing to disturb our own internal balance through our practice, it is appropriate to step back, release our desire to control and direct, and allow the results to unfold as they will. The evolution of our bodies and nerves may not proceed in the way that we expect or desire them to, but if we respect the innate intelligence of our body to integrate the "disturbance" that we give it via the sequence of asanas, and we allow our bodily intelligence to integrate that disturbance into a new structural framework at its own pace, we will eventually emerge on the other side of the transformative process in a state that is stable and balanced.

The tendency to always move towards balance, stability, or homeostasis is another important feature of complex living systems. When the system is disturbed—i.e., new information, elements or features are added to it—the system will temporarily be pushed out of balance as it attempts to integrate the new input into its organization framework. The phenomena of being temporarily pushed out of balance accounts for the various stiffnesses, aches and pains, etc., that we experience when we add new asanas, or move deeper into existing asanas in our practice. The new asanas, or the experience of attaining new depth in an asana, "disturbs" our internal state of balance. The important thing to understand is that the choice of adding new features to our practice is where our ability to consciously influence the result ends. We are in control of whether we add new asanas or not, or whether we push ourselves to attain new depths in an asana. Beyond that initial choice, we have no control or ability to direct how this disturbance will influence or change our internal organizational patterns. The mature and wise practitioner will step back and simply allow the results to play out within themselves. It may take days, weeks, or months for a new state of balance or internal homeostasis to manifest. Once this new balance or homeostasis is attained, it then becomes time to disturb the system again by adding more new postures, and then to again step back and allow the innate intelligence within us to sort things out. This is the cyclical process of self-evolution via the Ashtanga practice in a nutshell.

A mature teacher understands this process and watches for the stages of integration and rebalancing in his students. When we add new asanas to a student's practice, or we take a student deeper into asanas, it is normal to witness a period of destabilization in the student's body and practice. A patient teacher understands that this destabilization must be given time and space to play out, and that it is not necessarily appropriate to attempt to "fix" any discomfort that the student may experience during this process. When a student reports discomfort or stiffness, my response is nearly always to acknowledge that this phenomenon is "okay" to experience and to encourage the student to respect the process of integration that he is going through, rather than reactively attempting to apply quick fixes to make the discomfort or stiffness go away. There certainly are cases where we do need to make mechanical changes to the structure or form of the student's practice, but usually this simply involves a scaling back of intensity in order to create space for the body to incorporate and accommodate the process of structural evolution.

For one who has undertaken the commitment to a long term, daily Ashtanga practice, I feel that an understanding of the nature of complex systems is essential.

When one experientially understands the process of disturbance—discomfort—rebalancing within oneself, a deep respect for the intelligence inherent in nature should develop. The innate self-organizing intelligence of the human organism is a manifestation of the intelligence of nature. Self-healing (rebalancing) is an inherent feature of natural intelligence, and once we experience this phenomenon inside ourselves, we can more readily see it happening everywhere in nature. Have you ever watched how quickly a dog with an injured leg adapts to its condition? Or how a deeply disturbed ecosystem eventually finds a new balance, within which it can support life and flourish? Nearly every human attempt to engineer an ecosystem produces unintended and often negative consequences. Yet, if left alone, an ecosystem will always move towards health and homeostasis. The self-organizing intelligence inherent in nature is vastly superior to the rational, analytic intelligence of human beings. Undoubtedly, the rational human mind has invented and discovered wonderful things over our species evolutionary history. But none of these human inventions come close to the complexity and functionality of what nature itself has designed. Our experiments in tinkering with nature over the past few centuries have elucidated this inferiority. Unfortunately, our modern techno-industrial culture has not understood this important aspect of reality, and we continue to make devastating mistakes in our attempts to direct and control natural complex systems. Imagining that we can control the population growth cycle of a seasonal respiratory virus through totalitarianism is a recent example of this sort of mistake. This mistake is born from the same philosophical position that imagines it can hack the internal rebalancing process which arises through the Ashtanga practice.

My approach, which I believe is in resonance with the laws and properties inherent in nature and natural intelligence, is one of surrender. I actively and consciously choose how and when to disturb things and then I surrender to allow the effects of that disturbance to play out. The wisdom lies in knowing when to step forward and exert our will to disturb something, and when to step back and surrender to allow nature to take its own course. This is the ultimate balance I strive for in my practice and in my life. The Ashtanga practice is a wonderful teacher which guides my experiential understanding of the laws of nature.

Part 6: Final Backbending Sequence
- Urdhva Danurasana x 3
- Drop back and stand up x 3
- Tick Tocks x 3
- Vrichikasana
- Catching
- Paschimottanasana

In the Ashtanga system of asana, we practice the backbending sequence following the completion of whichever core series (Primary, Intermediate or Advanced) we have practiced on that day. Just as *Surya Namaskar A & B* and the Standing Sequence are always practiced before the core series, the backbending sequence is always practiced afterwards. Backbending serves as an intense and somewhat dramatic conclusion to the deep work of the core series, before we move into the final finishing postures.

The structure of the backbending sequence remains the same, regardless of whether one is practicing Primary, Intermediate, or Advanced series. The backbending sequence is gradually built up, and elements are added to it after certain milestones are reached in our progression through the various core series.

Urdhva Danurasana is usually added to the end of one's core series practice at some point during the first half of Primary series. Exactly which point in Primary series the backbending is brought in at, will vary depending on the unique strengths and weaknesses of each practitioner. By the time one has reached the *Marichyasana* sequence, it is usually appropriate to also be practicing *Urdhva Danurasana*.

The next element to be added to the backbending sequence is dropping back into and standing up from *Urdhva Danurasana*. This is usually initiated when a student is at or near the end of Primary series, though it can be added earlier for students who are naturally proficient in backbending. It is important NOT to begin forcing drop backs with a student who is not ready to do so. There are significant risk and effort involved in working on dropping back and standing up prematurely—for both the student and teacher—with little benefit to be gained. Attempting to drop back and stand up before the necessary prerequisites are developed will often lead to excessive pain and inflammation, and potentially more serious injury for the practitioner. It is also very taxing for the teacher, who would have to bear the entire weight of the student, if the student is not able to at least partially support himself during the movement up and down.

It is more appropriate and productive to begin cultivating the necessary skills to support dropping back and standing up while practicing *Urdhva Danurasana* on the ground. One should easily be able to straighten the arms in *Urdhva Danurasana*, and also to comfortably walk the hands in towards the feet. If one can straighten the arms and then walk the hands in at least half of the initial distance between the hands and the feet, then one likely has the requisite level of flexibility to attempt dropping back and standing up.

Strength and stability are also important factors to cultivate. Some practitioners are flexible, and can easily walk the hands in towards the feet, but are wobbly and cannot sustain a backbend without squirming around or coming down prematurely. I like to test a student's stability in *Urdhva Danurasana* by placing my hands on the two iliac crests of the pelvis, and pressing down on them while asking the student to push up against my hands. If a student can easily meet my pressing downwards with an equal amount of counter pressure upwards, and can sustain this resistance for a significant length of time, then I usually become confident that the student has sufficient strength in both the arms and the legs to support the dropping back and standing up movement. Another good test of a student's stability is whether he can follow a leisurely paced vinyasa count in the three backbends at the end of a led Primary series class. If a student cannot hold *Urdhva Danurasana* for a somewhat slow count to five, three times in a row (without lowering to the ground) at the end of led Primary series class, then that student is not ready to benefit from dropping back and standing up. I've witnessed students who are working on Intermediate series, and yet cannot sustain the vinyasas count for *Urdhva Danurasana* at the end of a led Primary series class. This is a recipe for disaster.

Standing up from and dropping back into *Urdhva Danurasana* without assistance is considered to be a prerequisite for beginning to learn Intermediate series. Learning to drop back and stand up at the end of Primary series ensures that a certain degree of flexibility, strength and control are developed for the backbending movement, and that the nerves become habituated to the *pranic* stimulation of the nervous system during the backbending sequence. If this prerequisite is firmly established while a student is still practicing Primary series, the subsequent process of learning Intermediate series will be smoother and less shocking to the body and nervous system.

Catching the legs with the hands can be added at any point in Primary or Intermediate series as the final element of the backbending sequence. Needless to say, one must be able to drop back and stand up with ease, in order to begin catching. One should also be able to easily walk the hands all the way to the heels while in *Urdhva Danurasana* on the ground. The legs must be strong, stable and grounded in order to support the catching position safely. To test this, I first ask a student to walk his hands all the way to his heels while in *Urdhva Danurasana* on the ground, and then to keep the hands and feet firmly engaged with the ground while I push down on their iliac bones with my hands. If I can feel the student's legs confidently engage to push back against my hands in this position, then I usually feel comfortable to start working on catching with this student.

It should be emphasized that adding catching as the final element should not be rushed, and some students may never be ready to do so. Catching is an extreme posture and should only be attempted by those who have put in the necessary effort and dedication in practice over a period of months or years to cultivate the necessary skills to attempt it safely. Usually, by the time one has fully integrated *Kapotasana* in Intermediate series, it will be possible to begin working on catching.

Within the catching posture itself, there are also varying degrees of depth one can work at, and it is customary to gradually work a student's hands higher up on the legs as their proficiency in the posture develops. One can hold the legs anywhere from the lower ankles to the lower thighs. In my last trip to Mysore, I experienced Sharathji putting my hands on my lower thighs, completely above my kneecaps, for the first time. I discussed this experience in the essay about my last trip in Mysore. In the video of my home practice, my hands are on my upper calves, just below the kneecaps.

The final two elements of the backbending sequence—*tick tocks* and *Vrischkasana*, are not added until one has completed Intermediate series, and sometimes not until one has practiced at least a few postures into Advanced A series. These movements are practiced after dropping back and standing up, and before catching. They both add deeper elements of strength, coordination and flexibility. *Vrischkasana* was the most difficult element of the backbending sequence for me to develop, and it was only in January 2021 that I was able to fully place the entirety of my feet on my head, with my heels pressed together. When the video was filmed—in September 2020—I could touch my head with my toes, but not with the bottom part of my feet.

I practice the full backbending sequence as described above—and as shown in the video—on the three or four days (Mondays–Thursdays) that I practice Advanced series. On Sundays, when I practice Intermediate series, my backbending consists of *Urdhva Danurasana*, drop backs, and then low catching at the ankles (no *tick tocks*, *Vrischkasana* or higher catching). On Fridays, when I practice Primary series, my backbending consists of three *Urdhva Danurasana* on the ground, followed by *Chakrasana* and *Paschimottanasana*, as in a traditional led Primary series class. I don't practice the other elements of backbending on Fridays.

It is important for practitioners to understand that there is a vinyasa count for the entire backbending sequence. The sequence should be practiced fluidly and seamlessly, in coordination with the breath, according to the vinyasa count. It is natural to need a few extra breaths to prepare for *Urdhva Danurasana*, and perhaps in between each of the different elements of the backbending sequence. In the video, you can see that I do take some extra breaths in between each element of the sequence.

As a teacher, I often see students abandon the vinyasa method completely when they practice the backbending sequence. It is common to see students lying on their mat for long periods of time before, or in between repetitions of *Urdhva Danurasana*, or adding in extra stretches to help prepare, etc. I have seen students literally take 20 minutes to complete three *Urdhva Danurasana* on the ground, and just as long to complete three drop backs. The backbending sequence should be practiced with the same focused flow of body and breath as one practices the core series. It should take no longer than a few minutes to practice the full backbending sequence. In the video, it is done in six minutes from start to finish, including nearly one third of that time spent in *Paschimottanasana*.

* * * * *

SUSTAINING A DAILY PRACTICE OF THE ASHANGA SYSTEM

A daily practice of the Ashtanga system of asana is difficult to maintain, especially when one does not have the support of a teacher and shala. Digging deeply into oneself and finding the willpower and motivation to persist in completing one's practice to the best of one's ability—each and every day—is the field where significant growth, evolution and progress arises from. It is only through cultivating the ability to maintain a strong and consistent personal practice in the face of adversity, that one can expect to realize one's full potential.

As a teacher based in Bali, I work predominantly with visiting students who practice with me for a temporary duration of time. There are a number of students who I see once or twice per year, for periods of time ranging from a few weeks to a few months. Of these returning students, there are three basic types. One type of student practices deeply, working at their edge consistently, year-round, whether they are practicing in my shala, or whether they are elsewhere working on their own or with another teacher. When this type of student visits me, I can clearly see the progress that has been made in their practice during the time period that they have been away from Bali. A second type of student practices deeply when they are in my shala, but when they are elsewhere, they maintain only a basic or rudimentary level of practice. When this type of student visits me, it is usually as if they are picking up where they left off on their previous visit with me. There has not been any progress during the time they were elsewhere, but there has also not been regress. The third type of student practices deeply when they are in my shala, but when they are elsewhere, they stop practicing altogether, or they practice only sporadically. This type of student usually regresses between trips to practice with me, and when they return it takes a few weeks or a few months of practice, just to attain to the same level they were at when they left at the end of their previous trip.

All students are welcome at my shala, whether they are consistent practitioners or not. I make the above distinctions to outline the fact that continuous application of effort to encounter one's edge is necessary to make deep and long-lasting progress in the Ashtanga system. Furthermore, cultivating the ability to find one's edge when one is alone, with fewer external motivating factors than one would have in a shala, brings a certain level of depth and self-understanding that cannot be found when practicing in a shala with a teacher. This is not easy to do, and the reality is that many Ashtanga teachers do not practice deeply themselves. We all experience situations where, for one reason or another, it becomes necessary to back off from the intensity of our practice for a period of time. There is, however, a big difference between taking a temporary respite from stronger practice, and simply lacking the motivation or willpower to engage in deep practice at all.

My practice is not effortless, and I struggle nearly every day. Awakening for practice at a time of the night when some people are just going to bed is difficult. Stepping onto my mat in those dark hours of the morning, regardless of how I feel, requires strength of will. More often than not, I begin my practice while being assailed by thoughts such as "there is no way I can do this today." I always give myself an out, by telling myself that if things end up going very badly in my practice, I will revert to "only Primary" or cut my practice short regardless of which series I am practicing on that day. More than 99 percent of the time, I do end up completing my intended practice for that day, and I almost always feel great at the end of my practice. The consistency of this outcome helps to generate the motivation to begin practice each morning. The process of dropping into my embodied experience in each moment, each vinyasa and each breath—and attempting to confine my awareness to each of these moments—is key. When one learns how to be fully present and absorbed within each posture and within each breath, it becomes natural to work deeply at one's edge in each vinyasa and in each posture, for the duration of one's entire practice, on each and every morning. This is an exercise in sustained embodied focus and concentration.

Success in the endeavor of maintaining a strong daily practice over a long period of time is empowering. One gains familiarity with the process of overcoming the unique and idiosyncratic obstacles that one encounters within oneself. Self-empowerment is one of the main benefits of long-term practice of the Ashtanga system. A system which necessitates reliance on external forces or authorities to derive benefit leads to disempowerment and enslavement. A system which necessitates the cultivation of self-motivation and self-reliance leads to self-empowerment and freedom. The main difference between a true teacher and a predatory leader is that the former attempts to transmit independence and self-reliance through their teachings, while the latter manipulates their students into codependence and enslavement.

At present, in human societies all over the planet, there are significant forces at work which are acting to disempower people. There are large-scale attempts to coerce people into surrendering their autonomy and freedom and to outsource the responsibility for their own health and wellbeing to external authorities. I'll refrain from a digression into global politics, but I will conclude by emphatically stating that I find the self-empowering nature of my personal practice to be more important than ever under the present conditions which persist in human society.

ASHTANGA, EMBODIMENT & COMPLEX SYSTEMS

INDEX

A

Abhyanga 179
Adho Mukha Svanasana 332
Advanced series 350
A Guide to Better Movement [book] 261
Ahamkara 225
Alf Nachemson 157, 168
Aligned, Relaxed and Resilient [book] 240
Alignment 155
Allen Enrique 243, 255, 258
Andreas Weber 186
Andy Davis 221, 317
Animate Earth [book] 139
Apana 335
Apanic body movement 67
Ardha Matsyendrasana 80
Aristotle 225, 226
Arne Naess 131, 218
Aṣṭāṅga Yoga as It Is [book] 90
Autopoiesis 188, 275
Ayurveda 312

B

Baddha Konasana 111, 344
Bakasana 80, 344
Bandha 74, 94, 117, 124, 129, 149, 151, 159, 227, 239, 264, 328, 334
Becoming Animal [book] 48
Bhagavad Gita 66, 225
Bhakti 19
Bharadvajasana 80
Bhekasana 112
Bhuja Dandasana 67
Bliss 42
Brahma 198
Brahmacharya 183
Breath and Bandha 239
Brendan Brazier 309
Buddha 40, 133, 200
Buddhism 215, 217

C

Carl Sagan 131
Chakrasana 369
Chaturanga 78, 84, 258, 332, 344
Chronic Pain 274
Conscious-Self 39

D

David Abram 48, 132, 139
David Eagleman 131
Descartes 272, 326
Desikachar 227
Dhamma 133
Dharana 323
Dharma 117
Dhyana 323
Diana Alstad 199, 211
Diet 178, 309, 312
Digasana 306
Discomfort 233
Disembodied Practice 180
Disempowerment 220, 373
Divide Between Us and Nature, The 62
Drishti 227
Duality and Separateness 198
Dwi Pada Sirsasana 25, 66, 95, 107, 342, 344, 355, 359
Dynamics of the Ashtanga System 330

E

Eastern Cosmology 199
Ekam 167
Eka Pada Bakasana 293, 344
Eka Pada Rajakapotasana 358
Eka Pada Sirsasana 25, 80, 342, 355
Embodied Practice 115, 180
Embodied Understanding 283
Empowerment 373

F

Feeling-Self 39
Fermented Food 309
Fifth series 34
Fight or Flight 270
Fourth series 23, 100

Francisco Varela 188, 361

G

Gaia 144, 207
Gandha Berundasana 281, 294, 351, 356, 358
Garbha Pindasana 106, 358
Gokulam 285
Gomukhasana 351
Greg Lehman 155, 262, 273

H

Half Primary 113
Hanumanasana 306
Homo Sapien 190
Humberto Maturana 188, 361

I

Imagination 224
Inflammation 316
Injury 21, 32, 86, 180, 181, 264
Interconnectedness 199
Intermediate series 18, 67, 89, 170, 228, 297, 325, 334, 341, 358
Iyengar 34, 164, 179

J

Joel Kramer 199, 211
Judgmental (being -) 202
Jung, Carl 213, 247

K

Kapotasana 18, 112, 171, 355, 359, 369
Karandavasana 67, 76, 95, 302, 344, 359
Katy Bowman 261
Koundinyasana 293
KPJAYI 12, 65, 95
Krishnamacharya 164, 227

L

Lakshmipuram 12, 34, 95
Liberal Ashtanga 111
Lifestyle 313
Lyn Margulis 131

M

Marichasana 29, 106, 358
Mark Darby 12, 23
Massage 179
Matthew Remski 39
Matthew Sweeney 90
Mayurasana 344
Movement Homeopathy 273
Movement Matters [book] 261
Mula Bandha 149, 151, 244, 334
Mysore 11, 23, 65
Mysore-Style Ashtanga 222, 227

N

Nakrasana 344
Nature Spirits 205

O

Organic Intelligence 115

P

Pain 21, 32, 40, 43, 66, 80, 92, 235, 269, 274, 280
Panchasila 183, 217
Parshvakonasana 342
Paschimottanasana 299, 354, 370
Patanjali 22, 64, 183, 217, 317
Pattabhi Jois 12, 227
Pincha Mayurasana 68, 69, 82
Playing With Movement [book] 262
Prana 335
Pranayama 18, 311
Preaching 209
Primary series 170, 334
Purna Matsyendrasana 351
Purvottanasana 340

R

Rajakapotasana 358
Recovery Strategies: A Pain Guidebook [book] 262
Reinhold Messner 53
Richard Freeman 13
Rolfing 91, 240

Rolf Naujokat 13, 23, 34, 35, 65, 95, 308

S

Sadhana 37
Samadhi 198, 319, 323
Samasthiti 161, 255, 357
Sampajanna 314
Samskara 64, 214, 225, 270, 274, 290, 318, 349
Sangha 133
Sankhara 41, 43, 132, 214, 270
Sarvangasana 81
Satipatthana Sutta 41
Savasana 179
Sayanasana 67
Sensation and Imagination 224
Setubandhasana 340
Shaktipat 42
Sharath Jois 15, 23, 65, 109, 285, 325, 347, 369
Sirsasana 81
SKPJ 24, 33, 95
Sleep 314
Standing Sequence 333
Stephan Harding 139
Sthira 149, 240, 307
Sukha 149, 240
Supta Kurmasana 85, 353, 354
Supta Vajrasana 18, 289
Surya Aamaskar 167
Surya Namaskara 330, 366
Sushumna Nadi 152
Systems Perspective 183

T

Teaching 209
Tensegrity 100, 115, 159, 173
The Biology of Wonder [book] 186
The Ecology of Wisdom [book] 218
The Guru Papers [book] 211
Third Series Practice 89, 329
Thrive Diet [book] 309
Tick Tock 369
Tightness 316
Tiredness 316

Tittibhasana 70, 82
Todd Hargrove 261
Tolkien, J.R.R. 202
Traditional Practice Instructions 20
Transcending the Physical 200
Trauma 274
Tree of Bandha 239
Trikonasana 151, 342

U

Uddiyana Bandha 151
Urdhva Danurasana 112, 243, 339, 354, 366
Urdhva Kukkutasana 98
Urdhva Mukha Svanasana 332
Utpluthi 167, 257, 258

V

Vasisthasana 342
Viparita Dandasana 301
Viparita Salabhasana 98, 300, 351, 358, 359, 360
Vipassana 40, 122, 123, 132, 133, 197, 320
Viranchyasana 351
Visvamitrasana 97, 342
Vrichikasana 360
Vrischkasana 369

W

Wellbeing 233
Western Cosmology 199
Will Johnson 240, 318

Y

Yama and Niyama 217
Yoga Mala 227
Yoga Mudra 81
Yoga Nidra 313
Yoga Nidrasana 82
Yoga Sutra 225

Discovery Publisher is a multimedia publisher whose mission is to inspire and support personal transformation, spiritual growth and awakening. We strive with every title to preserve the essential wisdom of the author, spiritual teacher, thinker, healer, and visionary artist.

www.ingramcontent.com/pod-product-compliance
Lightning Source LLC
Chambersburg PA
CBHW011944150426
43192CB00016B/2771